atlas of Cardiovascular Pathology

for the clinician

atlas of Cardiovascular

Pathology

for the clinician

volume editor
Bruce M. McManus, PhD, MD, FCAP, FACC, FRCPC
Professor and Head
Department and Head of Pathology and Laboratory Medicine
University of British Columbia;
Director, Cardiovascular Research Laboratory and Registry
St. Paul's Hospital–Providence Health Care
Vancouver, BC
Canada

series editor
Eugene Braunwald, MD, MD (Hon), ScD (Hon)
Distinguished Hersey Professor of Medicine
Faculty Dean for Academic Programs at Brigham and Women's
  Hospital and Massachusetts General Hospital
Harvard Medical School;
Vice President for Academic Programs
Partners HealthCare System
Boston, Massachusetts

With 30 contributors

Developed by Current Medicine, Inc., Philadelphia

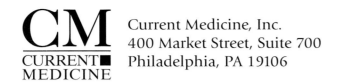

Current Medicine, Inc.
400 Market Street, Suite 700
Philadelphia, PA 19106

Developmental Editor	Elise M. Paxson
Director of Product Development	Charles Field
Books Supervisor	Fran Klass
Editorial Assistant	Annmarie D'Ortona
Art Director	Wendy Vetter
Cover Design	Jerilyn Kauffman, Christine Keller-Quirk
Design and Layout	Christine Keller-Quirk
Illustration Director	Ann Saydlowski
Illustrators	Larry Ward, Ann Saydlowski, Marie Dean
Production Manager	Lori Holland
Assistant Production Manager	Simon Dickey
Indexing	Holly Lukens

Atlas of cardiovascular pathology for the clinician / editor, Bruce M. McManus.
   p. ; cm
  Includes bibliographical references and index.
  ISBN 1-57340-160-9
  1. Cardiovascular system—Diseases—Atlases. I. McManus, Bruce M.
  [DNLM: 1. Cardiovascular Diseases—pathology—Atlases. WG 17 A88155 2000]
RC669.9.A834 2000
616.1'0022'2—dc21

00-057052

Library of Congress Cataloging-in-Publication Data

Printed in the United States by Imago

10 9 8 7 6 5 4 3 2 1

For more information please call 1-800-427-1796 or e-mail us at inquiry@phl.cursci.com
www.current-science-group.com

PREFACE

Great progress has been made over recent decades in our understanding of the causes and mechanisms of cardiovascular diseases, and the strategies for detection, treatment, and prevention. Scientific inquiry founded on advancing technologies has thus provided an ever-improving capability to establish the basis of cellular and systemic pathogenesis, the relationship between genes and the environment in disease processes, and how dynamic in vivo images can reflect features of abnormal structure. Classic pathologic observations themselves have bolstered the accelerated progress, and in an interesting way the new tools for assessing disease in vivo have driven the search for more refined and meaningful approaches to pathologic characterization. At times the extraction of new insights about the pathologic substrate for disease has come from revisitation of known lesions with renewed attention to detail, and, indeed, by more revealing and accurate photographic and artistic representation of lesions. On other occasions, progress has been augmented greatly by the application of relatively new techniques, such as molecular genetic manipulations in animal models, in situ hybridization for mRNA of expressed endogenous genes or chromosomal abnormalities, or molecular pursuit of exogenous genes such as those of viruses, and through correlation with indices such as electrophysiologic maps.

The *Atlas of Cardiovascular Pathology for the Clinician* reflects an attempt to capture the pathologic essence of cardiovascular lesions in the context of contemporary biology, on a backdrop of normal cardiovascular structure, focusing on details of structure from macro to micro, and from infancy to old age. A pathology atlas of relevance to cardiovascular medicine must define a scope, which, while demarcated, captures what is important in the relationship between cardiologic and surgical problems and their pathologic substrates. Only the range, experience, and insight of the chapter authors can account for the clarity and relevance of visual messages we have attempted to achieve here. Thus, highly selected images impart the central messages, while words link each photograph or drawing to a biologic or clinical context.

In chapter 1, Kishore Pasumarthi and Loren Field provide a lucid synopsis of genetically manipulated model systems that reflect unprecedented advances in understanding how the heart is formed and how such formation may go awry, and how genetic mechanisms may serve as a basis of heart development and congenital heart lesions. The model systems are then placed in a clinical context in chapter 2 by Paul Weinberg, who depicts vividly the major pathologic features of structural congenital heart conditions. A special category of congenital cardiovascular lesion is the anomalous vessel. In chapter 3, William Roberts contributes his life's experience and unique perspectives on anomalous coronary arteries in a fashion not possible by any other observer.

The problem of atherosclerosis is being attacked clinically with ferocious intensity, but remains a major cause of death and disability in developed societies, and stands to challenge the cardiovascular health of developing societies. As well, in our aging societies, more and more people will be faced with the sequelae of atherosclerosis. Thus, atherosclerosis is not leaving the planet anytime soon. We are fortunate to have two highly complementary contributions to this atlas on the pathology of atherosclerotic disease. First, chapter 4, by Peter Anderson and James Atkinson, presents a complete spectrum of pathological findings in atheromatous conditions, both as occur "naturally" and as manipulated clinically. This work is then placed in the perspective of atherosclerotic lesion development in chapter 5, wherein J. Fredrick Cornhill and Edward Herderick have written a topographic essay of the natural history of atherosclerosis in coronary arteries and aortae of young adults, whose vessels were contributed from the Pathobiological Determinants of Atherosclerosis in Youth (PDAY) Study. The pathology of other important vascular diseases, including a range of hereditary and acquired diseases of the aorta and the pulmonary circulation, are addressed in chapter 17 by Stanley Radio, Timothy Baxter, and Maurice Godfrey, and in chapter 8, by John English. The importance of ischemic myocardial injury as a consequence of coronary arterial lesions is given full emphasis in chapter 6 by Keith Reimer and Robert Jennings. In chapter 7, Jeffery Isner and Marianne Kearney similarly offer an extremely contemporary discussion of pathologic substrates and stimuli underlying angiogenesis in reparative processes that affect blood vessels and heart muscle.

H. Thomas Aretz provides, in chapter 9, a compilation of images and messages regarding the pathology of certain genetically and toxically determined cardiomyopathies, as well as a number of heart muscle diseases of unknown etiology. In chapter 10, Glenn Taylor and E. Rene Rodriguez present a detailed morphologic and molecular discussion of metabolic and other biochemical myopathies with associated cardiac involvement. The enigma of human myocarditis, often linked to cardiotropic viruses, is conveyed in chapter 11 by Reinhard Kandolf and myself. Other contemporary inflammatory and, at times, infectious challenges in the pathologic anatomy of heart allografts, at biopsy, at explant and autopsy, are addressed in chapter 12 by Gayle Winters. Dysrhythmias may attend all heart muscle diseases, and may be problems of immense consequence. Today, electrophysiologic-pathologic correlation has never been so feasible or so clinically relevant. In chapter 16, Jeffrey Saffitz, Frank Zimmerman, and Bruce Lindsay provide a thorough photographic illustration and discussion of the pathology and biology of heart muscle that may underlie rhythm disturbances.

Valvular heart disease remains a major clinical problem. The pathological features of native valve disease are documented in chapter 13 by Jagdish Butany and Avrum Gotlieb, and the special issues faced in understanding prosthetic valves and other clinically valuable implant materials are addressed in chapter 14 by Frederick Schoen. Finally, in chapter 15, Renu Virmani and Allen Burke illustrate a scholarly treatise on the pathology of tumors that can involve and impair the heart and blood vessels.

I am greatly indebted to every author in this book. Their extraordinary efforts to provide "custom-made" visual essays in a timely fashion, and for some, under challenging professional circumstances, will long be appreciated. I am also deeply aware of the persistent and collegial efforts of Ms. Shelly Wood and Ms. Salima Harji in my laboratory who in many ways assured that the volume would be finished and of substantial value. Similarly, the relentless vigilance and steady and constant guidance of Ms. Elise Paxson at Current Medicine ensured that we would succeed. Mr. Abe Krieger offered his essential energy and belief in the project. I remain honored at the opportunity to have edited this unique volume, a privilege bestowed by one of my most brilliant and thoughtful mentors, Eugene Braunwald.

To my wife, Janet, and the children, Cate, Amity, and Alex, I am thankful for their presence in my life, and for their patience and belief in our journey.

Bruce M. McManus

CONTRIBUTORS

Peter G. Anderson, DVM, PhD

Associate Professor of Pathology
University of Alabama at Birmingham
Birmingham, Alabama

H. Thomas Aretz, MD

Associate Professor of Pathology
Harvard Medical School;
Director, Cardiovascular Pathology
Massachusetts General Hospital
Boston, Massachusetts

James B. Atkinson, MD, PhD

Professor of Pathology
Director, Surgical Pathology
Vanderbilt University
Nashville, Tennessee

Timothy Baxter, MD

Associate Professor
Department of Surgery
University of Nebraska Medical Center
Omaha, Nebraska

Allen Burke, MD

Department of Cardiovascular Pathology
Armed Forces Institute of Pathology
Washington, DC

Jagdish Butany, MBBS, MS, FRCPC

Associate Professor of Laboratory Medicine and
Pathobiology
University of Toronto;
Staff Pathologist
Toronto General Hospital
Toronto, Ontario, Canada

J. Fredrick Cornhill, D.Phil.

Chair, Department of Biomedical Engineering
Lerner Research Institute
The Cleveland Clinic Foundation
Cleveland, Ohio

John C. English, MD, FRCPC

Clinical Assistant Professor of Pathology
University of British Columbia;
Consultant Pathologist
Vancouver General Hospital
Vancouver, British Columbia, Canada

Loren J. Field, PhD

Professor of Medicine and Pediatrics
Indiana University School of Medicine
Indianapolis, Indiana

Avrum I. Gotlieb, MDCM, FRCPC

Professor and Chair
Department of Laboratory Medicine and Pathobiology
University of Toronto;
Pathologist
University Health Network
Toronto, Ontario, Canada

Maurice Godfrey, MD

Associate Professor
Department of Pediatrics
University of Nebraska Medical Center
Omaha, Nebraska

Edward E. Herderick, BSc

Department of Biomedical Engineering
Ohio State University
Columbus, Ohio

Jeffrey M. Isner, MD

Professor of Medicine and Pathology
Tufts University School of Medicine;
Chief, Vascular Medicine and Cardiovascular Research
St. Elizabeth's Medical Center
Boston, Massachusetts

Robert B. Jennings, MS, MD

James B. Duke Professor of Pathology
Duke University
Durham, North Carolina

Reinhard Kandolf, MD, PhD

Professor and Director
Institute for Molecular Pathology
University of Tübingen
Tübingen, Germany

Marianne Kearney, BS

Supervisor, Cardiovascular Research
St. Elizabeth's Medical Center
Boston, Massachusetts

Bruce D. Lindsay, MD

Associate Professor of Medicine
Department of Cardiology
Washington University School of Medicine;
Director, Clinical Electrophysiology Laboratory
Barnes–Jewish Hospital
St. Louis, Missouri

Bruce M. McManus, MD, PhD, FCAP, FACC, FRCPC

Professor and Head
Department of Pathology and Laboratory Medicine
University of British Columbia;
Director, Cardiovascular Research Laboratory
Providence Health Care
St. Paul's Hospital
Vancouver, British Columbia, Canada

Kishore B.S. Pasumarthi, PhD

Post Doctoral Fellow
Department of Medicine
Indiana University School of Medicine
Indianapolis, Indiana

Stanley J. Radio, MD

Associate Professor of Pathology and Microbiology
University of Nebraska College of Medicine;
Active Academic/Clinical Pathologist
University Medical Associates
Omaha, Nebraska

Keith A. Reimer, MD, PhD

Professor of Pathology
Duke University
Durham, North Carolina

William Clifford Roberts, MD

Dean, A. Webb Roberts Center for Continuing Education
Baylor University Medical Center;
Medical Director
Baylor Cardiovascular Institute
Dallas, Texas

E. Rene Rodriguez, MD

Associate Professor
Department of Pathology
Johns Hopkins Hospital
Baltimore, Maryland

Jeffrey Saffitz, MD, PhD

Paul E. Lacy and Ellen Lacy Professor of Pathology
Department of Pathology
Washington University School of Medicine;
Staff Pathologist and Director of Autopsy Service
Barnes–Jewish Hospital
St. Louis, Missouri

Frederick J. Schoen, MD, PhD

Professor of Pathology
Harvard Medical School;
Vice Chair, Department of Pathology
Brigham and Women's Hospital
Boston, Massachusetts

Glenn P. Taylor, MD

Associate Professor of Pathology
University of British Columbia;
Pathologist
British Columbia Children's Hospital
Vancouver, British Columbia, Canada

Paul M. Weinberg, MD

Associate Professor of Pediatrics and Radiology
University of Pennsylvania;
Senior Cardiologist
Director of Cardiac Registry
The Children's Hospital of Philadelphia
Philadelphia, Pennsylvania

Gayle L. Winters, MD

Associate Professor of Pathology
Harvard Medical School;
Cardiovascular Pathologist and Director of Autopsy
Division
Brigham and Women's Hospital
Boston, Massachusetts

Renu Virmani, MD

Chair, Department of Cardiovascular Pathology
Armed Forces Institute of Pathology
Washington, DC

Frank Zimmerman, MD

Instructor
Department of Pediatrics
Washington University School of Medicine;
Director, Electrophysiology Service
St. Louis Children's Hospital
St. Louis, Missouri

In memory of my father and in love and appreciation of my mother.
–Bruce M. McManus

CONTENTS

Genetic Models of Cardiovascular Pathophysiology

Kishore B.S. Pasumarthi
Loren J. Field

Advances in molecular biology and mammalian embryology now make it possible to introduce defined genetic modifications into the germ line, thereby creating a transgenic animal. The genetic modification can result in either a gain of function (*ie,* the expression of an additional gene product in an otherwise normal genetic background) or a loss of function (*ie,* the ablation or modification of an endogenous gene). Because these modifications segregate in accordance with mendelian genetics, one can generate families of experimental and control animals that differ only by a specific genetic alteration. Transgenic animals thus constitute an extremely powerful experimental system that can be used to make unequivocal correlations between gene expression and a given physiologic trait simply by comparing the transgenic animals to their nontransgenic siblings.

Gain-of-function transgenic animals typically use a recombinant DNA molecule that employs a cell lineage–specific transcriptional regulatory element (*ie,* a promoter) to target expression of the desired gene product. The recombinant DNA molecule (known as the transgene) is delivered into the pronucleus of one-cell embryos by direct microinjection. The microinjected embryos are then implanted into the oviduct of a surrogate mother and allowed to develop to term. After the animals are born, molecular analysis of DNA prepared from biopsied material is used to identify the transgenic animals, which typically comprise 20% of the pups born. When the transgenic animals reach sexual maturity, they are bred with nontransgenic mates to establish families of transgenic mice. The entire process used for the generation of gain of function transgenic animals is shown in Figure 1-1. Hogan [1] has compiled an excellent laboratory manual that describes in detail the practical aspects of producing transgenic animals. It should be noted that many factors may influence the ultimate outcome of a given transgenic experiment. These include the use of cDNA versus genomic sequences, inclusion of heterologous introns in the transgene, the presence of bacterial vector sequences in the transgene, the genetic background used for embryogenesis, and so on [2]. Although gain-of-function transgenic technology has been used predominantly in mice, transgenic animals have been generated in many other species, including rats, pigs, sheep, and cows.

Advances in embryonic stem (ES) cell technology and homologous recombination have led to the ability to generate loss-of-function transgenic models. ES cells are totipotent cell lines. When injected into a surrogate blastocyst, ES cells can contribute to all tissue lineages, including the germ line. If the ES cells are modified genetically before blastocyst injection, the genetic modification can be passed on to subsequent generations, provided that the germ line is colonized. Homologous recombination is used to generate modifications that result in the loss of function of a specific gene. When mammalian cells are transfected with DNA, the vast majority of integration events occur at random sites. However, a small percentage of the integration events occur at the site homologous to the transfected DNA. Mansour *et al.* [3] devised a scheme that greatly facilitates the identification of homologous recombination events. The approach uses targeting vectors composed of genomic sequences from the gene one wishes to inactivate, as well as a combination of expression cassettes that permit both positive and negative selection. Typically, a neo^r (neomycin resistance) expression cassette is subcloned within the coding sequences of the target gene. The neo^r expression cassette provides a positive selection screen for transfected cells, as well as disruption of the coding sequences in the target gene. A second expression cassette, typically HSV–thymidine kinase (*HSV-TK*), is inserted at a site distal to the target gene sequences. In most random integration events, the targeting vector integrates intact, and the resulting transfectants will be resistant to neomycin (because of the presence of the neo^r expression cassette) and sensitive to ganciclovir (because of the *HSV-TK* gene). In contrast,

during homologous recombination events the internal neo^r expression cassette is retained but the flanking HSV-thymidine kinase sequences are lost. Consequently, the resulting transfectants are resistant to both neomycin and ganciclovir. By prescreening for neomycin-resistant and ganciclovir-resistant ES cells, the majority of the cells with random integration events are eliminated, thereby greatly reducing the molecular analyses required to identify correctly targeted clones.

After correctly targeted ES cells are identified, they are injected into host blastocysts, which are then surgically implanted into the uterus of a surrogate mother and allowed to develop to term. The resulting animals are chimeric, composed in part of cells deriving from the host blastocyst and in part from the genetically modified ES cells. If the modified ES cells colonize the germ line, the targeted mutation can be transmitted to subsequent generations. Interbreeding of mice heterozygous for the targeted mutation will produce homozygous mutant animals at a frequency of 25%. The entire process typically used for the generation of loss-of-function transgenic animals is shown in Figure 1-2. Robertson and Elizabeth [4] and Sedivy and Joyner [5] compiled excellent texts dealing with practical issues relating to gene targeting and the generation of chimeric animals with genetically modified ES cells.

The information provided here and shown in Figures 1-1 and 1-2 provides an introduction into the technical aspects of generating gain- and loss-of-function transgenic mice. However, the main focus of this chapter is to illustrate the ways that transgenesis has been used to alter cardiovascular structure and function. Accordingly, the remainder of the chapter provides examples of both gain- and loss-of-function studies wherein myocardial development, development of the cardiac conduction system, cardiomyocyte terminal differentiation, or cardiac hypertrophy have been altered by genetic manipulation. In addition to these limited examples, it should be noted that many excellent reviews have been published recently that summarize various cardiovascular perturbations in transgenic animals. These include reviews of gain-of-function models affecting blood pressure regulation, plasma lipoprotein metabolism and atherogenesis, as well as a catalog of promoters suitable for cardiovascular transgenic experiments [6–13]. In addition, several excellent review articles are available that describe loss-of-function transgenic models exhibiting altered cardiovascular function [14–19].

TYPICAL APPROACHES USED FOR THE GENERATION OF GAIN-OF-FUNCTION AND LOSS-OF-FUNCTION TRANSGENIC ANIMALS

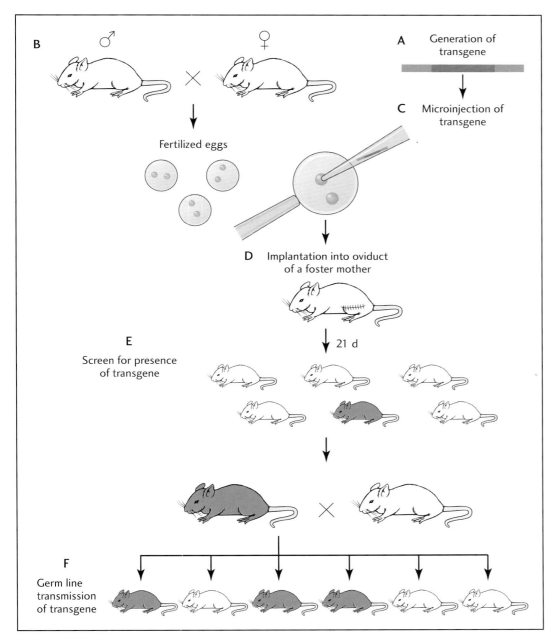

Figure 1-1.

General approach used to generate gain-of-function transgenic animals. The first step entails the generation of the transgene (**A**), which is designed to target expression of the desired gene product to the desired cell type or types. After the transgene is obtained, female mice are treated with follicle-stimulating hormone (FSH) and leuteinizing hormone (LH) to increase the yield of embryos during ovulation. The females are then mated with male mice (**B**), and the resulting embryos are harvested before pronuclear fusion (typically 12 hours after copulation). The embryos are visualized under Hoffman or Nomarski optics, and a solution containing the transgene is microinjected directly into either the male or female pronucleus using a microinjection pipette (**C**). After microinjection, the embryos are surgically implanted into the oviduct of a surrogate mother (*ie*, a mouse that is hormonally competent to accept the embryos [**D**]). The embryos are then allowed to develop to term. Shortly after birth, a small piece of tissue is biopsied and analyzed for the presence of the transgene (**E**). This usually entails either Southern blot analyses or polymerase chain reaction amplification using oligonucleotide primers specific for the transgene. More than 20% of the pups obtained from microinjected embryos will carry the transgene. The transgenic animals are then crossed with nontransgenic mates, and in most instances the transgene is passed onto subsequent generations in a mendelian fashion (**F**) [1,4,5].

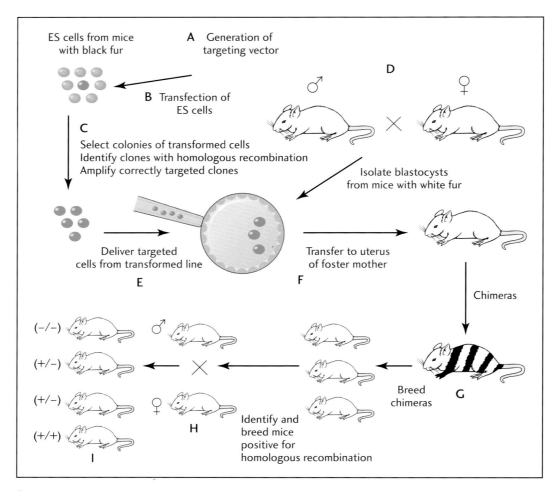

Figure 1-2.

General approach used to generate loss-of-function transgenic animals. The first step entails
the generation of the targeting vector that incorporates positive and negative drug selection
schemes for the enrichment of correctly targeted clones (**A**). The targeting vector is introduced into totipotent embryonic stem (ES) cells through electroporation or DNA/calcium
phosphate transfection (**B**). Neomycin- and ganciclovir-resistant clones are identified and
amplified. DNA is prepared from these clones and analytical Southern blotting is used to
identify those with correctly targeted homologous recombination events (**C**). These clones
are then used to generate transgenic animals. To produce host blastocysts, male and female
mice are mated and the resulting embryos are harvested 3.5 days after copulation (**D**). ES
clones carrying a correctly targeted gene are then injected into the blastoceal cavity (typically
10 to 15 ES cells per blastocyst [**E**]). The injected blastocysts are then surgically implanted
into the uterus of a surrogate mother and allowed to develop to term (**F**). Differences in
coat colors between the ES cells (black fur in this example) and the host blastocyst (white
fur in this example) are used to facilitate the degree of stem cell contribution to the resulting
chimeric mice. Animals derived largely from the ES cells (as evidenced by a preponderance
of black fur [**G**]) are mated, and the transmission of the targeted locus to the resulting pups
is monitored by molecular analysis (diagnostic Southern blotting or polymerase chain reaction amplification; coat color transmission cannot be used at this point because of independent assortment). After the targeted locus is transmitted, animals heterozygous for the targeted alleles are interbred to generate homozygous mutant animals (**H** and **I**).

Use of Gain-of-function Modification to Alter Cardiac Development

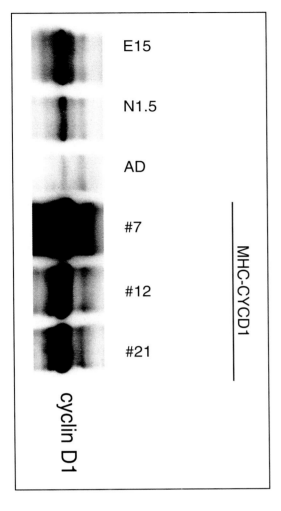

Figure 1-3.

During fetal life, increases in cardiac mass result from cardiomyocyte hyperplasia. At birth, cardiomyocyte proliferation ceases and subsequent increase in cardiac mass results from hypertrophy. Decreased expression of many cell-cycle regulatory genes (including members of the D-type cyclin gene family) accompanies cardiomyocyte cell-cycle withdrawal. In this study, Soonpaa *et al.* [20] generated transgenic mice that continued to express cyclin D1 during the period of cardiomyocyte cell-cycle withdrawal. Surprisingly, sustained expression of cyclin D1 was sufficient to increase cardiomyocyte multinucleation and promote sustained DNA synthesis in adult animals. Mice carrying the *MHC-CYCD1* (myosin heavy chain–cyclin D1) transgene express high levels of cyclin D1 in the adult heart. Protein was prepared from the hearts of three *MHC-CYCD1* adult mice (from transgenic lineages 7, 12, and 21). Control samples were prepared from nontransgenic embryonic (E15), neonatal (N15), and adult (AD) mice. The samples were resolved on polyacrylamide gels, transferred to nitrocellulose, and incubated with an anti–cyclin-D1 antibody. The sample was then incubated with a horseradish peroxidase–conjugated secondary antibody and signal was visualized using the enzyme-linked chemiluminescence system. Cyclin D1 is expressed at high levels in nontransgenic embryonic hearts, at intermediate levels in nontransgenic neonatal hearts, and at very low levels in nontransgenic adult hearts. In contrast, high levels of cyclin D1 were detected in the hearts of the adult transgenic mice. (*From* Soonpaa and coworkers [20]; with permission.)

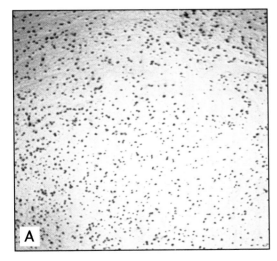

Figure 1-4.

Cardiomyocytes in adult *MHC-CYCD1* (myosin heavy chain–cyclin D1) transgenic mice. These cardiomyocytes continue to synthesize DNA. A thymidine incorporation assay was used to monitor cardiomyocyte DNA synthesis in the adult *MHC-CYCD1* transgenic animals. This assay used a second transgenic mouse model (designated *MHC-nLAC*) that expresses a nuclear-localized β-galactosidase (βGAL) reporter gene exclusively in the myocardium. Accurate cardiomyocyte DNA synthesis indices can be obtained readily with these animals simply by injecting tritiated thymidine, followed by screening for colocalization of βGAL activity, which appears blue after staining with X-GAL (5-bromo-4-chloro-3-indolyl-β-D-galactopyranoside) and silver grains in autoradiographs of heart sections. Accordingly, *MHC-CYCD1* mice were crossed with *MHC-nLAC* mice, and animals carrying the *MHC-nLAC* transgene alone or both the *MHC-nLAC* and the *MHC-CYCD1* transgenes were identified and sequestered. At 3 months of age, the mice received a single injection of tritiated thymidine, and the hearts were harvested, sectioned, stained with X-GAL (to identify the cardiomyocyte nuclei), and subjected to autoradiography (to identify nuclei synthesizing DNA). **A,** A survey photomicrograph of the ventricular septum of an adult *MHC-nLAC* transgenic mouse stained with X-GAL. Note the relative density of the cardiomyocyte nuclei (*blue staining*). (*continued on next page*)

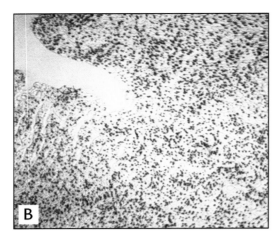

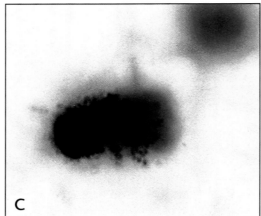

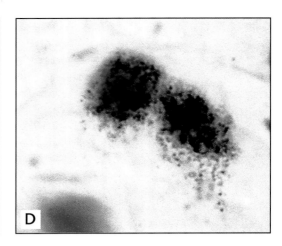

Figure 1-4. (*continued*)

B, A survey micrograph of the ventricular septum of an adult mouse carrying both the *MHC-nLAC* and the *MHC-CYCD1* transgenes, stained with X-GAL. Note the marked increase in nuclear density compared with the control litter mate shown in *panel A*. **C** and **D,** Autoradiographs of sections prepared from transgenic mice carrying both the *MHC-nLAC* and the *MHC-CYCD1* transgenes. Cardiomyocyte DNA synthesis is readily observed in the hearts of the adult transgenic mice; note the presence of silver grains over the blue nuclei. Two putative daughter cardiomyocyte nuclei can be seen in *panel D* (note that the silver grain intensity is approximately half that observed for synthetic nucleus depicted in *panel C*), suggestive of karyokinesis. Regional rates of DNA synthesis as high as 2% have been observed in these animals. (*From* Soonpaa and coworkers [20]; with permission.)

USE OF LOSS-OF-FUNCTION MODIFICATION TO ALTER CARDIAC DEVELOPMENT

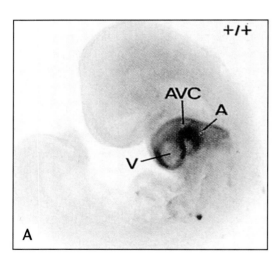

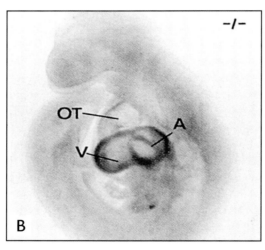

Figure 1-5.

Members of the NK class of homeodomain proteins play a pivotal role in the development of myogenic lineages during embryogenesis. In fruit flies, the homeodomain protein "Tinman" is required for determination of the cardiogenic lineage. Nkx2-5 is a mammalian homologue of Tinman. The elegant study by Lyons *et al.* [21] demonstrated that targeted disruption of Nkx2-5 results in abnormal heart morphogenesis, growth retardation, and ultimately embryonic lethality by embryonic day 10. Cardiac defects in Nkx2.5$^{-/-}$ embryos: the embryos were processed by whole mount in situ hybridization with an α-cardiac actin probe. **A,** A wild-type embryo. **B,** A mutant embryo. Both embryos were analyzed at 9.5 days postcoitum. The wild-type embryo exhibited the expected rightward looping of the heart tube that marks the beginning of chamber formation. In contrast, no tubular heart looping was observed in the mutant embryo. The mutant heart retained a linear confirmation with a narrow ventricular outflow tract (OT) and an open atrioventricular chamber lacking an atrioventricular canal (AVC). (*continued on next page*)

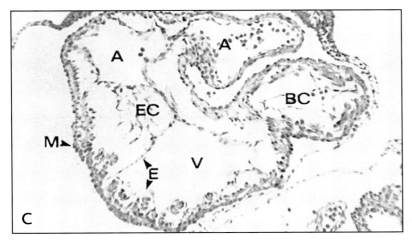

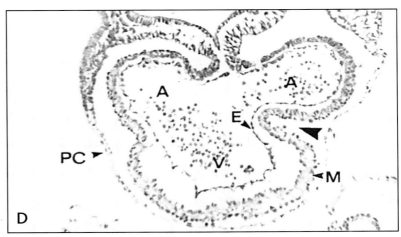

Figure 1-5. (*continued*)

Defects in cardiac development in the Nkx2-5–deficient embryos were further characterized by histologic analyses. Examination of wild-type embryos at the 22-somite stage of development (*panel C*) revealed the presence of a well-looped heart with normal endocardial cushion formation (EC) and ventricular trabeculation. The presence of myocardial (M) and endocardial (E) layers separated by cardiac jelly was readily apparent. In mutant embryos at the 20-somite stage (*panel D*), no cardiac looping was observed, consistent with the macroscopic analyses (see *panel B*). The *arrowhead* indicates the cleft between the presumptive atrial and ventricular chambers. A—atrium; PC—pericardium. (*From* Lyons and coworkers [21]; with permission.)

USE OF GAIN-OF-FUNCTION MODIFICATION TO ALTER THE CARDIAC CONDUCTION SYSTEM

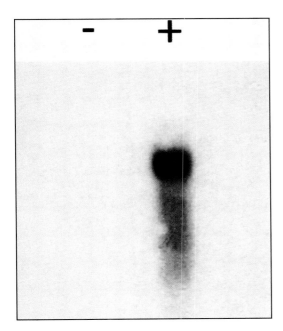

Figure 1-6.

This figure shows high levels of nerve growth factor (NGF) transcripts in *MHC-NGF* (myosin heavy chain–nerve growth factor) transgenic mice. During development, the relative levels of neutrophic agents such as NGF will determine the ultimate extent of innervation in the adult organ. In an effort to increase the level of cardiac innervation, Hassankhani *et al.* [22] used the α-cardiac MHC promoter to target high levels of NGF expression in the myocardium of transgenic mice. The adult transgenic animals exhibited cardiac hypertrophy that was concomitant with constitutively elevated levels of catacholamine and the infiltration of cells with apparent neural origins. RNA prepared from the hearts of an adult *MHC-NGF* transgenic mouse (*plus sign*) and a nontransgenic litter mate (*minus sign*) was displayed on an agarose gel, transferred to Genescreen (NEN Research Products, Boston) and hybridized to a radiolabeled probe prepared from human NGF exon 4. This probe reacts with human NGF sequences but not with mouse sequences. High levels of NGF expression are detected in the adult transgenic mouse heart, but not in the heart from the nontransgenic litter mate.

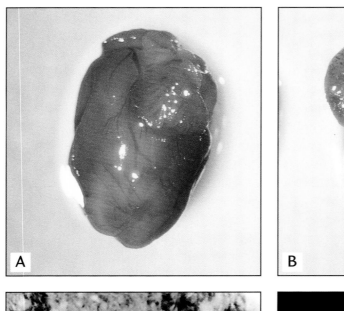

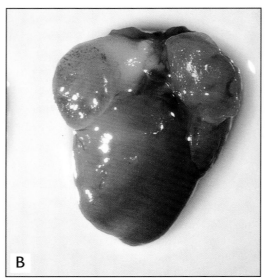

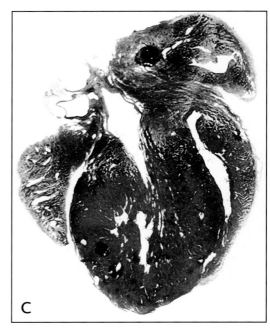

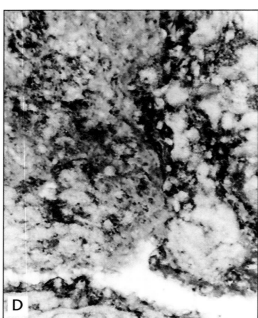

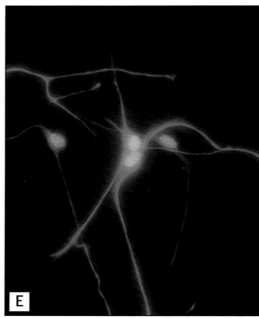

infiltration of cells at the base of the heart. **D,** Immune cytologic analysis of an adult *MHC-NGF* transgenic heart. The image was photographed near the base of the heart; the atrial appendage is visible in the *upper portion* of the image. The section was reacted with an anti-GFAP (glial fibrillary acidic protein) (blue signal from an alkaline phosphatase-conjugated secondary antibody) and anti-S100 (brown signal from a horseradish peroxidase–conjugated secondary antibody). Cells of both neuronal and glial origin are present in the infiltrate at the base of the hearts. **E,** A cultured cell prepared from the *MHC-NGF* transgenic hearts. The sample was reacted with an anti-TH (tyrosine hydroxylase) antibody, followed by a rhodamine-conjugated secondary antibody and visualized under fluorescence illumination. The presence of numerous TH-positive bipolar cells in primary cultures is consistent with the notion that NGF overexpression promotes hyperinnervation in the transgenic hearts. (Part C *from* Hassankhani and coworkers [22]; with permission.)

▌**Figure 1-7.**
Cardiomegaly and hyperinnervation in transgenic hearts that overexpress nerve growth factor (NGF). **A,** A gross view of the heart dissected from a nontransgenic mouse. **B,** A gross view of the heart dissected from an *MHC-NGF* (myosin heavy chain–nerve growth factor) transgenic litter mate. Note the marked increase in cardiac mass in the heart of the transgenic animal. **C,** A survey micrograph of the same *MHC-NGF* transgenic heart depicted in *panel B.* The section was stained with Masson's trichrome. Note the pronounced

USE OF LOSS-OF-FUNCTION MODIFICATION TO ALTER THE CARDIAC CONDUCTION SYSTEM

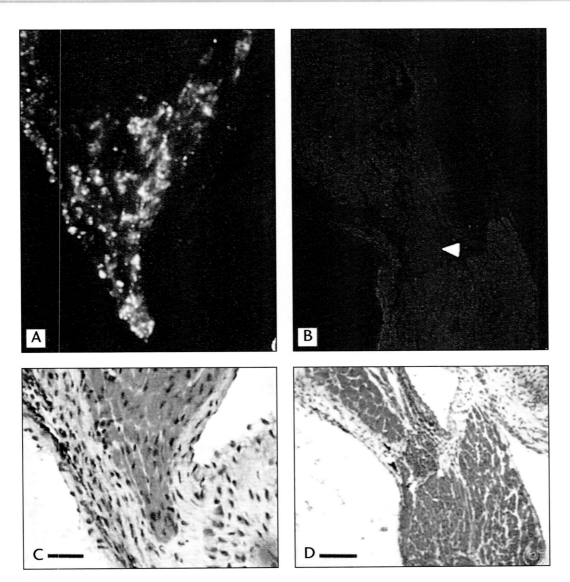

Figure 1-8.

Cx40 is a prominent gap junction protein found in the AV node and Purkinje fibers of the cardiac conduction system. To establish the functional role of Cx40, Simon *et al.* [23] disrupted the gene in transgenic mice. Although homozygous mutant animals are viable, surface ECG analysis revealed that the loss of Cx40 results in cardiac conduction abnormalities characteristic of atrioventricular block with associated bundle branch block. These results confirm that Cx40 is required for conduction system action potential propagation, and raise the possibility that anomalies in Cx40 may underlie some forms of cardiac arrhythmia in humans. This figure shows Cx40 expression in the His–Purkinjë system of wild-type mice and Cx40[-/+] mice: frozen sections of hearts from wild-type and Cx40[-/-] mice were subjected to immune histologic analyses with an anti-Cx40 antibody followed by rhodamine conjugated secondary antibody (*panels A and B*). Adjacent sections (*panels C and D*) were stained for AChE (acetylcholinesterase activity, brown signal) to identify cells of conduction system origin. Cx40 immune reactivity was restricted to AChE-positive Purkinjë fibers in wild-type heart (*panel A*). In contrast, no Cx40 was detected in AChE-positive fibers from Cx40[-/-] animals (*panel B*; *arrowhead*). The *bars* indicate 50 μm in *panel C* and 150 μm in *panel D*. (*From* Simon and coworkers [23]; with permission.)

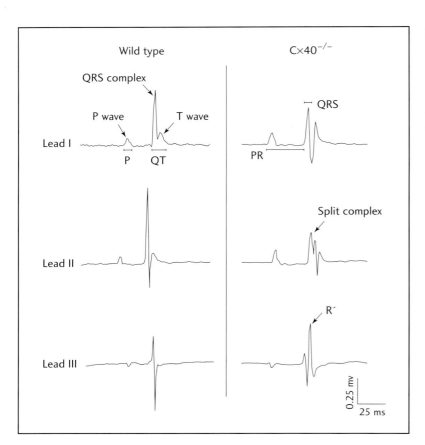

Figure 1-9.

Electrocardiographic (ECG) analyses revealing the presence of conduction anomalies in Cx40$^{-/+}$ transgenic mice. Three-lead ECGs were recorded from wild-type and Cx40$^{-/-}$ mice. Both PR and QRS intervals were prolonged in Cx40$^{-/-}$ mice compared with wild-type controls, indicating that both atrioventricular and intraventricular conduction was delayed in mutant animals. ECGs recorded from the Cx40$^{-/-}$ mutant animals also exhibited split QRS complexes in lead II, rSR' morphology in lead III, and wide S waves in lead I, indicating uncoordinated ventricular activation. Collectively, these results underscore the importance of Cx40 function in activation of cardiac depolarization. (*Adapted from* Simon and coworkers [23]; with permission.)

USE OF GAIN-OF-FUNCTION MODIFICATION TO ALTER CARDIOMYOCYTE TERMINAL DIFFERENTIATION

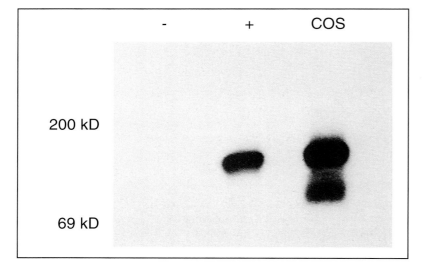

Figure 1-10.

SV40 T-Antigen (T-Ag) has been widely used to induce cell lineage–specific tumors in transgenic animals. When expressed in the fetal heart, T-Ag expression was sufficient to block terminal differentiation in both atrial and ventricular cardiomyocytes, thereby resulting in the formation of cardiac tumors comprising differentiated, proliferating cardiomyocytes. The resulting tumors were subsequently used to generate differentiated cell lines. This figure shows expression of large T antigen (T-Ag) in atrium in ANF-TAG (atrial natriuretic factor–SV40 T-Ag) transgenic mice: total protein prepared from the atria of nontransgenic (-) and transgenic (+) adult ANF-TAG atria was displayed on a polyacrylamide gel, transferred to nitrocellulose, and reacted with an anti–T-Ag antibody, followed by radiolabeled protein A. Protein prepared from COS cells (an SV40-transformed cell line) was used as a positive control for T-Ag. Abundant expression of T-Ag (molecular weight, 92 kD) was detected in the sample prepared from the ANF-TAG atria, but not from the nontransgenic control. (*From* Field [24]; with permission.)

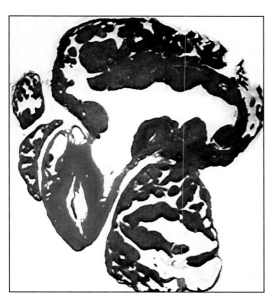

Figure 1-11.

Large T-antigen (T-Ag) expression resulting in atrial tumorigenesis in adult ANF-TAG (atrial natriuretic factor–large T-antigen) transgenic mice. A survey photomicrograph of a section stained with hematoxylin and eosin prepared from an adult ANF-TAG heart is shown. Fulminate right atrial tumorigenesis is apparent, as is a limited degree of left atrial tumorigenesis. The ventricles are not affected, which was expected, because the ANF promoter is not transcriptionally active in the adult ventricles. Note that T-Ag expression resulted in uniform atrial hyperplasia, as opposed to focal outgrowths. This suggests that T-Ag expression alone is sufficient to drive atrial cardiomyocyte proliferation (*ie*, secondary mutation in cooperating proto-oncogenes does not appear to be required for tumor progression in this model). (*From* Field [24]; with permission.)

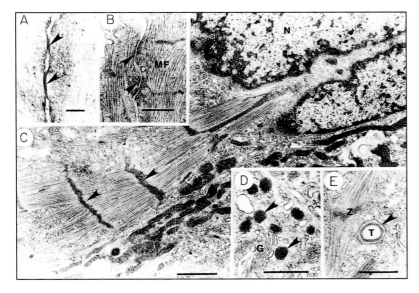

Figure 1-12.

A high plating efficiency and a limited capacity for proliferation in vitro are exhibited in AT-1 cardiomyocytes, a transplantable tumor lineage derived from primary ANF-TAG (atrial natriuretic factor–large T-antigen) tumors. During the course of a series of syngeneic transplantation studies, a transplantable tumor lineage designated AT-1 was obtained. AT-1 tumors can attain a large mass (10 to 20 g) when grown in a suitable host. In primary culture, AT-1 cardiomyocytes exhibit a highly differentiated phenotype and a limited capacity for proliferation. Shown is an AT-1 cardiomyocyte in the process of cytokinesis. The sample was reacted with an anti-sarcomeric myosin heavy chain antibody followed by a fluorescein isothiocyanate–conjugated secondary antibody and visualized under fluorescent illumination. Well-developed myofibers are apparent in the cytoplasm of the cell. Moreover, primary cultures of AT-1 cardiomyocytes exhibit spontaneous contractile activity.

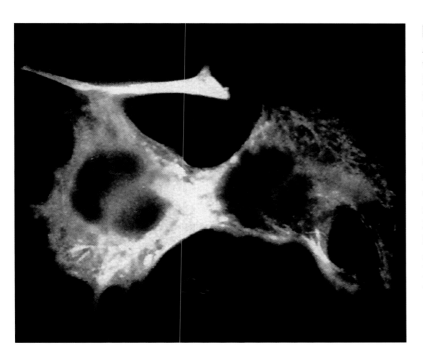

Figure 1-13.

Survey electron micrograph of cultured atrial cardiomyocytes derived from a transplant tumor. Primary cultures of AT-1 cardiomyocytes were processed from transmission electron microscopic analysis using standardized approaches. Shown are the junctional complexes that connect adjacent AT-1 cardiomyocytes. Desmosomes (**A**) and gap junctions (**B**) are observed, as would be expected because of the synchronous beating seen in these cultures. A well-developed myofiber network is also apparent, with prominent Z bands (**C** [*arrows*]). Secretory granules (which contain atrial natriuretic factor [**D**]) and a prominent T-tubule system (**E**) also are present throughout the cultured AT-1 cardiomyocytes. (*From* Steinhelper and coworkers [25]; with permission.)

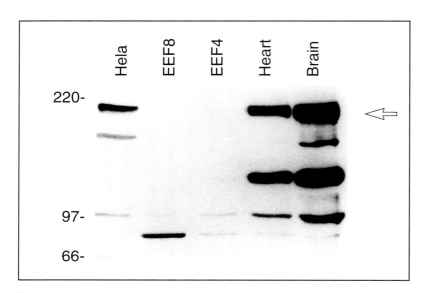

Figure 1-14.

Tuberous sclerosis complex (TSC) is characterized by the appearance of nonmalignant tumors that affect a wide spectrum of organs, including the heart. TSC disease-causing genes have been identified on chromosomes 9 (*TSC1*) and 16. Pajak *et al.* [26] took advantage of the observation that Eker rats carry a germline *TSC2* mutation. Rats heterozygous for the mutation (*TSC2$^{EK/+}$*) are predisposed to renal carcinoma, whereas animals homozygous for the mutation (*TSC2$^{EK/EK}$*) die in utero during midgestation. Spontaneously contractile cardiomyocytes were observed after multiple passages of whole-embryo cultures prepared from embryonic day 12.5 *TSC2$^{EK/EK}$* fetuses, but not from *TSC2^{EK+}* or *TSC2$^{+/+}$* fetuses. The *TSC2$^{EK/EK}$* cardiomyocytes continued to actively synthesize DNA after as many as eight passages, indicating that the *TSC2* gene product is required for normal cardiomyocyte cell-cycle withdrawal and terminal differentiation. Although this model exploits a naturally occurring mutation (not one introduced by transgenesis), it is included here because it demonstrates how loss-of-function mutations can block cardiomyocyte terminal differentiation: analogous mouse mutants at the *TSC2* locus have recently been generated using homologous recombination. Whole embryo cultures generated from *TSC2$^{EK/EK}$* embryos do not express tuberin, the protein encoded by the *TSC2* locus: heterozygous Eker rats (*TSC2$^{EK/+}$*) were intercrossed to produce homozygous mutant embryos. The embryos were harvested at day 12 of development and whole embryo cultures were generated. Total protein from the *TSC2$^{EK/EK}$* whole embryo cultures (designated *EEF8* and *EEF4*) was fractionated on a 7.5% polyacrylamide gel, transferred to Immobilon, and probed with an anti-tuberin antibody. Signal was visualized by the enzyme-linked chemiluminescence (ECL) method. Protein from HeLa cells, as well as from normal fetal rat heart and brain, was included as positive controls. Molecular weight markers are indicated on the *left*; the position of tuberin is indicated on the *right*. Tuberin was readily detected in the positive control samples. However, tuberin was not expressed in the *TSC2$^{EK/EK}$* whole embryo cultures. (*From* Pajak and coworkers [26]; with permission.)

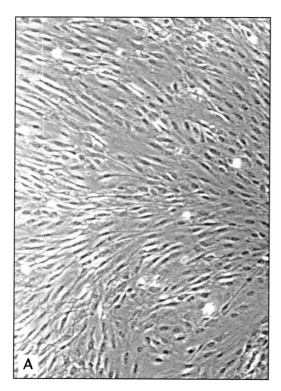

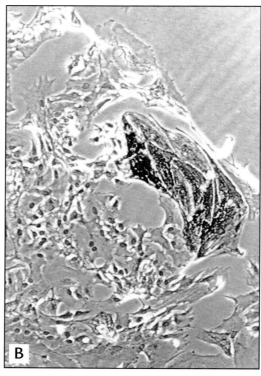

Figure 1-15.

Cells expressing sarcomeric myosin heavy chain (MHC) are present in the passage 4 *TSC2$^{EK/EK}$* whole embryo cultures but not in *TSC2$^{+/+}$* or *TSC2$^{EK/+}$* cultures. Passage 4 cultures were fixed and reacted with anti-sarcomeric MHC antibody MF20, followed by an HRP-conjugated anti-mouse secondary antibody. MHC expression (*brown signal*) was detected with a diaminobenzidine-based reaction. Clusters of MHC-positive cells were apparent throughout the *TSC2$^{EK/EK}$* whole embryo cultures but not in *TSC2$^{+/+}$* or *TSC2$^{EK/+}$* cultures. Moreover, these clusters of MHC-positive cells exhibited spontaneous and rhythmic contractile activity, indicating that they are likely of myocardial origin. This was subsequently proven by molecular, cytologic, and ultrastructural analyses. (*From* Pajak and coworkers [26]; with permission.)

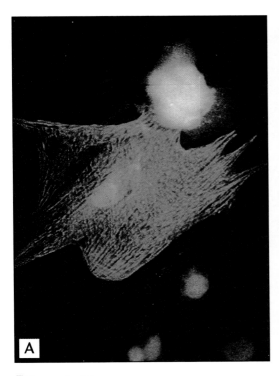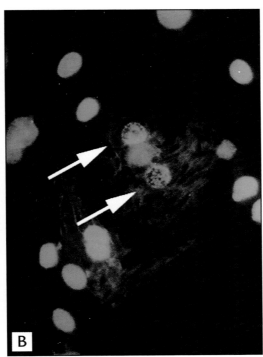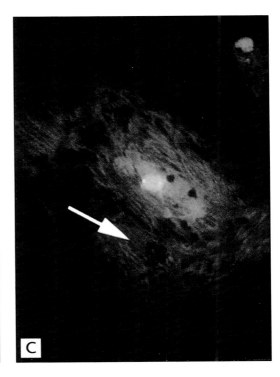

Figure 1-16.

Sustained cardiomyocyte DNA synthesis in passage 8 *TSC2^{EK/EK}* whole embryo cultures. *TSC2^{EK/EK}* cultures were incubated with tritiated thymidine for 2 hours. The cells were then fixed and reacted with an anti-MHC antibody, followed by an FITC-conjugated secondary antibody (*green signal* when visualized under fluorescent illumination [**A–C**]). After immune cytologic processing, the samples were subjected to autoradiography to permit identifica-

tion of cells actively synthesizing DNA (signal visualized as nuclear *silver grains* [**B** and **C**]). Finally, the samples were counterstained with Hoechst 33342 to visualize nuclei (*blue signal* under fluorescent illumination [**A–C**]). The presence of nuclear silver grains in MHC-expressing cells (*arrows*) indicates that the cardiomyocytes in passage 8 *TSC2^{EK/EK}* whole embryo cultures continue to synthesize DNA. (*From* Pajak and coworkers [26]; with permission.)

USE OF GAIN-OF-FUNCTION MODIFICATION TO INDUCE CARDIAC HYPERTROPHY

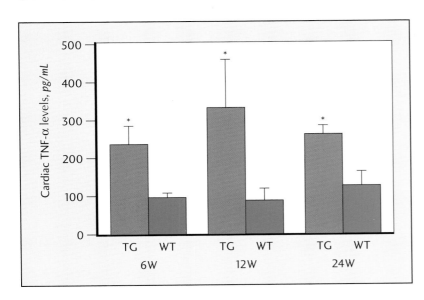

Figure 1-17.

Several studies have shown that the failing myocardium expresses TNF-α, an important proinflammatory cytokine. To elucidate cause–effect relationships between TNF-α expression and the pathogenesis of heart failure, Kubota *et al.* [27] generated transgenic mice that overexpressed this cytokine in the heart. Mice overexpressing TNF-α developed progressive cardiac hypertrophy resulting in recapitulated the phenotype of congestive heart failure, ultimately giving rise to dilated cardiomyopathy. TG and wild-type (WT) mice were sacrificed at 6, 12, and 24 weeks of age, and cardiac TNF-α levels were determined by enzyme-linked immunosorbent assay. As expected, TNF-α levels were higher in TG mice than in the nontransgenic controls at all ages analyzed. Values are expressed as mean ± SD. *Asterisks* indicate $P < 0.001$. (*Adapted from* Kubota and coworkers [27].)

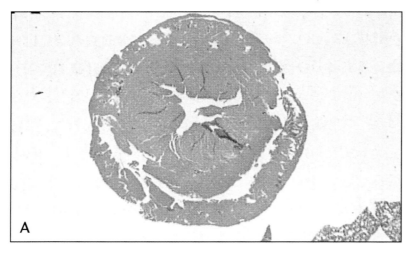

Figure 1-18.

Cardiac hypertrophy in tumor necrosis factor (TNF)-α transgenic mice. Formalin-fixed sections of age-matched (24 weeks old) wild-type (*panel A*) and transgenic (*panel B*) hearts were stained with hematoxylin and eosin (magnification, × 5). Sections were taken at the midventricular level, as evidenced by the presence of papillary muscle in the cavity and the semicircular shape of the right ventricular free wall. The TNF-α transgenic hearts exhibited eccentric hypertrophy (*panel B*), as well as patchy interstitial fibrosis and interstitial inflammation (not shown). None of these histopathologic anomalies was present in the nontransgenic controls. (*From* Kubota and coworkers [27]; with permission.)

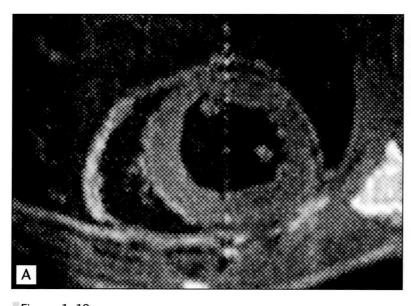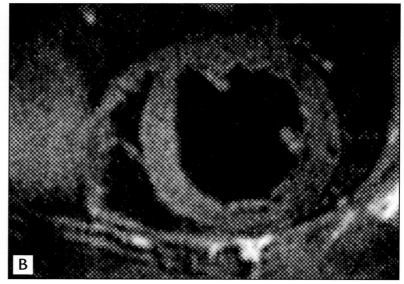

Figure 1-19.

Progression of cardiac hypertrophy in the tumor necrosis factor (TNF)-α mice progresses to dilated cardiomyopathy as revealed by in vivo magnetic resonance (MR) analyses. MR images were recorded from age-matched wild-type (*panel A*) and TNF-α (*panel B*) mice; representative midventricular short-axis views captured at the end of diastole are shown. The transgenic heart was markedly dilated as compared with the nontransgenic control. *Bars* indicate 2.5 mm. (*From* Kubota and coworkers [27]; with permission.)

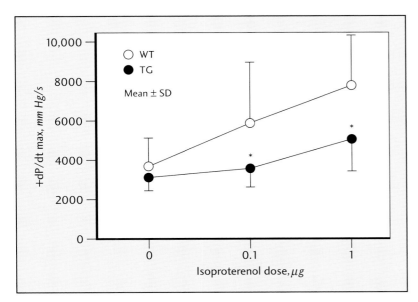

Figure 1-20.

Depressed contractile response to isoproterenol challenge in vivo among tumor necrosis factor-α, transgenic (TG) mice. Left ventricular dP/dt max (recorded via an intraventricular 1.4-F micromanometer catheter) was used as an index of contractility before and after isoproterenol injections. Although left ventricular dP/dt max for transgenic and wild-type (WT) mice was similar at baseline, its responsiveness to isoproterenol was blunted in the transgenic animals (*asterisk* indicates $P < 0.05$). This observation is consistent with decreased cardiac function in the transgenic mice, which may contribute to the development of hypertrophy and ultimately dilated cardiomyopathy in these animals. Values are mean ± SD. (*Adapted from* Kubota and coworkers [27].)

USE OF HOMOLOGOUS RECOMBINATION TO INTRODUCE A SPECIFIC AMINO ACID ALTERATION IN MYOSIN HEAVY CHAIN

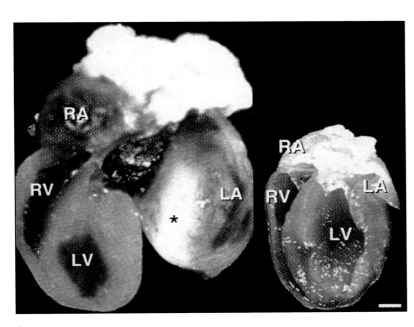

Figure 1-21.

Familial hypertrophic cardiomyopathy (FHC) is an autosomal dominant disease characterized by cardiac hypertrophy with cardiomyocyte disarray. Genetic analyses of FHC patients revealed that the disease is caused by mutations in genes encoding cardiac myofiber proteins. Thus far mutations in cardiac MHC, actin, or tropomyosin genes have been identified in MHC patients. Geisterfer-Lowrance *et al.* [28] generated a mouse model of FHC by introducing an R403Q mutation (*ie*, a substitution of Arg to Gln at amino acid residue 403) into the α-cardiac *MHC* gene: an analogous mutation in the β-MHC has been identified in humans with FHC. Although sedentary heterozygous mutant mice survived for 1 year, their exercise capacity was compromised and histologic analyses of the heats revealed pathologies similar to that seen in FHC patients. Gross sections of hearts from a 15-week-old α-MHC[403/+] (*left side*) and control mice (*right side*) are shown: the mice had been subjected to an exercise regimen. The α-MHC[403/+] heart exhibits asymmetrical hypertrophy of the left ventricle. Moreover, pronounced left atrial enlargement was apparent. Fresh blood clots were apparent in all chambers, and an organized thrombus (*asterisk*) was observed in the left atrium (LA). In contrast, no gross abnormalities were apparent in the wild-type control mouse (WT). The *bar* indicates 1 mm. LA—left atrium; LV—left ventricle; RA—right atrium; RV—right ventricle. (*From* Geisterfer-Lowrance and coworkers [28]; with permission.)

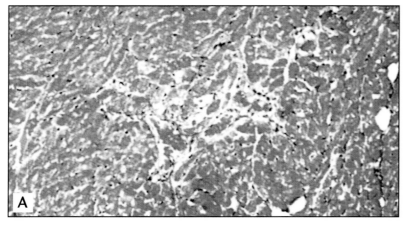

Figure 1-22.

Histopathology in sections prepared from α-MHC[403/+] mice. Hearts were sectioned transversely at the midventricular level and stained with Masson's trichrome stain. Progressive fibrosis was evident by collagen staining (*blue*) in 15-week-old (*panel A*) and 30- week-old (*panel B*) α-MHC[403/+] mice. Extensive myofiber disarray was also evident. In contrast, no fibrosis or myofiber disarray were observed in the hearts from wild-type mice (not shown). (*From* Geisterfer-Lowrance and coworkers [28]; with permission.)

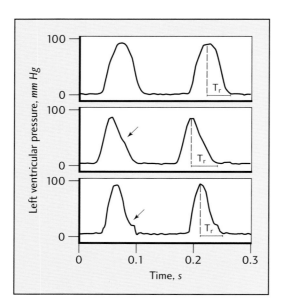

Figure 1-23.

Functional anomalies in working heart preparations of α-MHC[403/+] mice. Pressure tracings were recorded from wild-type (5 weeks old [*top panel*]) and α-MHC[403/+] (5 and 15 weeks old [*middle and bottom panels*], respectively) mice. Although the maximum left ventricular pressures generated by wild-type and MHC[403/+] hearts were similar, the profiles of their pressure curves differed significantly. Most notably, anomalies in cardiac relaxation were apparent in the hearts from mutant animals (*arrows*). (*Adapted from* Geisterfer-Lowrance and coworkers [28].)

REFERENCES

1. Hogan B: *Manipulating the Mouse Embryo*. Plainview, NY: Cold Spring Harbor Laboratory Press; 1994.

2. Field LJ: Transgenic mice in cardiovascular research. *Ann Rev Physiol* 1993, 55:97–114.

3. Mansour SL, Thomas KR, Capecchi MR: Disruption of the proto-oncogene int-2 in mouse embryo-derived stem cells: a general strategy for targeting mutations to non-selectable genes. *Nature* 1988, 336:348–352.

4. Robertson EJ, Elizabeth J: *Teratocarcinomas and Embryonic Stem Cells*. Washington, DC: IRL Press; 1987.

5. Sedivy JM, Joyner AL: *Gene Targeting*. New York: WH Freeman; 1992.

6. Koh GY, Klug MG, Field LJ: Atrial natriuretic factor and transgenic mice. *Hypertension* 1993, 22:634 –639.

7. Yang CW, Striker LJ, Kopchick JJ, *et al.*: Glomerulosclerosis in mice transgenic for native or mutated bovine growth hormone gene. *Kidney Int* 1993, 39(suppl):90–94.

8. Striker LJ, Doi T, Striker GE: Transgenic mice in renal research. *Adv Nephrol Necker Hosp* 1991, 20:91–108.

9. Suzuki T, Hayashi M, Sofuni T: Initial experiences and future directions for transgenic mouse mutation assays. *Mutation Res* 1994, 307: 489–494.

10. Breslow JL: Lipoprotein metabolism and atherosclerosis susceptibility in transgenic mice. *Curr Opin Lipidol* 1994, 5:175–184.

11. Hunter JJ, Zhu H, Lee KJ, *et al.*: Targeting gene expression to specific cardiovascular cell types in transgenic mice. *Hypertension* 1993, 22:608–617.

12. Grant FD, Reventos J, Kawabata S, *et al.*: Transgenic mouse models of vasopressin expression. *Hypertension* 1993, 22:640–645.

13. Franklin M, Field LJ: Use of transgenic animals in cardiovascular toxicology testing. In *Comprehensive Toxicology: Cardiovascular Toxicology*, vol 6. Edited by Bishop SP, Kerns WD (vol eds); Sipes IG, McQueen CA, Gandolfi AJ. 1997:197–208.

14. Lin MC, Rockman HA, Chien KR: Heart and lung disease in engineered mice. *Nat Med* 1995, 1:742–751.

15. Chien KR: Cardiac muscle diseases in genetically engineered mice: evolution of molecular physiology. *Am J Physiol* 1995, 269(suppl H):755–766.

16. Tamura K, Umemura S, Fukamizu A *et al*.: Recent advances in the study of renin and angiotensinogen genes: from molecules to the whole body. *Hypertension Res* 1995, 18:7–18.

17. Carmeliet PF: Physiological consequences of over- or under-expression of fibrinolytic system components in transgenic mice. *Baillieres Clin Haematol* 1995, 8:391–401.

18. Chien KR: Molecular advances in cardiovascular biology. *Science* 1993, 260:916–917.

19. Rossant J: Mouse mutants and cardiac development: new molecular insights into cardiogenesis. *Circ Res* 1996, 78:349–353.

20. Soonpaa MH, Koh GY, Pajak L, *et al*.: Cyclin D1 overexpression promotes cardiomyocyte DNA synthesis and multinucleation in transgenic mice. *J Clin Invest* 1997, 99:2644–2654.

21. Lyons I, Parsons LM, Hartley L, *et al*.: Myogenic and morphogenetic defects in the heart tubes of murine embryos lacking the homeo box gene Nkx2-5. *Genes Dev* 1995, 9:1654–1666.

22. Hassankhani A, Steinhelper ME, Soonpaa MH *et al*.: Overexpression of NGF within the heart of transgenic mice causes hyperinnervation, cardiac enlargement, and hyperplasia of ectopic cells. *Dev Biol* 1995, 169:309–321.

23. Simon AM, Goodenough DA, Paul DL: Mice lacking connexin have cardiac conduction abnormalities characteristic of atrioventricular block and bundle branch block. *Curr Biol* 1998, 8:295–298.

24. Field LJ: Atrial natriuretic factor-SV40 T antigen transgenes produce tumors and cardiac arrythmias in mice. *Science* 1988, 239:1029–1033.

25. Steinhelper ME, Lanson NA, Jr, Dresdner KP, *et al*.: Proliferation in vivo and in culture of differentiated adult atrial cardiomyocytes from transgenic mice. *Am J Physiol* 1990, 259(suppl H):1826–1834.

26. Pajak L, Jin F, Xiao G-H, *et al*.: Sustained cardiomyocyte DNA synthesis in whole embryo cultures lacking the TSC2 gene product. *Am J Physiol* 1997, 273 (suppl H):1619–1627.

27. Kubota T, McTiernan CF, Frye CS, *et al*.: Dilated cardiomyopathy in transgenic mice with cardiac-specific overexpression of tumor necrosis factor-alpha. *Circ Res* 1997, 81:627–635.

28. Geisterfer-Lowrance AAT, Christe M, Conner DA, *et al*.: A mouse model of familial hypertrophic cardiomyopathy. *Science* 1996, 272:731–734.

Congenital Heart Disease

Paul M. Weinberg

Congenital heart disease includes a group of abnormalities in which defects of spatial arrangement, internal organization, or chamber, valve, and vessel morphology are present at birth. Most of these abnormalities actually are present from the time of cardiac morphogenesis, between 21 and 56 days postovulation. However, because of impaired growth manifested by altered intracardiac or extracardiac blood flow, some abnormalities may appear or develop much later. Whereas a few lesions have long been known to be genetic, associated with major chromosomal abnormalities, more recent work has shown a genetic basis for a growing number of congenital heart defects. Other causes include maternal exposure to toxins such as drugs and infections, as well as maternal metabolic illnesses.

Cardiac morphology is best described using the segmental approach to diagnosis of Van Praagh [1]. After morphologic identification of each chamber and great artery, the spatial arrangements and intersegmental connections of the chambers and vessels are made. Finally, individual chamber, valve, and vessel abnormalities are described.

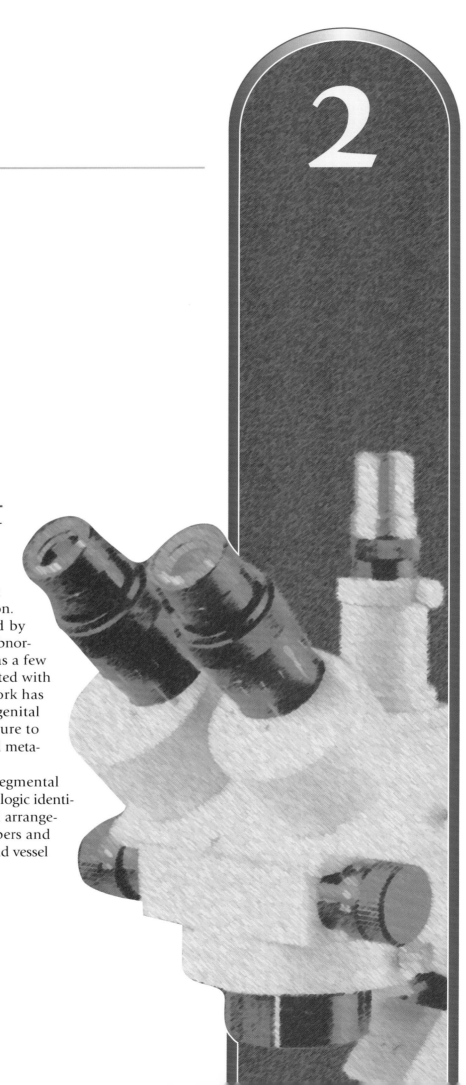

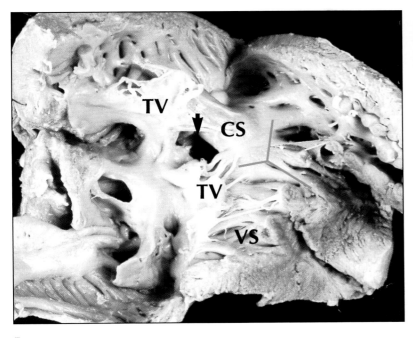

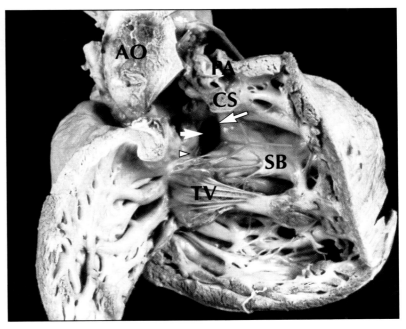

Figure 2-1.
Conoventricular/perimembranous ventricular septal defect (VSD).
Anterior views of opened right ventricle from a postmortem heart
specimen illustrate a conoventricular (also called perimembranous
or paramembranous) VSD (*arrow*) located between the infundibular (conal) septum (CS) and the trabeculated portion of septum
(VS), with the infundibular septum located *in* the fork of the Y of
the septal band. Typically, the tricuspid valve (TV) has chordal
attachments to the margins of the VSD. (*From* Weinberg [2].)

Figure 2-2.
Malalignment ventricular septal defect (VSD). Conal septal
malalignment type VSDs are located *in* the Y of the septal band
(SB) with the infundibular or conal septum (CS) present but in an
abnormal location, as shown here in a case of tetralogy of Fallot.
Note that the VSD (*arrow*) is beyond the tricuspid valve (TV)
chordal attachments (*arrowhead*), unlike the conoventricular VSD,
which may have chordal attachments to its rim. Displacement of
the CS relative to the remainder of the septum implies the presence of conotruncal anomalies (see Fig. 2-33). AO—aorta; PA—
pulmonary artery. (*From* Weinberg [2]; with permission.)

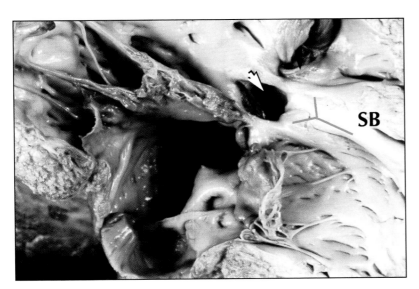

Figure 2-3.
Conal septal hypoplasia ventricular septal defect (VSD). Conal
septal hypoplasia VSDs (*arrow*) also may be located *in* the Y of the
septal band (SB), with either complete absence of the conal
septum (CS) or partial absence but with any remnants of the CS in
their normal plane. That is, the CS or the truncal septum (fibrous
ridge between semilunar valves seen when CS is completely
absent) is not displaced into the pulmonary or aortic outflow
tracts, as in tetralogy of Fallot or interrupted aortic arch. (*From*
Weinberg [2].)

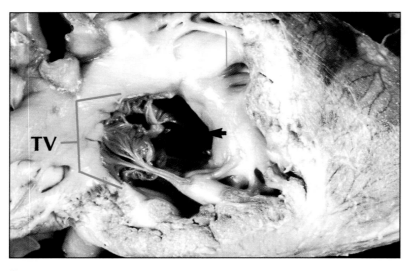

Figure 2-4.
Atrioventricular (AV) canal-type ventricular septal defect (VSD). An AV canal-type VSD (*arrow*) is found immediately beneath the annulus of the tricuspid valve (TV), running the full length of the septal leaflet of the TV or the diameter of the AV valve annulus, where it intersects the septal plane in the case of straddling tricuspid valve (shown here) or complete common AV canal. Like conoventricular VSDs, they may have chordal attachments to the crest of the VSD; however, conoventricular VSDs do not extend the full length of the septal leaflet, as do canal-type VSDs. (*From* Weinberg [2].)

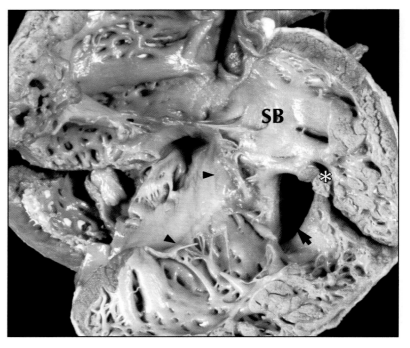

Figure 2-5.
Muscular ventricular septal defects (VSDs) are those located in the trabeculated portion of the ventricular septum. They can occur inferior to the septal band (SB) (mid-muscular), as shown here (*arrow*); anterior and superior to the SB (anterior muscular); anterior to the moderator band (*asterisk*) take-off (apical muscular); or beneath the septal leaflet of the tricuspid valve (*arrowheads*) but separated from the annulus by muscle (posterior muscular). (*From* Weinberg [2]; with permission.)

ATRIAL SEPTAL DEFECTS

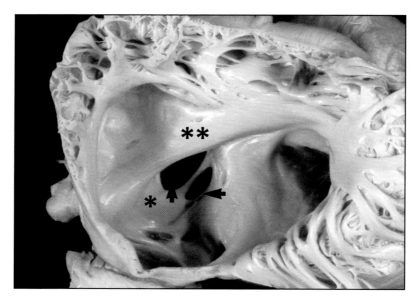

Figure 2-6.
Ostium secundum atrial septal defect (ASD). Right lateral views of opened right atrium from postmortem heart specimen illustrate an ostium secundum-type ASD (*arrows*) located within the septum primum (*single asterisk*) or flap valve of foramen ovale. In some cases, this defect may represent a total absence of that structure. Sometimes, as shown here, there are multiple defects separated by strands of septum primum tissue. The *double asterisk* indicates the septum secundum. (*From* Weinberg [2]; with permission.)

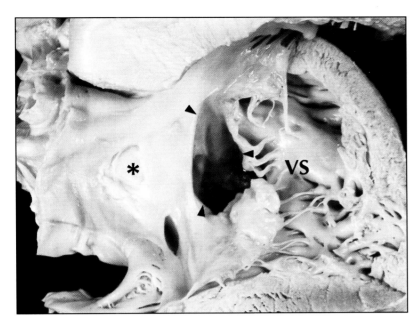

Figure 2-7.

Ostium primum atrial septal defect (ASD). Right lateral view of the atrial aspect of common atrioventricular (AV) valve with a commissural attachment of the superior leaflet to the crest of the ventricular septum (VS). This is the Rastelli type A form of complete common AV canal (see fig. 2-12). Note the normal appearance of septum primum (*asterisk*) and the anteriorly located ostium primum atrial septal defect (*arrowheads*). Note that there is no tissue between this ASD and the AV valve leaflets. Cases with a so-called common atrium may have a combination ostium secundum and ostium primum atrial septal defect. (*From* Weinberg [2]; with permission.)

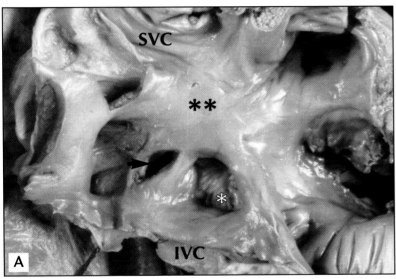

Figure 2-8.

Sinus venosus type atrial septal defect (ASD). Sinus venosus defects have two varieties. **A,** The more common variety is found posterior or superior to the septum primum (*single asterisk;* the so-called superior vena cava [SVC] variety), where a pulmonary vein essentially straddles the atrial septum, and the mouth of the pulmonary vein *is* the sinus venosus ASD. **B,** The second variety (*arrow;* the so-called inferior vena cava [IVC] variety) is similar, but with the IVC straddling the septum primum (*single asterisk*) inferiorly. Note that a foramen ovale also may be present between the septum primum and septum secundum (*double asterisk*). (*From* Weinberg [2].)

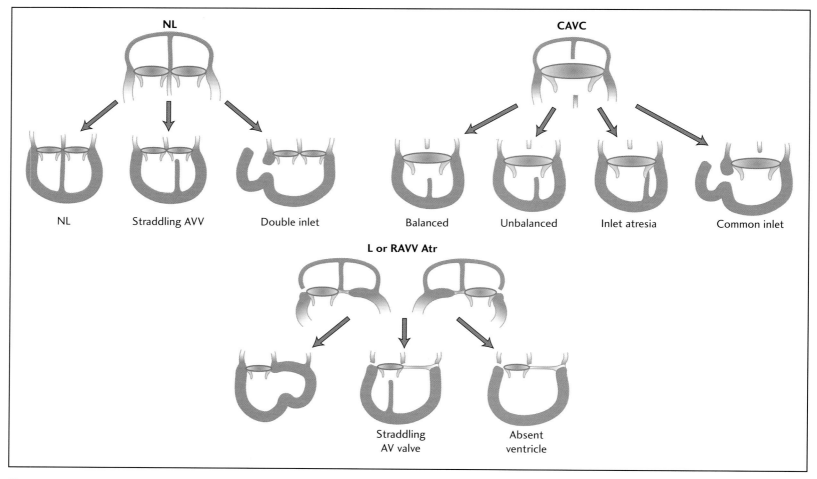

Figure 2-9.

Atrioventricular (AV) alignments. This intersegmental connection shows four atrial-to-AV valve connections: normal (NL), each atrium connected to a separate AV valve; common AV canal (CAVC), both atria connected to one AV valve; and left (L) or right AV valve atresia (RAVV Atr). This figure shows that for each atrial-to-AV valve connection, there are several possible AV valve (AVV)-to-ventricle connections.

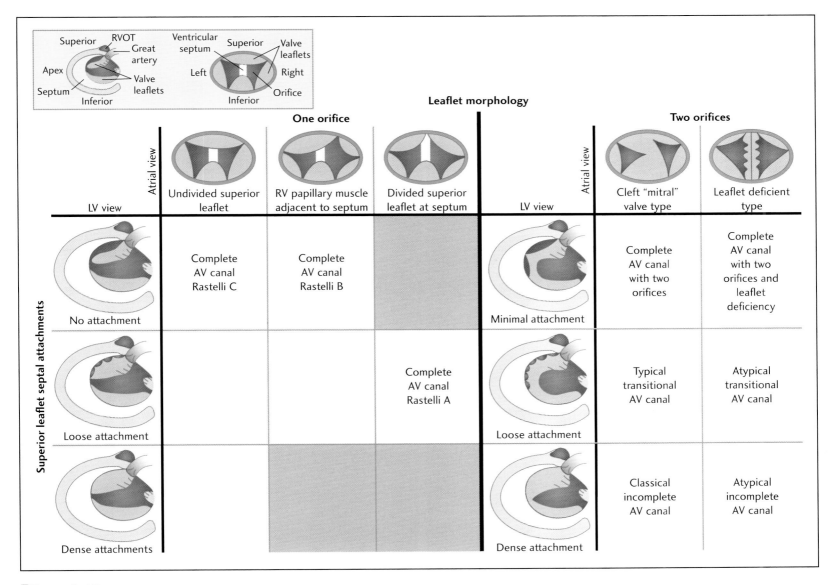

Figure 2-10.

Common atrioventricular (AV) canal. In all cases of common AV canal, there is a single large valve connected to both atria. This valve may have one or two major orifices, but has only one annulus. Valve morphology is determined in large part by the location of papillary and other commissural attachments and the degree of attachments to the ventricular septum. The classification of common AV canal is based on balance of the AV valve with respect to the ventricles, AV valve morphology, and the degree of attachment of the superior leaflet to the ventricular septal crest. This figure shows the various combinations of AV valve morphology and septal attachment for cases of balanced common AV canal; *ie,* the common AV valve empties nearly equally into both ventricles.

The three forms of superior leaflet attachment to ventricular septal crest, viewed *en face* from the left ventricular aspect, are shown in the columns labeled LV VIEW. Valve leaflet morphology (*top row of the figure*) is viewed from behind (Atrial view), looking toward the ventricles. Three forms with two major orifices (*left side of the figure*) and two forms with one major orifice (*right side of the figure*) are displayed. Keys to each diagram are shown at upper left. Classical or typical combinations are labeled accordingly. *Empty boxes* represent those combinations not covered by the Rastelli classification [3] of complete common AV canal. *Gray boxes* represent combinations that have not been described.

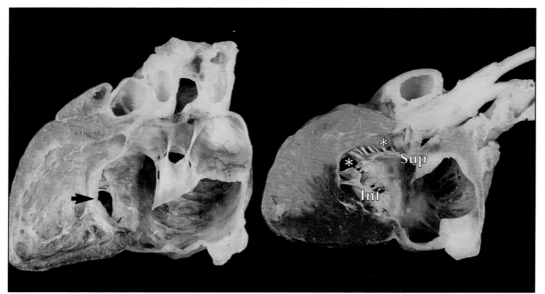

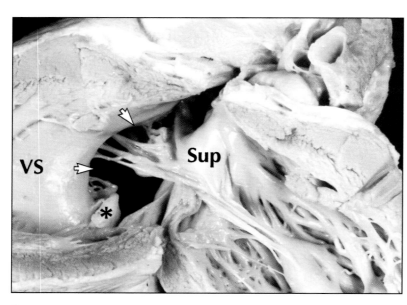

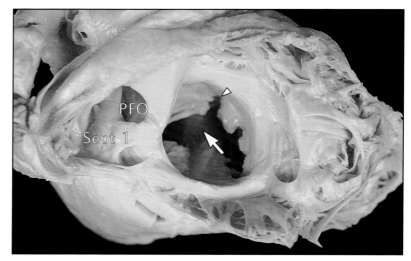

Figure 2-11.

Comparison of complete and incomplete atrioventricular (AV) canal. In cases with two major orifices, dense attachment of valve tissue over the full length of the septal crest effectively eliminates the ventricular septal defect (so-called incomplete common AV canal) despite deficiency of the canal (or inflow) portion of the ventricular septum. *Left,* An incomplete common AV canal with AV valve leaflet (*arrow*) densely adherent to the scooped out ventricular septal crest. *Right,* in contrast, a complete common AV canal shows both superior (Sup) and inferior (Inf) leaflets of the common AV valve above the crest of the ventricular septum; the intervening space constitutes the ventricular septal defect (*asterisks*). Note the deficiency of ventricular septum is similar in both cases. (*From* Weinberg [2].)

Figure 2-13.

Rastelli type B complete common atrioventricular (AV) canal, atrial view. The superior leaflet has a commissure (*arrowhead*) slightly to the right of the ventricular septal crest (*arrow*). The septum primum (Sept 1) portion of the atrial septum and a valve-incompetent patent foramen ovale (PFO) also are shown.

Figure 2-12.

Rastelli type A complete common arterioventricular (AV) canal (see Fig. 2-7 for atrial view). Left ventricular view of a pathologic specimen opened along the paraseptal incision, showing an example of one major valve orifice with the superior leaflet (Sup) loosely attached by chordae to the crest of the ventricular septum (VS). The ventricular septal defect (*white arrows*) occurs not only between the superior leaflet and the septal crest, but also between the superior and inferior (*asterisk*) leaflets. (*From* Weinberg [2].)

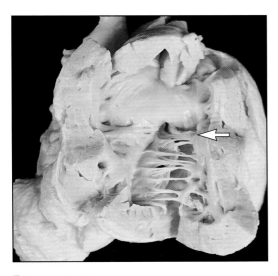

Figure 2-14.
Rastelli type B complete common atrioventricular (AV) canal, right ventricular view. View of the opened right ventricle in the case shown in Figure 2-13 demonstrates the unusually high take-off of the right ventricular papillary muscle (*arrow*) from the septal band. This corresponds to the commissure adjacent to the ventricular septal crest.

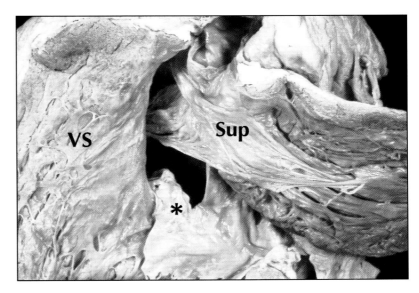

Figure 2-15.
Rastelli type C complete common atrioventricular (AV) canal. The left ventricle has been opened along a paraseptal incision and the freewall folded back to view the ventricular septal surface (VS). The superior leaflet (Sup) shows no attachment to the ventricular septal crest. The *asterisk* indicates inferior leaflet. (See also Fig. 2-21.) (*From* Weinberg [2].)

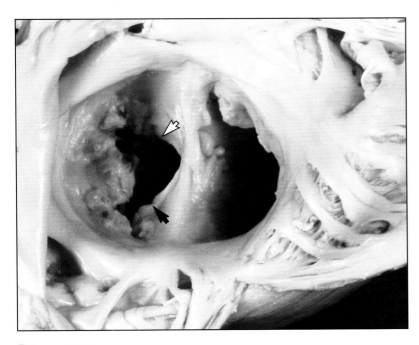

Figure 2-16.
Cleft "mitral" valve type of incomplete common atrioventricular (AV) canal, atrial view. In the two-orifice type of common AV canal (see right side of Fig. 2-10), a strip of valve tissue overlying the ventricular septal crest connects the superior and inferior leaflets. In most cases of common AV canal with two orifices, the superior (*white arrow*) and inferior (*black arrow*) leaflets on the LV side of the valve form a V or so-called cleft mitral valve with the apex of the V at the septal crest. (*From* Weinberg [2].)

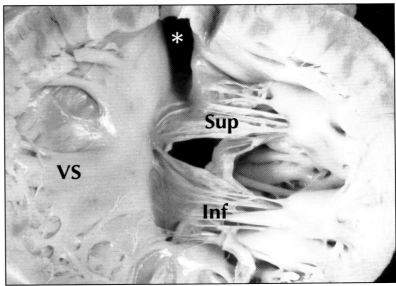

Figure 2-17.
Cleft "mitral" valve type of incomplete common atrioventricular (AV) canal, left ventricular view. A case with two major orifices has a dense attachment of the superior (Sup) and inferior (Inf) leaflets to the ventricular septal (VS) crest: so-called cleft mitral valve. The *asterisk* indicates left ventricular outflow tract. (*From* Weinberg [2].)

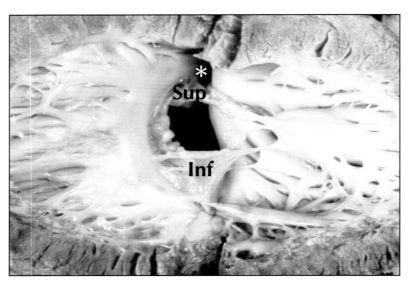

Figure 2-18.
Leaflet deficiency type of incomplete common atrioventricular (AV) canal. This case demonstrates leaflets that are densely adherent to the septal crest, but with wide separation of superior (Sup) and inferior (Inf) leaflets, in contrast with Figure 2-17. The deficiency of leaflet tissue over most of the septal crest usually causes severe AV valve regurgitation. The *asterisk* indicates left ventricular outflow tract. (*From* Weinberg [2].)

Figure 2-19.
Transitional common atrioventricular (AV) canal. This specimen illustrates a case of two major orifices created by tissue connecting the superior and inferior AV valve leaflets. A ventricular septal defect (*arrow*) is present beneath the leaflets, which are loosely attached to the ventricular septal (VS) crest. (*From* Weinberg [2].)

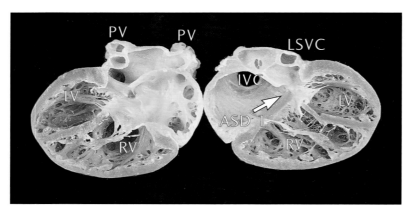

Figure 2-20.
Balanced atrioventricular (AV) canal (ventricular level). Paraffin-infiltrated postmortem specimen sectioned in a plane comparable to an echocardiographic subcostal four-chamber view with inferior half on the right and superior half on the left. This demonstrates the common AV valve entering the left ventricle (LV) and right ventricle (RV) equally. An ostium primum atrial septal defect (ASD 1) is noted immediately above the common AV valve. IVC—inferior vena cava; LSVC—left superior vena cava; PV—pulmonary vein.

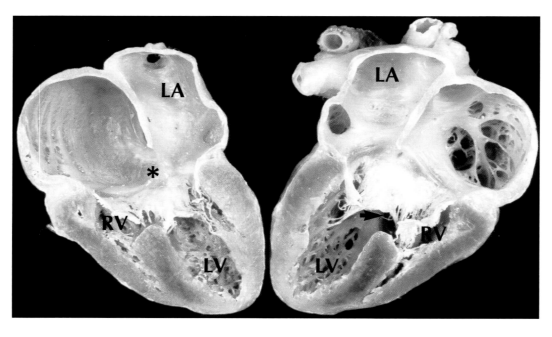

Figure 2-21.
Unbalanced atrioventricular (AV) canal (ventricular level). Paraffin-infiltrated postmortem specimen sectioned in a plane comparable to subcostal four-chamber view: inferior half on the left, superior half on the right. Note that the superior leaflet of the common AV valve passes through the AV canal-type ventricular septal defect (VSD; *arrow*) and is undivided. Most of the common AV valve opens into the left ventricle (LV), whereas only a few chordae are attached to the right ventricle (RV). The septum primum portion of the atrial septum is present posteriorly. The more anterior canal septum is deficient, resulting in an ostium primum atrial septal defect (*asterisk*). LA—left atrium. (*From* Weinberg [2].)

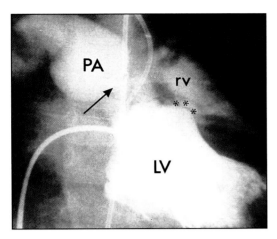

Figure 2-22.

Single left ventricle, left ventricular angiocardiogram. Contrast injection into the left ventricle (LV) demonstrates a small ventricular septal defect (*asterisks*) leading to the right ventricular outlet chamber (rv). The pulmonary artery (PA), which fills directly from the LV, in this case has a PA band (*arrow*). Recent information suggests that PA banding in the face of effective subaortic stenosis from a restrictive ventricular septal defect (VSD) in single LV is detrimental, because the decreased pulmonary blood flow results in decreased ventricular volume, further decrease in VSD size, and progressive outflow obstruction that leads to severe ventricular hypertrophy [4]. (*From* Freedom and Benson [5].)

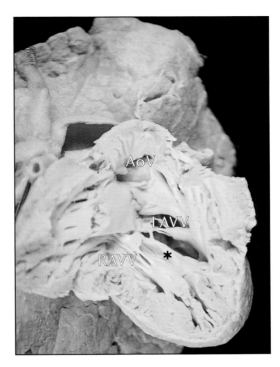

Figure 2-23.

Single right ventricle. Both right (RAVV) and left atrioventricular valves (LAVV) enter a morphologic right ventricle with coarse, parallel trabeculations. A prominent muscular ridge (*asterisk*) between the AV valves may be mistaken for a ventricular septum on echocardiography or angiocardiography. Note that in contrast to single left ventricle, there is no outlet chamber beneath the aortic valve (AoV). This patient had pulmonary atresia, and hence no pulmonary valve.

Figure 2-24.

Tricuspid atresia. The four morphologic types of tricuspid atresia are shown diagrammatically. The most common type is muscular with no valve remnant but a dimple in the floor of the right atrium (see Fig. 2-26). The membranous type represents the presence of the membranous atrioventricular (AV) septum in the floor of the right atrium; there are no chordal remnants, and the membrane is between the right atrium and left ventricle, not the right ventricle. The rare valvar and Ebstein types have presence of miniature, imperforate tricuspid valves that either hang down into the right ventricle or partially line the right ventricular sinus.

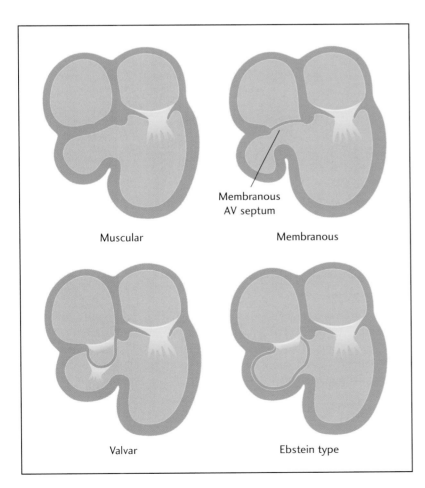

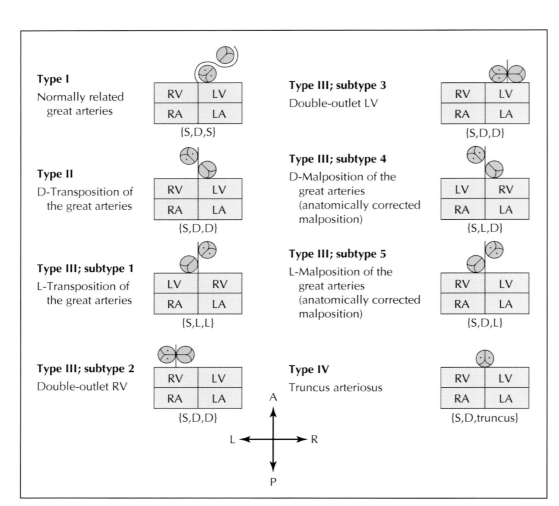

Type I
Normally related
great arteries

RV	LV
RA	LA

{S,D,S}

Type II
D-Transposition of
the great arteries

RV	LV
RA	LA

{S,D,D}

Type III; subtype 1
L-Transposition of
the great arteries

LV	RV
RA	LA

{S,L,L}

Type III; subtype 2
Double-outlet RV

RV	LV
RA	LA

{S,D,D}

Type III; subtype 3
Double-outlet LV

RV	LV
RA	LA

{S,D,D}

Type III; subtype 4
D-Malposition of the
great arteries
(anatomically corrected
malposition)

LV	RV
RA	LA

{S,L,D}

Type III; subtype 5
L-Malposition of the
great arteries
(anatomically corrected
malposition)

RV	LV
RA	LA

{S,D,L}

Type IV
Truncus arteriosus

RV	LV
RA	LA

{S,D,truncus}

A

L ←→ R

P

Figure 2-25.
The most commonly seen segmental
subsets with tricuspid atresia. Note that tricuspid atresia is usually right sided with a
right-sided right ventricle (RV), but can be
left sided with an L ventricular loop and
left-sided RV. Other combinations include
situs inversus of atria, *ie*, left-sided right
atrium (RA) and right-sided left atrium
(LA). Also, double-outlet right (DORV)
and left ventricle (DOLV) can occur with
segments {S,D,L} and {S,L,L}. A—anterior; L—left; LV—left ventricle; P—posterior; R—right. (*From* Rao [6].)

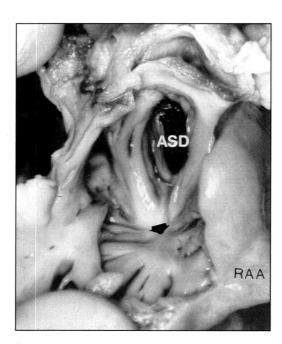

Figure 2-26.
Tricuspid atresia, right atrial view [6]. Pathologic heart specimen
with right atrium opened through right atrial appendage (RAA).
Note dimple (*arrow*) in the floor of the atrium seen in most cases
with muscular tricuspid atresia. The only exit from the right
atrium is an atrial septal defect (ASD). (*Adapted from* Rao and
coworkers [7], with permission.)

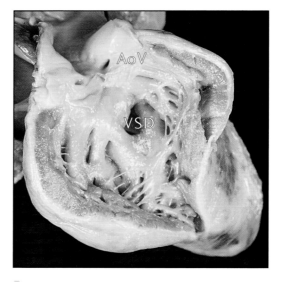

Figure 2-27.
Tricuspid atresia, right ventricular view with a large ventricular
septal defect (VSD). Pathologic heart specimen with relatively
large right ventricular remnant and a large VSD is seen giving rise
to the aortic valve (AoV) in a case of tricuspid atresia with transposition of the great arteries.

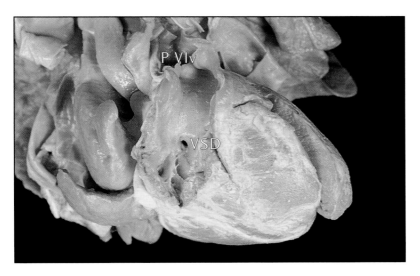

Figure 2-28.

Tricuspid atresia, right ventricular view with small ventricular septal defect (VSD). Pathologic specimen with opened right ventricular remnant showing "pinhole" VSD. The pulmonary valve (P Vlv) arises from the right ventricle in this case, with normally aligned great arteries. This muscular VSD was probably larger earlier in life.

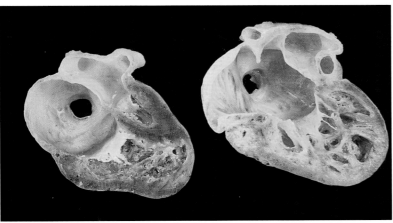

Right upper PV
Septum secundum
Septum primum
Left ventricle
Right atrium

Figure 2-29.

Mitral atresia versus hypoplasia with hypoplastic left heart. Inferior half of two postmortem specimens with hypoplastic left heart syndrome sectioned in planes comparable to subcostal four-chamber views. *Left,* Mitral valve hypoplasia and normal attachment of septum primum to the left side of the superior limbic band or septum secundum. *Right,* Leftward displacement of septum primum medial to the pulmonary vein entrances. In the latter case, usually associated with mitral and aortic atresia [8], note the separation between septum secundum and septum primum. The posterior portion of septum primum forms a hood or tunnel for the right upper pulmonary vein (PV) entrance. The more severe the displacement, the greater the tendency for the superior portion of septum primum to be horizontal. This, in the presence of mitral atresia, tends to force the septum primum against the roof of the left atrium, further obstructing left atrial outlet via the foramen ovale (see also Fig. 2-50). (*From* Weinberg [2].)

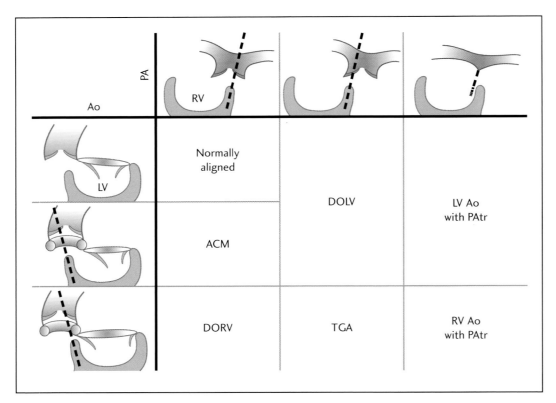

Figure 2-30.

Determinants of ventriculoarterial alignments. Ventriculoarterial alignments or the relationship of great arteries to ventricles are determined by a variety of factors. The presence of conus or infundibulum beneath a great artery generally causes that great artery to lie above the right ventricle, although rarely the infundibulum may be partly or totally related to the left ventricle, as in anatomically corrected malposition, some double-outlet left ventricles (DOLV) and, rarely, in transposition. Absence of conus beneath a great artery tends to result in that artery lying above the left ventricle. However, absence or hypoplasia of one or the other ventricle from early in embryonic development may force both great arteries to reside above the other ventricle, regardless of conal development.

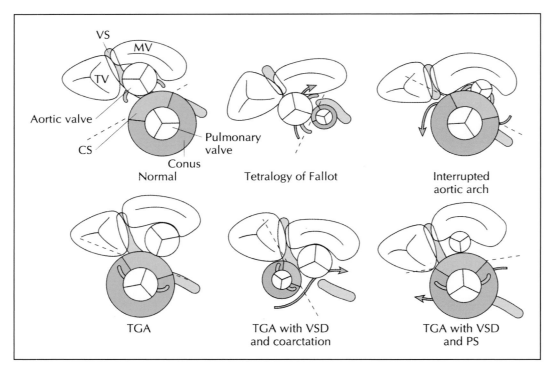

Figure 2-31.

Various conotruncal anomalies. The normal conotruncus consists of a fully expanded subpulmonary infundibulum (conus) arising from the right ventricle and the absence of subaortic infundibular free wall (resulting in mitral-aortic fibrous continuity) with a fully expanded subaortic area in the left ventricle. Conotruncal abnormalities consist of variations in the presence and length of subpulmonary and subaortic infundibulum or conus,

as well as the relative diameters of the subaortic and subpulmonary regions [9]. This figure shows normal conotruncus and several common conotruncal anomalies as viewed from above. The aortic valve is indicated by accompanying coronary arteries. The *dotted lines* show the plane of the infundibular or conal septum (CS) for comparison with the ventricular septum (VS). Note the leftward anterior deviation in tetralogy of Fallot relative to normal, the rightward anterior deviation in transposition of the great arteries (TGA) with ventricular septal defect (VSD) and coarctation, the posterior leftward deviation in interrupted aortic arch, and the posterior and rightward deviation in transposition with VSD and subpulmonary stenosis (PS) [10]. The *green arrows* represent the malalignment VSDs associated with displacement of the CS. (For pathologic specimens of representative conotruncal anomalies, see Fig. 2-2 [tetralogy of Fallot], Fig. 2-33 [interrupted aortic arch], Figs. 2-34 and 2-35 [TGA], Fig. 2-36 [TGA, VSD, coarctation of the aorta], Fig. 2-37 [TGA, VSD, PS].) MV—mitral valve; TV—tricuspid valve. (*From* Weinberg [2].)

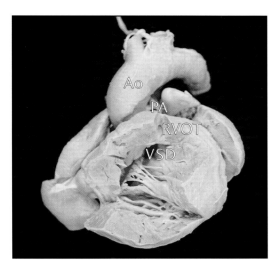

Figure 2-32.
Tetralogy of Fallot with pulmonary atresia. Pathologic specimen, anterior view of opened right ventricle shows malalignment ventricular septal defect (VSD) and diminutive right ventricular outflow tract (RVOT) to an atretic pulmonary valve. In many cases, no RVOT can be found and the infundibular septum (seen here separating RVOT from VSD) is presumed to be fused with the anterior free wall to of the right ventricle. Ao—aorta; PA—pulmonary artery.

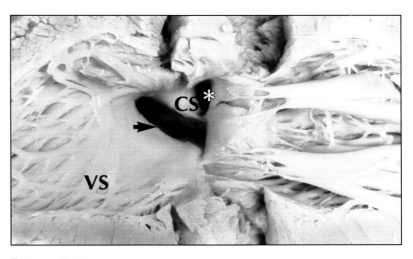

Figure 2-33.
Interrupted aortic arch. Interrupted aortic arch has subpulmonary without subaortic conus but with a poorly expanded subaortic region, causing subaortic stenosis. The malaligned infundibular or conal septum (CS) is shifted posteriorly and leftward so that it can be seen in the opened left ventricular (LV) view. The small subaortic LV outflow tract (*asterisk*) is bounded by the mitral valve and CS. The ventricular septal (VS) defect is marked by an *arrow*. (*From* Weinberg [2].)

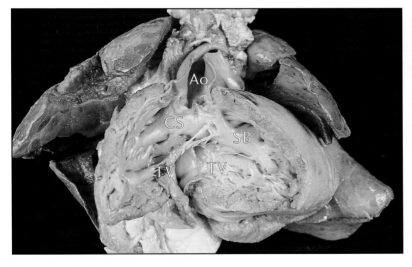

Figure 2-34.
Transposition of the great arteries, right ventricular view. Pathologic specimen of transposition of the great arteries with intact ventricular septum viewed from the right ventricle (RV). The conal or infundibular septum (CS) sits in the ϒ of the septal band (SB), but the aorta (Ao) arises farther to the right than does the pulmonary artery in the normal heart. TV—tricuspid valve.

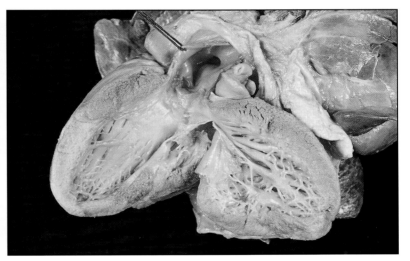

Figure 2-35.
Transposition of the great arteries, left ventricular view. Pathologic specimen of transposition of the great arteries with intact ventricular septum viewed from the left ventricle (LV). There is typically, but not necessarily, mitral valve (MV) to pulmonary valve fibrous continuity, indicating absence of subpulmonary conus. Because of the more leftward position of the pulmonary artery (PA) compared with the normal heart, the PA sits entirely above the LV cavity, rather than over the ventricular septum (VS) to a large extent, as with the normal aorta.

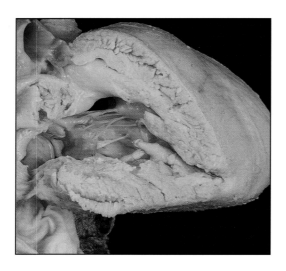

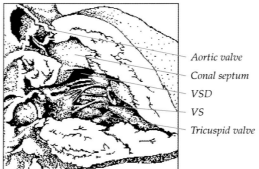

Aortic valve
Conal septum
VSD
VS
Tricuspid valve

Figure 2-36.

Transposition of the great arteries (TGA), ventricular septal defect (VSD), and coarctation of the aorta. With TGA, there is usually, but not always, subaortic conus without subpulmonary conus. If the subaortic conus is poorly expanded, as noted in this right ventricular view, there is TGA with VSD and coarctation of the aorta—actually aortic arch hypoplasia. The infundibular septum is deviated anteriorly, superiorly, and rightward relative to the septal band and ventricular septum (VS) so that the pulmonary valve (behind the conal septum) may override the VS. (*From* Weinberg [2].)

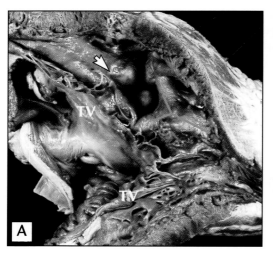

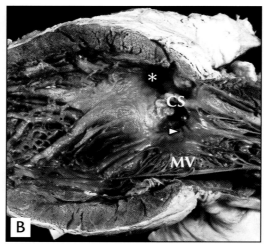

Figure 2-37.

Transposition of the great arteries (TGA), ventricular septal defect (VSD), and pulmonary stenosis. **A,** Right ventricular view of a specimen with TGA, VSD, and subpulmonary stenosis is shown here. A malalignment type VSD is noted *in the* Υ of the septal band and anterior to the tricuspid valve (TV). With posterior malalignment, the aortic valve (*arrow*) sits astride the VSD. **B,** Left ventricular view of the same case demonstrates the posteriorly deviated conal septum (CS). The pulmonary valve (*arrowhead*) is seen between the CS and the mitral valve (MV), with the malalignment VSD indicated by an *asterisk*. (*From* Weinberg [2].)

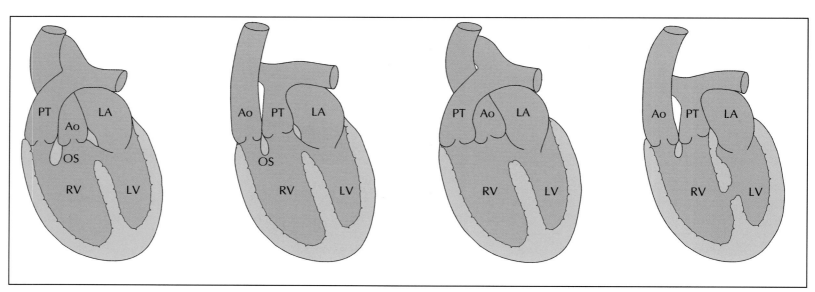

Figure 2-38.

Double-outlet right ventricle (DORV), great arteries relative to ventricular septal defect (VSD) [11]. In DORV, the VSD is the only outlet from the morphologic left ventricle (LV). Therefore, in cases where a two-ventricle repair is feasible, the type and size of the VSD is important in assessing the likelihood of residual or subsequently developed LV outflow obstruction. In addition to the morphologic description of the VSD, the proximity of great arteries to the VSD is important in determining which vessel will be connected to the LV. It is critical that the clinician understands that in DORV most VSDs are in the same place relative to other septal structures—usually in the Υ of septal band. However, because there is no good way of independently describing great artery position, the terms *subaortic*, *subpulmonary*, and *beneath both* or *doubly committed* VSD have been used. Thus, these terms refer to great artery position and not VSD position. So-called "beneath neither" or "uncommitted" VSDs are generally in another location, usually atrioventricular (AV) canal (or inlet) type or muscular. Ao—aorta; LA—left atrium; PT—pulmonary trunk; RV—right ventricle (*From* Rigby and Horowitz [11].)

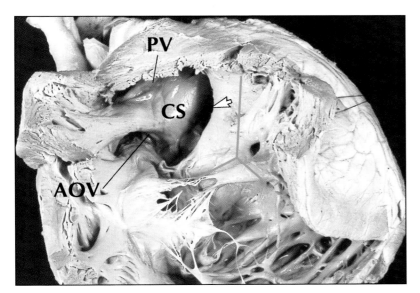

Figure 2-39.

Double-outlet right ventricle (DORV) with doubly committed ventricular septal defect (VSD). Conotruncal anomalies derive from varying degrees of bilateral presence or deficiency of sub-semilunar infundibulum (conus), in addition to varying degrees of subsemilunar stenosis. Factors such as ventricular size, orientation, and connection to infundibulum, together with the various conotruncal anomalies mentioned above, determine the spatial ventriculoarterial alignments: transposition, double-outlet ventricles, anatomically corrected malposition, and so forth. Bilateral infundibulum with full expansion of both subaortic and subpulmonary areas may result in malalignment of the infundibular or conal septum (CS), placing both the aortic valve (AoV) and the pulmonary valve (PV) above the right ventricle and equidistant from the VSD (*arrow*)(so-called "doubly committed" VSD); however, the morphologic VSD type is malalignment as seen in the other conotruncal anomalies above. (*From* Weinberg [2].)

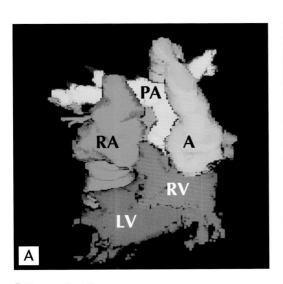 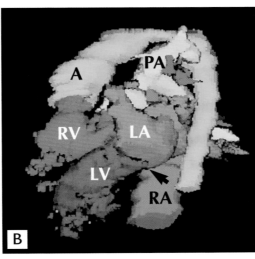

Figure 2-40.

Double-outlet right ventricle (DORV) with supero-inferior ventricles. Perhaps the most intriguing example of altered spatial relationships is that of supero-inferior ventricles with criss-crossing atrioventricular relations [12]. These are characterized by a small right ventricle (RV) sinus with a normal to large infundibulum with a fairly horizontal ventricular septum. **A,** A three-dimensional reconstruction from magnetic resonance imaging of a patient with DORV {S,D,L} (that is, situs solitus of viscera and atria, ventricular D loop, and L malposition of the great arteries) is viewed anteriorly with slight cranial angulation. Other thoracic structures plus the myocardium are removed, and a shaded surface display showing the cavities as solid surfaces is created by computerized post-processing. The right atrium (RA) connects to a superiorly situated RV, which in turn gives rise to the pulmonary artery (PA) and a leftward aorta (Ao). The RV shows right-handed or D-loop organization, as previously described [13], despite the fact that the majority of the RV cavity (the infundibular portion) is actually left sided. A portion of the inferiorly situated left ventricle (LV) is seen extending to the right. **B,** A left posterior oblique view of the same three-dimensional reconstruction with caudal angulation shows the left atrium (LA) connecting via the mitral valve (*arrow*) to the inferiorly located left ventricle. (*From* Weinberg [2].)

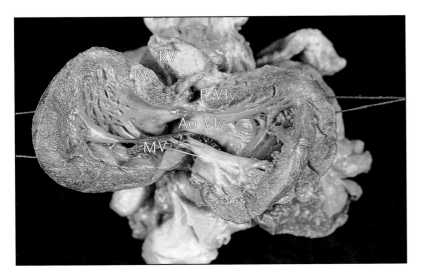

Figure 2-41.

Double-outlet left ventricle (DOLV) with tricuspid atresia. DOLV, like double-outlet right ventricle (DORV), is not a single entity, but rather a group of assorted lesions in which both great arteries are assigned to the morphologic left ventricle. View of the opened left ventricle (LV) of this pathologic specimen with tricuspid atresia has a markedly diminutive right ventricular remnant (RV), which is essentially a small pocket filling from the large LV through a ventricular septal defect. The aortic valve (Ao Vlv) is in fibrous continuity with the mitral valve (MV), and the pulmonary artery arises entirely from the LV. PV—pulmonary valve.

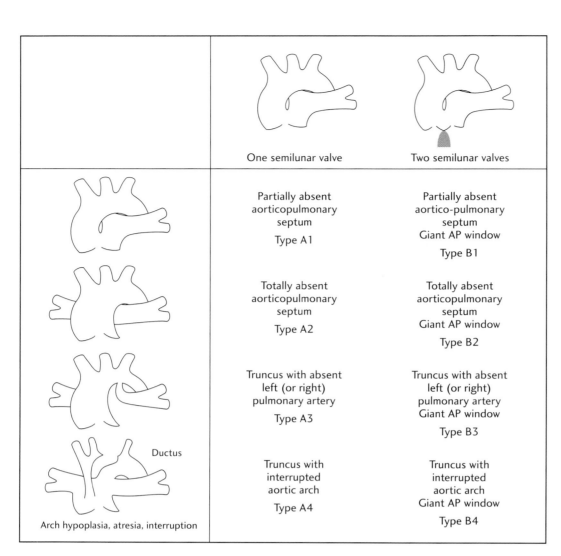

	One semilunar valve	Two semilunar valves
	Partially absent aorticopulmonary septum Type A1	Partially absent aortico-pulmonary septum Giant AP window Type B1
	Totally absent aorticopulmonary septum Type A2	Totally absent aorticopulmonary septum Giant AP window Type B2
	Truncus with absent left (or right) pulmonary artery Type A3	Truncus with absent left (or right) pulmonary artery Giant AP window Type B3
Ductus Arch hypoplasia, atresia, interruption	Truncus with interrupted aortic arch Type A4	Truncus with interrupted aortic arch Giant AP window Type B4

Figure 2-42.
Truncus arteriosus communis is a great artery abnormality in which a single great artery arises from the ventricular portion of the heart and gives rise to the aorta, at least one pulmonary artery, and at least one coronary artery. Typical truncus has a single semilunar valve. However, it is possible to have what is essentially a single or common vessel arise above two semilunar valves, usually with an intact ventricular septum. This group is called type B in the Van Praagh classification [13]. It also has been termed *giant aorticopulmonary window*. This figure shows the various subtypes of truncus based on the Van Praagh classification with the modification that the distinguishing feature is one or two semilunar valves rather than with or without ventricular septal defect (VSD).

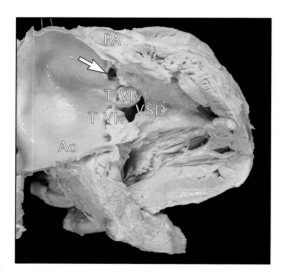

Figure 2-43.
Truncus arteriosus showing truncal valve and ventricular septal defect (VSD). Pathologic heart specimen of truncus arteriosus communis (TAC) type A1 in the Van Praagh classification [14]. The malalignment type of VSD is like other malalignment defects, situated in the Υ of the septal band. However, unlike the VSD typically seen in tetralogy, in TAC the posterior limb of the Υ is prominent and muscular, whereas in tetralogy there may be no posteromedial limb of the Υ. Note the thick, myxomatous leaflets of the truncal valve (T Vlv). The pulmonary artery (PA) arises from the truncus via a relatively small aorticopulmonary septal defect (*arrow*). Ao—aorta.

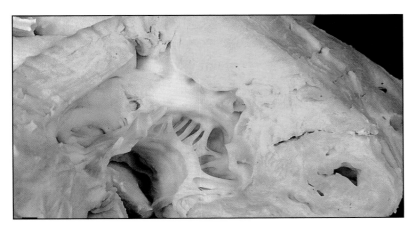

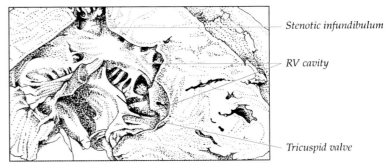

Stenotic infundibulum

RV cavity

Tricuspid valve

Figure 2-44.

Pulmonary atresia with small right ventricle [15]. A very small, muscle-bound right ventricular cavity with hypoplasia of the infundibulum and distal atresia. The tricuspid valve leaflets are thickened, as are the chordae tendineae. (*From* Zuberbuhler and Park [15].)

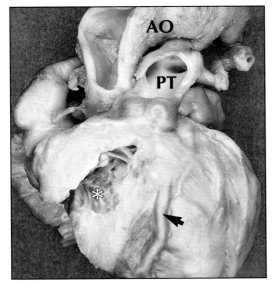

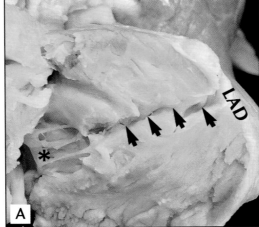

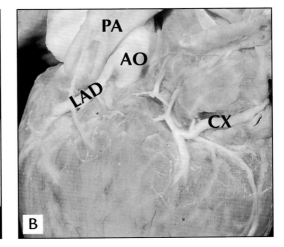

Figure 2-45.

Pulmonary atresia [15]. This exterior view of a pathologic specimen with pulmonary atresia demonstrates the typical appearance of a diminutive right ventricular chamber (*asterisk*) delimited by the anterior descending coronary artery (*arrow*), whose distal portion is deviated to the right of normal. Note the marked dilatation of the distal coronary, undoubtedly caused by a fistulous connection between the coronary and the right ventricular cavity. Also of note is the normal or nearly normal size of the pulmonary trunk (PT), in contrast to that seen when pulmonary atresia is part of a conotruncal anomaly such as tetralogy of Fallot. Ao—aorta. (*From* Zuberbuhler and Park [15]; with permission.)

Figure 2-46.

Pulmonary atresia and sinusoids [15]. Coronary artery abnormalities are seen frequently with pulmonary atresia, probably because of persistence of embryonic coronary-cameral connections maintained by the high right ventricular pressures. **A,** Coronary cameral fistulae opened from the suprasystemic right ventricular chamber (*asterisk*) to the left anterior descending coronary artery (LAD). **B,** In another case, the LAD arises from the aorta, but the circumflex coronary (CX) has no connection to the aorta and fills retrograde from right ventricular sinusoids instead. This situation precludes any intervention aimed at decompressing the right ventricle, such as outflow tract reconstruction, tricuspid valve occlusion, excision, or disruption by interventional catheterization. Ao—aorta; PA—pulmonary artery. (*From* Zuberbuhler and Park [15].)

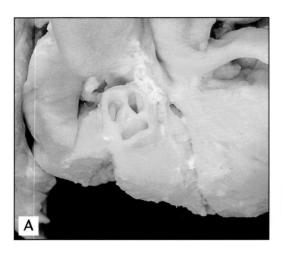

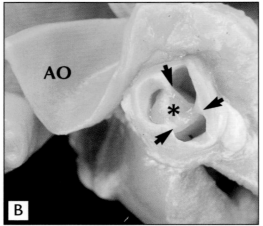

Figure 2-47.
Pulmonary atresia showing the pulmonary valve [15]. The valve in pulmonary atresia without conotruncal anomaly is typically tricommissural. **A,** Relatively long, thick, sealed commissures or raphes imply infundibular atresia. **B,** Shorter rudimentary commissures (*arrows*) with a doming central portion (*asterisk*) are more characteristic of cases with a patent outflow tract up to the valve plate. Ao—aorta. (*From* Zuberbuhler and Park [15].)

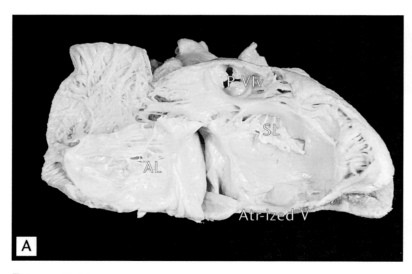

Figure 2-48.
Pulmonary atresia and large right ventricle with Ebstein's and Uhl's anomalies. Pulmonary atresia also occurs in patients with Ebstein's anomaly of the tricuspid valve. These cases show a markedly dilated right ventricle (RV) and have severe tricuspid regurgitation. The poor antegrade flow secondary to tricuspid regurgitation is responsible for the pulmonary valve leaflets sealing shut. This paraffin-infiltrated specimen is cut in a plane simulating an echocardiographic apical four-chamber view. The superior half is on the left and the inferior half on the right. The hallmarks of Ebstein's anomaly are the rudimentary septal leaflet (SL), the long, curtain-like anterior leaflet (AL), and the displacement of the posterior leaflet (*small unlabeled arrows*) downward into the RV relative to the annulus (*white arrow*). This case also displays the parchment-thin appearance of the RV free wall seen in Uhl's anomaly.

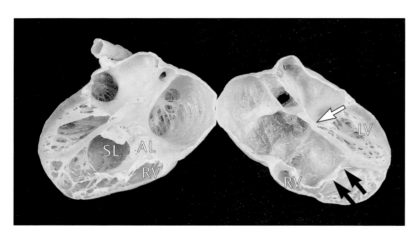

Figure 2-49.
Ebstein's anomaly of the tricuspid valve. **A,** Right anterior oblique view of opened right ventricle (RV) in a pathologic specimen of Ebstein's anomaly of the tricuspid valve with a patent pulmonary valve (P Vlv). The septal leaflet (SL) is rudimentary and the anterior leaflet (AL) is curtain-like. Note the atrialized portion of the right ventricle (Atr-ized V), a very thin, dysplastic area of right ventricular myocardium proximal to the displaced posterior leaflet

of the tricuspid valve. **B,** Anterior view of a different case with severe Ebstein's anomaly, showing the curtain-like AL of the tricuspid valve. Note how the AL extends all the way to the free wall of the right ventricle with virtually no chordae or papillary muscles. Because of the widespread direct attachment to the free wall, this type of valve is not amenable to direct repair.

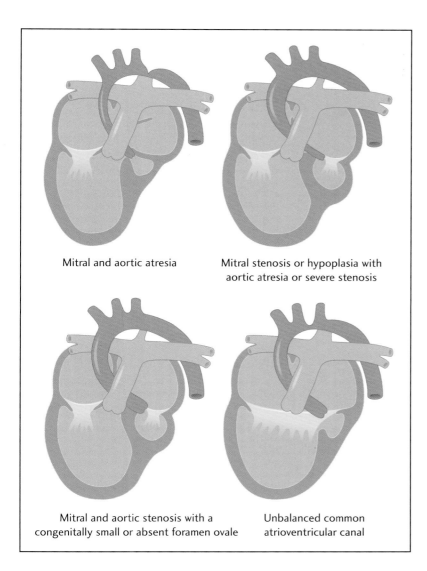

Mitral and aortic atresia

Mitral stenosis or hypoplasia with aortic atresia or severe stenosis

Mitral and aortic stenosis with a congenitally small or absent foramen ovale

Unbalanced common atrioventricular canal

Figure 2-50.

Several varieties of hypoplastic left heart syndrome. Hypoplastic left heart syndrome includes patients with normal cardiac segments, normally aligned great arteries, and hypoplasia or absence of the morphologic left ventricle. Mitral and aortic atresia commonly is associated with discrete coarctation of the aorta, where the ductal stream of blood divides to supply the proximal aorta retrograde and the distal aorta antegrade. There often is leftward displacement of the posterior portion of the septum primum (flap valve of foramen ovale), forming a hood over the right upper pulmonary vein. Mitral stenosis or hypoplasia with aortic atresia or severe stenosis often has endocardial fibroelastosis of the left ventricle, showing a small, round, thick-walled chamber, sometimes with coronary-cameral fistulae. A subgroup of mitral and aortic stenosis has a congenitally small or absent foramen ovale. The foramen ovale probably becomes sealed secondary to high left atrial pressures from left ventricular failure. The last group is that with unbalanced common atrioventricular canal (CAVC) with a hypoplastic left ventricle. This group is hemodynamically different from the others in that it lacks a restrictive interatrial communication leading to pulmonary over-circulation. All types of hypoplastic left heart are amenable to surgical palliation using the Norwood operation followed by staged cavopulmonary anastomosis (see Fig. 2-31). (*From* Weinberg and Cohen [16].)

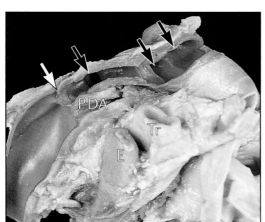

Figure 2-51.

Coarctation of the aorta. Right posterior oblique view of discrete coarctation of the aorta (*large white arrow*) in its typical contraductal location; ie, opposite the entrance of the patent ductus arteriosus (PDA). The take-off of the aortic arch vessels is shown (*three small arrows*). E—esophagus; Tr—trachea.

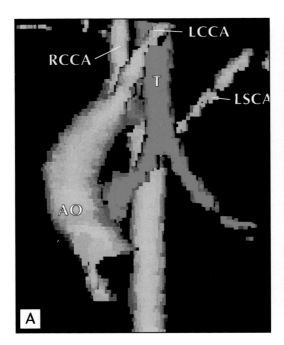
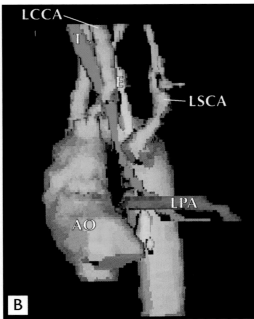

Figure 2-52.

Examples of right aortic arch anomalies are illustrated with shaded surface displays of three-dimensional reconstructions from magnetic resonance imaging. Other thoracic structures are removed and vessel lumina are shown as solid surfaces. **A,** This right aortic arch with retroesophageal left subclavian artery (LSCA) viewed from a slight left anterior oblique (LAO) position has a left common carotid artery (LCCA) as the first branch, then a right common carotid artery (RCCA), right subclavian, and finally the anomalous LSCA. No vascular ring is formed, but the LSCA does indent the esophagus (not shown but located behind trachea [T]) posteriorly. **B,** This right arch with retroesophageal diverticulum is viewed from a steep LAO position. This anomaly *is* a form of vascular ring because the diverticulum (*arrow*) gives rise to a left ductus arteriosus or, in this case, a ligamentum arteriosum (not visualized because there is no lumen) which, in turn, connects to the left pulmonary artery (LPA) trapping the trachea (T) and esophagus (E), whose lumina appear indented and interrupted, respectively, due to vascular compression. The diverticulum also fills the LSCA, the last arch vessel. This differs from the case in *panel A* in that there is a distinct change in the caliber of the retroesophageal vessel from diverticulum to LSCA (*ie*, after the take-off of the ligamentum). Similar to the case in *panel A*, the aorta (Ao) gives rise to the LCCA as the first arch vessel. (*From* Weinberg [17].)

REFERENCES

1. Van Praagh R: The segmental approach to diagnosis in congenital heart disease. In *Birth Defects: Original Article Series*, vol. 8, no. 5. Edited by Bergsma D. Baltimore: Williams & Wilkins; 1972:4–23.

2. Weinberg P: Morphology of congenital heart disease. In *Atlas of Heart Diseases*, vol. XII: Congenital Heart Disease. Philadelphia: Current Medicine; 1997:4.1–4.14.

3. Rastelli G, Kirklin JW, Titus JL: Anatomic observations on complete form of persistent common atrioventricular canal with special reference to atrioventricular valves. *Mayo Clin Proc* 1966, 41:296–308.

4. Donofrio MT, Jacobs ML, Norwood WI, Rychik J: Early changes in ventricular septal defect size and ventricular geometry in the single left ventricle after volume-unloading surgery. *J Am Coll Cardiol* 1995, 26:1008–1015.

5. Freedom RM, Benson LN: The Fontan operation: indications and scrutiny of operative criteria. In *Atlas of Heart Diseases*, vol. XII: *Congenital Heart Disease*. Edited by Freedom RM. Philadelphia: Current Medicine; 1997:17.1–17.10

6. Rao PS: Tricuspid atresia: anatomy, imaging, and natural history. In *Atlas of Heart Diseases*, vol. XII: *Congenital Heart Disease*. Edited by Freedom RM. Philadelphia: Current Medicine; 1997:14.1–14.14

7. Rao PS, Levy JM, Nikiciz E, Gilbert-Barness EF: Tricuspid atresia: association with persistent truncus arteriosus. *Am Heart J* 1991, 122:829–835.

8. Chin AJ, Weinberg PM, Barber G: Subcostal two-dimensional echocardiographic identification of anomalous attachment of septum primum in patients with left atrioventricular valve underdevelopment. *J Am Coll Cardiol* 1990, 15:678–681.

9. Van Praagh R, Weinberg PM, Smith SD, *et al.*: Malpositions of the heart. In *Moss' Heart Disease in Infants, Children, and Adolescents*, edn 4. Edited by Adams FH, Emmanouilides GC, Riemenschneider TA. Baltimore: Williams & Wilkins; 1989:530–580.

10. Van Praagh R, Weinberg PM, Calder AL, *et al.*: The transposition complexes: how many are there? In *Second Henry Ford Hospital International Symposium on Cardiac Surgery*. Edited by Davila JC. New York: Appleton-Century-Crofts; 1977:207–213.

11. Rigby ML, Horowitz ES: Double-outlet ventricle. In *Atlas of Heart Diseases*, vol. XII: *Congenital Heart Disease*. Edited by Freedom RM. Philadelphia: Current Medicine; 1997:20.1–20.9

12. Anderson RH, Shinebourne EA, Gerlis LM: Criss-cross atrioventricular relationships producing paradoxical atrioventricular concordance or discordance: their significance to nomenclature of congenital heart disease. *Circulation* 1974, 50:176–180.

13. Van Praagh S, LaCorte M, Fellows KE, *et al.*: Supero-inferior ventricles: anatomic and angiocardiographic findings in ten postmortem cases. In *Etiology and Morphogenesis of Congenital Heart Disease*. Edited by Van Praagh R, Takao A. Mount Kisco, NY: Futura Publishing; 1980:317–378.

14. Van Praagh R: Truncus arteriosus: what is it really and how should it be classified? *Eur J Cardiothorac Surg* 1987, 1:65–70.

15. Zuberbuhler JR, Park SC: Pulmonary atresia with intact ventricular septum. In *Atlas of Heart Diseases*, vol. XII: *Congenital Heart Disease*. Edited by Freedom RM. Philadelphia: Current Medicine; 1997:19.1–19.9.

16. Weinberg PM, Cohen MS: Hypoplastic left heart syndrome. In *Saunders Manual of Pediatric Practice*. Edited by Finberg L. Philadelphia: WB Saunders; 1998:540–543.

17. Weinberg PM: Aortic arch anomalies. In *Moss and Adams' Heart Disease in Infants, Children, and Adolescents, Including the Fetus and Young Adult*, edn 5. Edited by Emmanouilides GC, Riemenschneider TA, Allen HD, Gutgesell HP. Baltimore: Williams & Wilkins; 1994:810–837.

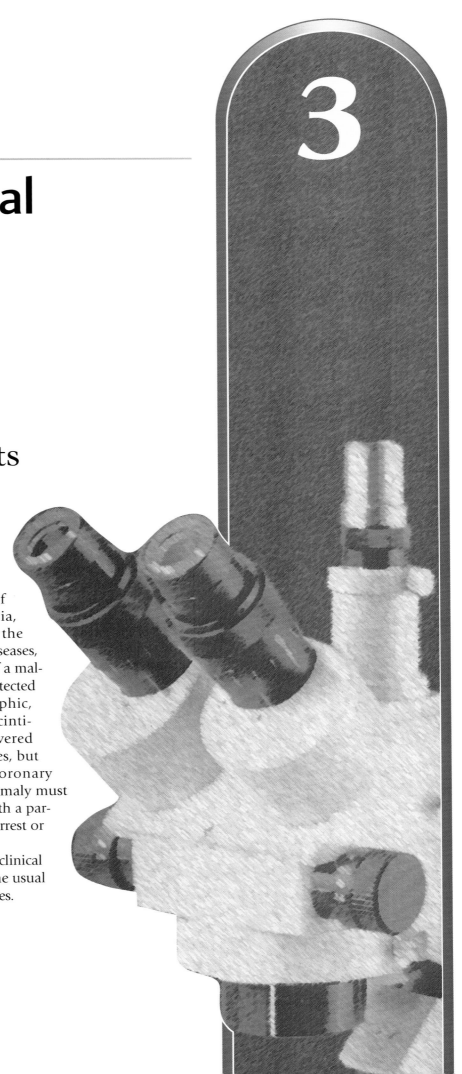

Coronary Arterial Anomalies

William Clifford Roberts

Congenital abnormalities of the heart are important causes of morbidity and mortality. Although less common than those structural derangements of the cardiac chamber and wall size, placement, and contour, and of the cardiac valves, coronary arterial anomalies must be considered across a wide range of ages and both sexes as a basis for myocardial ischemia, infarction, and sudden death, and as a challenge to the success of operative interventions for other coronary diseases, valve replacement, or for correction of the physiology of a malformed heart. Gross lesions of the heart are typically detected by imaging studies, whether radiographic, angiographic, echocardiographic, magnetic resonance–based, or scintigraphic. Coronary arterial anomalies may be discovered through careful and selective angiographic approaches, but may not be the first thought in the context of a coronary ischemic syndrome. Thus, the presence of such an anomaly must be suspected clinically, and, indeed, must be sought with a particular diligence at necropsy when unexpected cardiac arrest or fatalities occur.

This chapter illustrates coronary arterial anomalies of clinical relevance, and by these examples, attempts to convey the usual appearance and associated sequelae of these abnormalities.

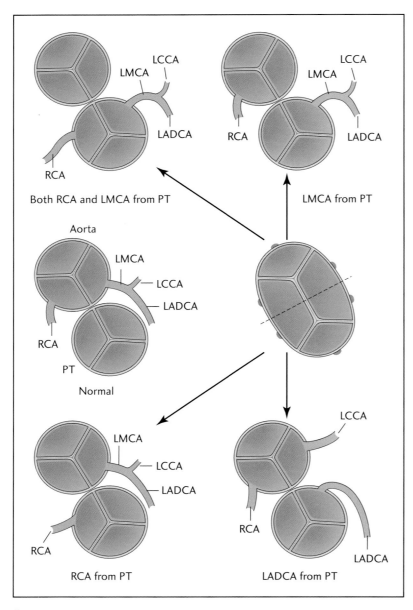

Figure 3-1.

The common arterial trunk arising from the heart and its early development, with six potential coronary arterial ostia and the possible coronary anomalies resulting when inappropriate ostia do not regress.

Top left, Both right left and right main coronary arteries (or single coronary artery) from the pulmonary trunk (PT) without a coronary artery from the aorta (type IA). This is an extremely rare anomaly; fewer than 20 patients have been reported with the disorder [1]. Most die during the first month of life, usually in the first 1 or 2 days. Most had other major anomalies of the heart or great arteries. For a patient with this anomaly to live, systemic pressure must be present in the PT. The presence of a ventricular septal defect can do that and so can an obstructive lesion on the left side of the heart (*eg*, in congenital mitral stenosis).*Top right*, Origin of the left main coronary artery (LMCA) from the PT and the right coronary artery (RCA) from the aorta (type IIA). This

anomaly was first described by Abbott [2] in 1908. Her patient, a woman who lived for 60 years, appears to be the oldest reported survivor with this anomaly. This anomaly is usually diagnosed in infants; in some quarters, it has been called Bland-White-Garland syndrome since 1933 [3]. Approximately 50% of patients with this anomaly die between ages 3 and 6 months, and about 80% die by age 12 months. The other 20% live longer than 15 years. The major cause of death during the first year of life is congestive heart failure, and the mode of death is usually sudden and unexpected if adulthood is reached. If a patient with this anomaly is able to survive the first year of life, the chances are good that the child will survive until adulthood. The reason some adults with anomalous origin of the LMCA from the PT die during the first year or so of life yet others survive into adulthood (without operative intervention) is related to the development of collaterals between the coronary artery attached to the ascending aorta (AA; the right one) and the coronary attached to the PT (the LMCA). At birth and during the first 2 months or so of life, the systolic and diastolic pressures in the AA and PT are similar; consequently, the LMCA is perfused with blood within the PT. At about 2 months of life, the pressure in the PT decreases so the systolic pressure in the PT is about a quarter of that in the aorta by 12 months of age. Survival depends on the development of collateral channels between the normally and abnormally arising coronary arteries so that flow in the anomalous LMCA is retrograde because it is supplied entirely by blood from the normally arising RCA [4,5]. The anomalous artery "steals" blood from the normally arising artery, placing considerable myocardium at risk of ischemia or necrosis. An extensive collateral system must develop for survival to occur. Death is common during the period of transition from antegrade to retrograde flow in the anomalously rising LMCA. In infants with this anomaly, the cardiac mass is increased and the ventricular cavities are dilated. The left ventricular (LV) papillary muscles appear to arise more cephalad than normally. The anterolateral papillary muscle is much smaller than the posteromedial papillary muscle. The endocardium of the LV may be thickened. In contrast to the appearance of the infant's heart, the survivors of this anomaly who live to adulthood have hearts that are distinguished primarily by the appearance of the coronary arteries. The right one is dilated and tortuous. In contrast, the branches of the LM are straighter and not as dilated but have a thinner wall (like a vein). Vascular channels connecting the RCA to the branches of the LMCA are visible on the surface of the heart. The ventricular mass is increased and the ventricular cavities are dilated. The anterolateral papillary muscle is usually scarred and calcified. The definitive diagnosis of this anomaly is by angiography with injection of contrast material into the lumen of the RCA (or aortic root) with drainage through the collaterals into the LM branches of the LMCA and visualization of the connection of the LM to the PT. LV angiography usually shows mitral regurgitation in addition to cavity dilatation. Operative treatment is either ligation of the LMCA at its attachment to the PT or attachment of the LMCA to the AA or to another arterial branch arising from an aorta [6]. (*continued on next page*)

Figure 3-1. (*continued*)

Bottom left, Origin of the RCA from the PT and the LMCA from the aorta (type IIB). This anomaly appears to be about 10 times less common than origin of the LMCA from the PT [7–9]. Whereas an increase in ventricular mass, LV scarring, anterolateral papillary muscle fibrosis, and calcification, right ventricular and LV dilatation, and diffuse LV endocardial fibroelastosis might be expected in cases of origin of the LMCA from the PT, none of these morphologic findings appear to be the consequence of origin of the RCA from the PT. Indeed, the only predictable morphologic finding is an increase in size of the LMCA and its branches and an increase (but less so) in size of the RCA with thinning of its walls (compared with normal). This anomaly usually produces no symptoms of cardiac dysfunction and no evidence of myocardial ischemia. Certain diagnosis is established by angiography with injection of contrast material into the LMCA arising from the aorta with visualization of RCA via collaterals from the branches of the LMCA and finally the appearance of contrast material in the PT. The operation of choice for this anomaly is transection of the RCA from the PT and direct anastomosis of the RCA to the aorta [10].

Bottom right, Left anterior descending coronary artery (LADCA) from the PT and right and left circumflex coronary arteries (LCCAs) from the aorta (type IIC). Fewer than 20 patients have been reported in whom the LADCA arose from the PT and both the RCA and the LCCA arose from the aorta [11]. Most patients with this anomaly develop symptoms of myocardial ischemia. They usually have precordial murmurs, which may be only systolic, only diastolic, or both systolic and diastolic. Heart size is usually normal. Right-sided pressures are normal. Coronary angiography with injection of contrast material into the RCA and LCCA usually provides the diagnosis in that each of these two arteries are large and occasionally tortuous and the LADCA is filled by extensive collateral vessels from the RCA and LCCA. Operation, usually warranted because of the presence of angina, usually consists of ligating the LADCA at its connection to the PT with insertion of a conduit from the AA to the LADCA.

No adults have been reported with the LCCA from the PT and the right LADCAs from the aorta (IID). The anomaly has been observed angiographically in a few children with other major anomalies of the heart or great arteries. (*Courtesy of* William C. Roberts, Baylor University Medical Center, Dallas.)

Figure 3-2.
The coronary anomalies not associated with the "coronary steal" phenomenon (type IIA) (*top*) and those associated with this phenomenon (*bottom*) (types IA, IB, IC, ID). LADCA—left anterior descending coronary artery; LMCA—left main coronary artery; PT—pulmonary trunk. (*Adapted from* Roberts [1].)

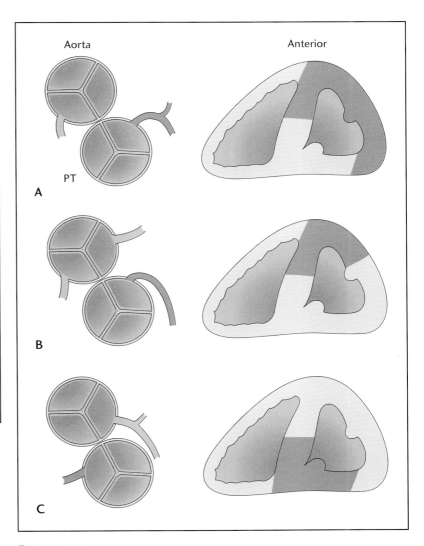

Figure 3-3.
The portion of left ventricular myocardium at risk of ischemia or necrosis when the left main coronary artery (**A**; type IA), left anterior descending coronary artery (**B**; type IC), or right coronary artery (**C**; type IB) arises from the pulmonary trunk. (*Adapted from* Roberts [1].)

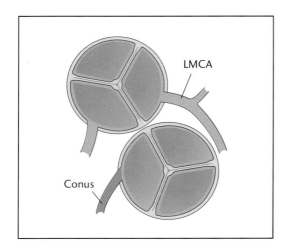

Figure 3-4.
The origin of the conus artery from the pulmonary trunk (PT) (type IIE). The most common accessory coronary artery arising from the PT is a conus artery. The origin of this small coronary artery from the PT is of no functional significance. LMCA—left main coronary artery. (*Adapted from* Roberts [1].)

ANOMALOUS ORIGIN OF ONE OR MORE CORONARY ARTERIES FROM THE AORTA WITHOUT ORIGIN OF A CORONARY ARTERY FROM THE PULMONARY TRUNK

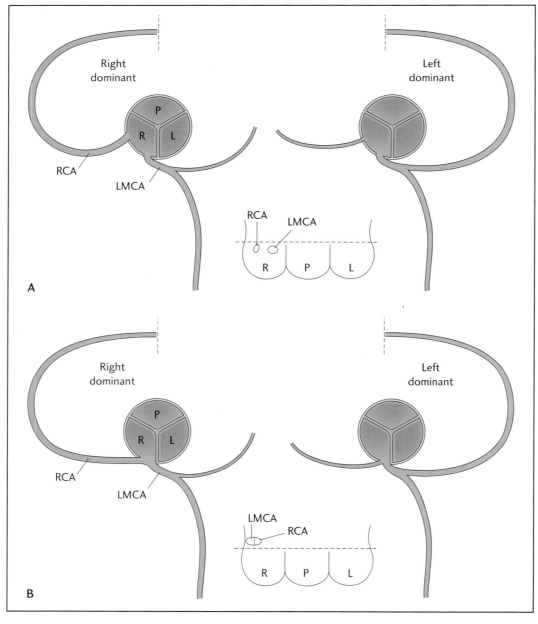

Figure 3-5.
The coronary anatomy in cases of anomalous origin of the left main coronary artery (LMCA) from the aorta, illustrating both right coronary artery (RCA) and left circumflex coronary artery (LCCA) dominance with coursing of the anomalously arising LMCA in the groove between the ascending aorta and PT (type IIIA2). **A,** Both coronary ostia are located within the right sinus. **B,** Both are located in a common ostium located above the sino-tubular junction, which is an imaginary line at the most cephalad extension of the lateral attachments (commissures) of the aortic valve and separates the sinus portion from the tubular portion of aorta. Indicated is the importance of knowing which artery in the atrioventricular sulcus is the dominant one. On the *left*, the RCA is dominant and the LCCA is hypoplastic; on the *right*, the LCCA is dominant and the RCA is hypoplastic. The situation on the *right* is far more dangerous than the situation on the *left*. This anomaly, however, is a very dangerous one and is frequently associated with sudden death in teenagers. It is more common in males than in females. The usual scenario is fainting during physical activity. When the diagnosis is made, proper therapy is operative; it includes insertion of bypass conduits from the aorta into both the left anterior descending coronary artery (LADCA) and the LCCA or movement of the LMCA to insert into the left sinus of Valsalva. L—left; P—posterior; R—right. (*Adapted from* Kragel and Roberts [20].)

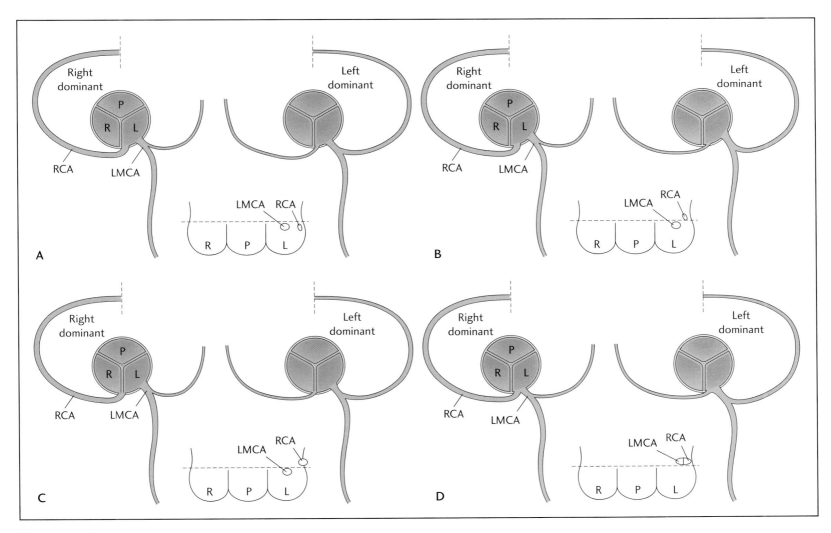

Figure 3-6.

Coronary anatomy in patients with anomalous origin of the right coronary artery (RCA) from the aorta with coursing of the anomalously arising coronary artery between the PT and aorta (type IIIB2). **A** and **B,** The right coronary ostium is slitlike. In *panel A,* it arises within the sinus; in *panel B,* it arises above the sinotubular junction. **C,** The RCA arises just cephalad to the sinotubular junction. **D,** Both the RCA and the left main coronary artery (LMCA) have a common origin above the sinotubular junction. This anomaly is usually clinically silent. A few patients have been reported who have developed evidence of myocardial ischemia. That situation occurs only when the RCA is dominant and does not occur when the RCA is hypoplastic.

The author has studied at necropsy 32 patients in whom either the LMCA arose from the right aortic sinus and coursed between the PT and aorta or the RCA arose from the left aortic sinus and coursed between the PT and ascending aorta [15,16]. In seven (22%) of the 32 patients, the LMCA arose abnormally and then coursed between aorta and PT before reaching the left side [17]. The ages of these seven patients ranged from 13 to 81 years (mean, 38 years). Four were men and three were women. In five of the seven patients, the anomaly was considered the cause of death. All of these five patients had signs or symptoms of cardiac disease during life: two had angina pectoris, three had one or more episodes of syncope, one had abnormal electrocardiogram findings, and one had congestive heart failure. Both coronary ostia arose from the right sinus of Valsalva in six patients and in one patient, as a single coronary ostium, which divided immediately to form the RCA and LMCA, which straddled the right sinus of Valsalva

and the commissure between the right and left cusps. The ostium of the LMCA was slitlike in at least four patients. The RCA was dominant in six patients, and the LCCA was dominant in one patient. Grossly visible foci of left or right ventricular wall necrosis were absent in all seven patients, but four had grossly visible left ventricular scars, only one of whom had significant coronary narrowing (> 75% cross-sectional area) by atherosclerotic plaque of one or more coronary arteries.

In 25 (78%) of the 32 patients, the RCA arose anomalistically and then coursed between the aorta and PT [15,16,20]. The ages of these 25 patients ranged from 4 months to 74 years (mean, 39 years). Five were female and 20 were male. The anomaly was considered the cause of death in eight patients. Of these, five had no signs or symptoms of cardiac disease during life; two had angina pectoris; two had abnormal electrocardiogram findings, and one had recurrent ventricular tachycardia with a nonfatal cardiac arrest followed by a fatal cardiac arrest. Four others had evidence of myocardial ischemia during life; in three of them, necropsy disclosed more than 75% cross-sectional area narrowing of one or more major coronary arteries by atherosclerotic plaques; one of the four patients had hypertrophic cardiomyopathy. The ostium of the RCA arose from within the left sinus of Valsalva in eight patients; from above the left sinus of Valsalva in five patients; directly above the commissure between the right and left cusps in 10 patients; and as a single ostium, which straddled the left sinus of Valsalva and the commissure between the right and left cusps, in two patients. Of the 25 patients, the ostium of the RCA was slitlike in 14, oval in seven, and not determined in four. (*continued on next page*)

Figure 3-6. (*continued*)

The LCCA was dominant in seven patients,, the RCA was dominant in 10 patients, and both the RCA and the LCCA were small and neither artery coursed to the crux of the heart in one patient. The LCCA was not dominant in any patients in whom the anomaly was clinically significant. Seven patients had more than 75% cross-sectional area narrowing by atherosclerotic plaque of one or more major coronary arteries. Grossly visible foci of left ventricular necrosis were present in two patients, one of whom had significant coronary arterial atherosclerosis; the other had evulsion of the RCA from the aorta by aortic dissection. Grossly visible left ventricular scars were present in five patients, two of whom had one or more major epicardial coronary arteries significantly narrowed by plaque. Abnormalities of the aortic valve were present in four patients, one of whom had a congenitally bicuspid aortic valve; the other three had partial fusion of one or more of the three commissures.

Anatomic classification of anomalous origin of the LMCA and RCA from the aorta with subsequent coursing of the anomalously arising coronary artery between the aorta and PT is complex. It is not sufficient, as has been done in the past, to classify the anomaly as "origin of the RCA from the left sinus of Valsalva" and "origin of the LMCA from the right sinus of Valsalva." The LMCA may arise from either behind the right sinus of Valsalva or from a common ostium with the RCA straddling the right-to-left commissure and the left sinus of Valsalva. The RCA may arise from behind or above the left sinus of Valsalva, from above the commissure between the right and left cusps, or from a common ostium at the LMCA, which straddles the commissure between the right and left sinus of Valsalva. Subclassification of the anomalies does not appear, however, to predict the clinical significance of the anomaly.

The shape of the ostium of the anomalously arising coronary artery is not helpful in predicting the clinical significance of the anomaly. In cases in which the anomaly was considered to be the cause of death, the anomalistically arising artery was slitlike in some instances; in others, the ostium was round. When anomalous origin of the LMCA alone is considered, four of six patients had slitlike ostia, and the anomaly was fatal in all four. In 21 patients with anomalous origin of the RCA in which the ostial shape was determined, the ostium was slitlike in 14 (67%); in six of them (42%); the anomaly was fatal. In seven patients (33%) the ostium was round, and the anomaly was fatal in two (29%).

Coronary dominance was important in separating clinically significant from clinically insignificant anomalies. In seven patients with anomalous origin of the RCA from the left sinus of Valsalva, the LCCA was dominant; the anomaly was not clinically significant in any of them. In one patient, both the LCCA and RCA were hypoplastic (neither was dominant), and the anomaly was considered the cause of death. In the seven patients with anomalous origin of the LMCA, the LCCA was dominant in only one; in the other six patients, the LCCA was nondominant (the RCA was dominant). In four, the anomaly was clinically significant; it was not clinically significant in two patients. Thus, in the case of anomalous origin of the LMCA, whereas LCCA dominance is probably always clinically significant or at least potentially significant, RCA dominance is usually but not always clinically significant. L—left; P—posterior; R—right. (*Adapted from* Kragel and Roberts [14].)

Figure 3-7.

The mechanism by which origin of the right coronary artery (RCA) arising from the left sinus of Valsalva may cause myocardial ischemia (IIIB). **A,** Normally, a stick placed in either the RCA or left main coronary artery (LMCA) tends to point to the central portion of the aorta. However, when the RCA arises from the left aortic sinus and then courses between the pulomnary trunk (PT) and aorta, a stick placed within the RCA points directly to the aortic wall. With exercise, both the ascending aorta (AA) and PT dilate; with the dilatation, the slitlike orifice of the anomalously arising artery tends to become quite narrowed or to close off. The same situation occurs when the LMCA arises from the right sinus and courses between the PT and AA. It appears that the compression at the ostium of the anomalously arising coronary artery (rather than compression of the anomalous artery in its course between the AA and the PT) produces the sudden myocardial ischemia. L—left; P—posterior; R—right. (*Adapted from* Roberts and coworkers [13].)

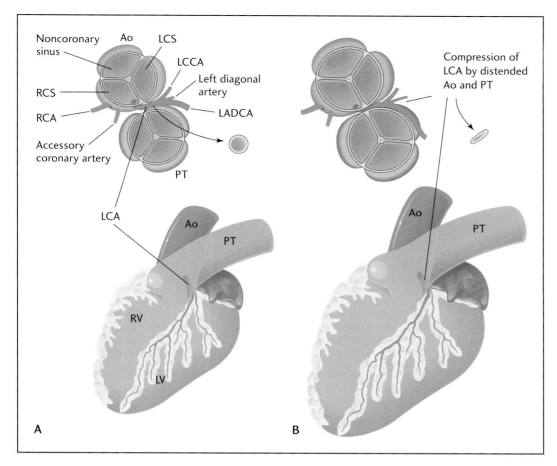

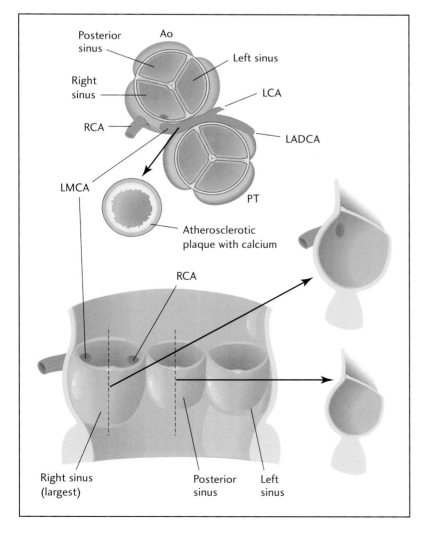

Figure 3-8.

A proposed mechanism by which origin of the left main coronary artery (LMCA) from the right sinus of Valsalva causes non-fatal or fatal myocardial ischemia (IIIA). The ostium of the anomalously arising artery is closed off by the dilatation of both the ascending aorta and pulmonary trunk during exercise. Ao—aorta; LADCA—left anterior descending coronary artery; LCA—left coronary artery; LCCA—left circumflex coronary artery; LCS—left coronary sinus; RCA—right coronary artery; RCS—right coronary sinus. (*Adapted from* Roberts [1].)

Figure 3-9.

An anomalously arising left main coronary artery (LMCA) from the right sinus of Valsalva is shown in an 81-year-old man who never had evidence of myocardial ischemia and who died of a noncardiac condition (IIIA). In this patient, the wall of the anomalously arising LMCA is heavily calcified. It is not clear how he survived to this old age. LADCA—left anterior descending coronary artery; LCCA—left circumflex coronary artery; RCA—right coronary artery. (*Adapted from* Barth and Roberts [16].)

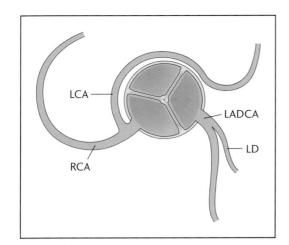

Figure 3-10.

The origin of the left circumflex coronary artery (LCCA) as the first branch of the right coronary artery (RCA) and its coursing posterior to the aorta before reaching the left atrioventricular sulcus (IIID). This is the most common anomalous coronary artery; in this circumstance, it has no functional significance. It has been estimated to occur in one in 300 people [9,21]. If, however, the LCCA arises directly from the right aortic sinus, on rare occasion, myocardial ischemia can result, presumably because the ostium of the anomalously arising artery is compressed when the ascending aorta dilates. This appeared to be the situation in one of 22 patients seen by the author with this anomaly at necropsy. If the LCCA arises directly from the RCA, no such compression can occur. In both circumstances, the left anterior descending coronary artery (LADCA) usually arises directly from the left sinus. This anomaly occurs mainly in males. If the LCCA arises directly from the RCA, the most proximal portion of the RCA (before the LCCA arises from it) becomes the equivalent of the LMCA in that it supplies two major coronary arteries [23]. In addition, the LCCA arises directly from the RCA with a retroaortic course; the LADCA may also arise from the RCA and course to the left side of the heart either anterior to the right ventricle or beneath the right ventricular outflow tract in the crista supraventricularis [24]. (*Adapted from* Roberts [1].)

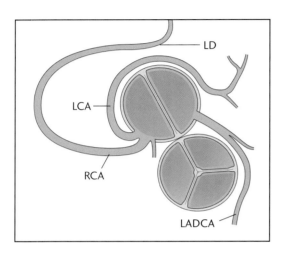

Figure 3-11.

The left circumflex coronary artery (LCCA) arises directly from what would be the right sinus of Valsalva, but this patient has a congenitally bicuspid aortic valve (IIID). The LCCA courses in a retroaortic position before reaching the left atrioventricular sulcus; the left anterior descending coronary artery (LADCA) arises from the left aortic sinus. Coronary anomalies are far more common in patients with congenitally malformed aortic or pulmonic valves than in patients with normally formed aortic and pulmonic valves. Shown is the anomaly in a 43-year-old man who died of complications of severe coronary atherosclerosis. The coronary anomaly caused no clinical dysfunction, and the congenitally bicuspid aortic valve had functioned normally during life. (*Adapted from* Roberts [1].)

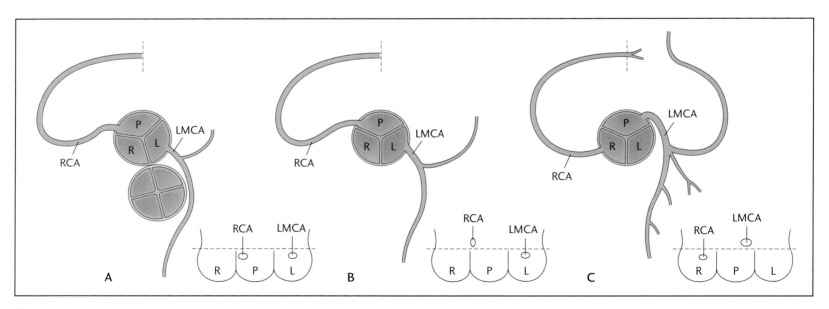

Figure 3-12.

Origin of the right coronary artery (RCA) or left main coronary artery (LMCA) from the posterior aortic valve cusp is an exceedingly uncommon circumstance. **A,** Origin of the RCA was observed in a 19-year-old man who died suddenly while playing basketball. The cause of his sudden death was not determined. It is unclear whether the coronary anomaly played a role in his sudden death. The pulmonic valve was congenitally malformed, being quadricuspid. It appeared not to have caused any dysfunction. This is another example of an abnormality of a semilunar valve in association with a coronary anomaly. **B,** The ostium of the anomalously arising RCA, which arose cephalad to the sinotubular junction, was slitlike. **C,** The LMCA arose from the posterior aortic sinus also above the sinotubular junction. L—left; P—posterior; R—right. (*Adapted from* Roberts and Kragel [20].)

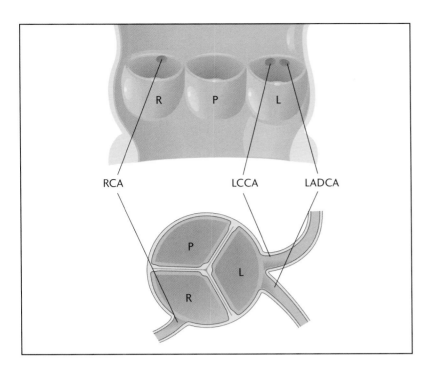

Figure 3-13.

The aorta shows origin of both the left circumflex coronary artery (LCCA) and the left anterior descending coronary artery (LADCA) arising from a separate ostium in the left aortic sinus (type IIIH). This anomaly causes no myocardial ischemia or cardiac dysfunction. Attention is called to this anomaly because it cannot be recognized at angiography, and operation could potentially lead to serious consequences. If contrast material is injected into only one or the other of the two arteries arising from the left aortic sinus during coronary angiography, the noninjected artery might mistakenly be interpreted as being totally occluded at its origin from the left main coronary artery (LMCA). If either the LADCA or LCCA is not visualized by selective injection of contrast material, injection into the sinuses of Valsalva may prevent confusing an anomalously arising coronary artery with a totally occluded coronary artery. If either ostium is not perfused at the time of cardiopulmonary bypass, a portion of the left ventricular myocardium might not be adequately oxygenated, as observed in a patient described by Ogden [27]. A theoretical advantage of a separate ostium of both the LADCA and LCCA from the left aortic sinus is the inability to have complications resulting from narrowing of the LMCA. Two of four patients with separate origin of the LADCA and LCCA studied by the author had severe (> 75% cross-sectional area) narrowing of both LDCA and LCCA proximal to any major branches and, therefore, had so-called "LM equivalent" narrowing. This coronary anomaly does not appear to accelerate atherosclerosis in either of the separately arising coronary arteries [23]. L—left; P—posterior; R—right. (*Adapted from* Dicicco and coworkers [23].)

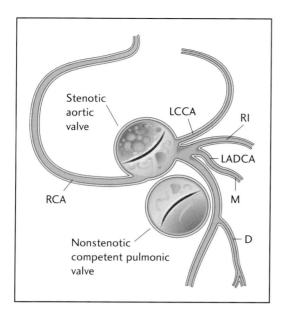

Figure 3-14.

Origin of both left-sided coronary arteries directly from the left side of the aorta is shown in a 60-year-old man in whom both semilunar valves were congenitally bicuspid and the aortic valve also stenotic (type IIIH). This case is another example showing congenital malformation of one or both semilunar valves in association with a coronary anomaly. LADCA—left anterior descending coronary artery; LCCA—left circumflex coronary artery; D—diagonal; R—right; RI—ramus intermedius. (*Adapted from* Roberts [1].)

ANOMALOUS ORIGIN OF ONE CORONARY ARTERY FROM ANOTHER CORONARY ARTERY

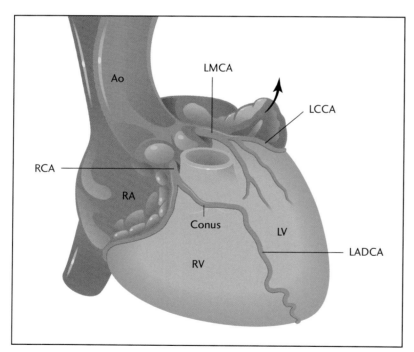

Figure 3-15.

An example of anomalous origin of one or more coronary arteries from the aorta. In this case, the left anterior descending coronary artery (LADCA) arose from the conus artery passing anterior to the right ventricular outflow tract. The proximal portion of the LADCA arose from the left main coronary artery (LMCA), but that artery stopped when the more distal portion of the LADCA arose from the conus. This patient was a 60-year-old man who died from consequences of severe coronary atherosclerosis. The coronary anomaly caused no cardiac dysfunction or myocardial ischemia. Ao—aorta; LV—left ventricle; R—right; RA—right atrium; RV—right ventricle. (*Adapted from* Roberts and coworkers [18].)

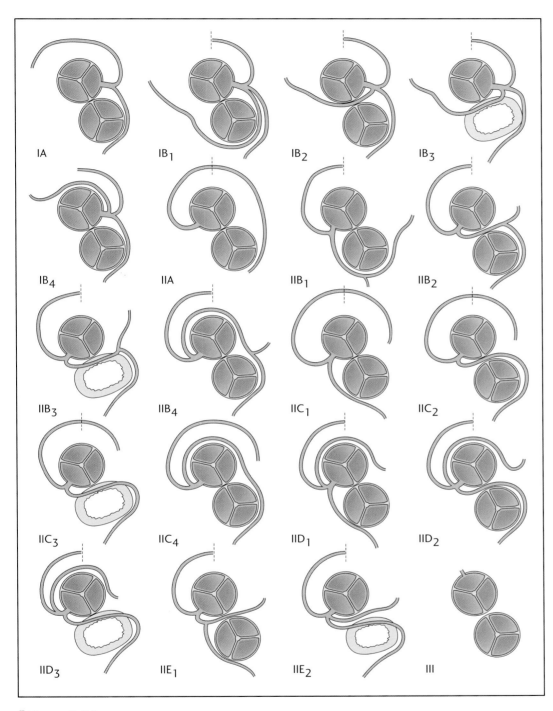

IA   IB₁   IB₂   IB₃   IB₄   IIA   IIB₁   IIB₂   IIB₃   IIB₄   IIC₁   IIC₂   IIC₃   IIC₄   IID₁   IID₂   IID₃   IIE₁   IIE₂   III

Figure 3-16.

The origin and pattern of distribution of various types of solitary coronary ostium in the aorta. Origin of only one coronary artery from the aorta without origin of a coronary artery from the pulmonary trunk (PT; single coronary ostia) (type IV). Solitary coronary ostium in the aorta, in the absence of other major congenital cardiovascular anomalies, is rare. Only about 40 necropsied patients with this cardiac anomaly have been reported, and just more than 50 with this anomaly at coronary angiography [24]. The largest necropsy study of this anomaly included only 10 patients [24]. None of these 10 patients with solitary coronary ostium in the aorta were associated with origin of a coronary artery from the PT, and none had other major congenital cardiovascular anomalies. Using clinical and morphologic data from these 10 patients and from previously published reports, Shirani and Roberts [24] developed a classification for single coronary ostium in the aorta unassociated with other

major congenital cardiovascular anomalies. That classification is shown here.

The 10 patients ranged in age from 5 to 78 years; seven were male and three were female. The coronary anomaly did not cause any symptoms or signs of myocardial ischemia in any of the 10 patients. The solitary coronary ostium was located in the left aortic sinus in four patients and in the right aortic sinus in six patients. When the solitary coronary ostium was located in the left aortic sinus, three of four patients had an "anatomic single coronary artery" in which the left main coroanry artery (LMCA) divided normally into the left anterior descending coronary artery (LADCA) and left circumflex coronary artery (LCCA) with the LCCA coursing in the left atrioventricular groove to reach the crux and to continue in the right atrioventricular groove as the right coronary artery (RCA). In the remaining patient, the LMCA trifurcated into the LADCA, LCCA, and an aberrant-coursing artery that coursed anterior to the right ventricle to reach the right atrioventricular groove and from there on continued as an otherwise normal RCA.

An aberrant-coursing artery was present in all six patients whose solitary coronary ostium was located in the right aortic sinus. Of these aberrant coursing arteries, four were the LMCA and two were the LADCA. The aberrant-coursing LMCA reached the left side of the heart (to divide into the LADCA and the LCCA) by coursing anterior to the right ventricle in one patient, in between the PT and ascending aorta in one patient, and dorsal to ascending aorta in two patients. In two patients, the aberrant-coursing artery was the LADCA, which reached the anterior ventricular groove by coursing between the right ventricular outflow tract within the superior portion of the ventricular septum.

Shirani and Roberts [24] also summarized findings in 87 previously reported patients with solitary coronary ostium in the aorta. The diagnosis was made at necropsy in 35 patients and by coronary angiography in 52. On the basis of morphologic and angiographic findings, using the 87 previously reported patients and their 10 patients, Shirani and Roberts produced a simple (*continued on next page*)

Figure 3-16. (*continued*)

practical classification for single aortic coronary ostium. The location or the solitary coronary ostium in relation to the aortic sinus, the presence or absence of an aberrant-coursing coronary artery, and the course taken by the aberrant-coursing coronary artery (when present) formed the basis of the classification. The most frequently seen anomaly type is type IA, of which 28 cases have been reported. The other anomaly types have each been reported in 10 or fewer patients. Types IIC4, IID1, IIE1, IIE2, and III have not been reported.

Information regarding the presence or absence of significant luminal narrowing in the major coronary arteries by atherosclerotic plaque was available in 85 of the 97 patients reviewed. Of these 85 patients, 32 (38%) had atherosclerotic coronary artery disease (nine at necropsy) and 23 by angiography; eight (15%) patients (aged 13 to 65 years old at death or at the time of coronary angiography) had clinical evidence of myocardial ischemia attributable to the coronary anomaly. Four of the eight had angina pectoris, five had acute myocardial infarction, and three had positive exercise stress tests results. Two patients died as a direct result of the coronary anomaly: a 13-year-old boy had a solitary ostium in the right aortic sinus and an aberrant-coursing LMCA that originated from the RCA and crossed to the opposite side of the heart between PT and aorta. Another patient had an anatomic single RCA. He was a professional basketball player for many years and did not have symptoms of myocardial ischemia. He died suddenly at age 40 years on the basketball court. His heart weighed 560 g, and all cardiac chambers were dilated. The myocardium of the anterior left ventricular wall was extensively scarred. The LADCA in this patient was a continuation of the LCCA and had a very small diameter. Another patient had an anatomic single left coronary artery: he was 21 years old and took part in vigorous physical activity during adolescence without any symptoms of cardiac dysfunction; acute myocardial infarction was diagnosed after an episode of exertional dizziness. In four of the eight patients, an aberrant-coursing coronary artery originated from the RCA (three patients) or the LMCA (one patient) and crossed to the opposite side between the ascending aorta and PT. One of these four patients, a 65-year-old man, had severe exertional angina and

pacing-induced electrocardiographic changes of myocardial ischemia. Another patient had an aberrant-coursing RCA originating from the LADCA; it coursed in the superior portion of the ventricular septum to reach the right side of the heart; angina pectoris and myocardial ischemia were present in this 50-year-old woman. Finally, in a 25-year-old woman, the LMCA originated from the RCA and then coursed to the left side of the heart anterior to the right ventricular wall; acute myocardial infarction (anterior left ventricular wall) occurred despite the absence of narrowing of the coronary arteries by angiography.

Solitary coronary ostium in the aorta was first reported in 1841 [25]. According to Hrytl's postulate at that time, a single coronary artery is present when the entire heart is supplied by either the LMCA or the RCA in the absence of any aberrant-coursing branches. Three further attempts at classification were made as various other types of single coronary arteries were recognized. In 1950, Smith [26] recognized three different types of single coronary arteries: type 1, or anatomic single coronary artery; type 2, in which an aberrant-coursing coronary artery followed the usual distribution of the "missing" coronary artery after originating from a solitary coronary ostium located in the opposite aortic sinus; and type 3, which included atypical cases that could not be classified as type 1 or as type 2. Recognizing the inadequacy of such broad categories, Ogden and Goodyear [27] proposed a more complete classification of single coronary arteries in 1970. They classified the single coronary artery into 14 basic distribution patterns. The type C of Shirani and Roberts [24] (aberrant-coursing coronary artery crossing to the other side of the heart in the crista supraventricularis) was not included in their classification. Moreover, patients with associated major anomalies of the heart and great vessels and those with coronary atresia were not separated. In 1979, Lipton *et al.* [28] described nine angiographic patterns of an isolated single coronary artery. Type C anomalies again were not included. One of the 10 patients reported by Shirani and Roberts [24] was not classified by the angiographic patterns described (type IID2 is the classification). In summary, the anatomic classification presented here is useful both clinically and surgically. (*Adapted from* Shirani and Roberts [24].)

CONGENITAL CORONARY ARTERIAL ANOMALIES UNASSOCIATED WITH OTHER MAJOR ANOMALIES OF THE HEART OR GREAT ARTERIES

Origin of one or more coronary arteries from the PT without origin of a coronary artery from the aorta

RCA and LMCA from the PT*

"Single coronary artery" from the PT*

Origin of one or more coronary arteries from the PT and one or more coronary arteries from the aorta (within a sinus or immediately cephalad to it)

LMCA from the PT

RCA from the PT

LADCA from the PT

LCCA from the PT

Accessory coronary artery from the PT

Anomalous origin of one or more coronary arteries from the aorta (within a sinus or immediately cephalad to it) without origin of a coronary artery from the PT

Both the LMCA and RCA from the right aortic sinus with the LMCA coursing to the left side via one of four routes

Anterior to the RV (type a)

Between the PT and AA (type b)[†]

In the CS (type c)

Dorsal to the AA (type d)

Both the LMCA and RCA from the left aortic sinus with the RCA coursing to the right side via one of two routes

Anterior to the RV (type a)

Between the PT and AA (type b)[†]

Both the LMCA and RCA from the posterior aortic sinus

RCA and LCCA from the right aortic sinus (or LCCA from RCA) with retroaortic course of the LCCA and LADCA from the left sinus

RCA from the posterior aortic sinus and the LMCA from the left aortic sinus

LMCA from the posterior aortic sinus and the RCA from the left aortic sinus

LADCA and LCCA from a separate ostium in the left aortic sinus and the RCA from right aortic sinus

Origin of only one coronary artery from the aorta (within the sinus or immediately cephalad to it) without origin of a coronary artery from the PT (single coronary ostium)

In the right aortic sinus

Without an aberrant-coursing coronary artery (anatomic single RCA)

LMCA from the RCA with coursing to the left side via one of four routes before dividing into the LADCA and the LCCA

Anterior to the RV (type a)

Between the PT and the AA (type b)[†]

In the CS (type c)

Dorsal to the AA (type d)

LADCA from the RCA with 1 coursing to the left side via one of four routes (RCA arises normally and continues in the atrioventricular sulcus past the crux to form the LCCA

Anterior to the RV (type a)

Between the PT and ascending aorta (type b)[†]

In the CS (type c)

Dorsal to the AA (type d)

LCCA from the RCA with 2 coursing to the left side dorsal to the AA; LADCA from the RCA with 3 coursing to the left side via one of three routes

Anterior to the RV (type a)

Between the PT and the AA (type b)[†]

In the CS (type c)

In left aortic sinus

Without with an aberrent-coursing coronary artery (anatomic single left coronary artery)

RCA arises from the LMCA or from the LADCA and courses to the right atrioventricular sulcus via four routes:

Anterior to the RV (type a)

Between the PT and the AA (type b)

In the CS (type c)

Dorsal to the AA (type d)

In posterior aortic sinus (not reported)

Coronary arterial aneurysm[†]

Coronary arterial fistula[†]

High take off coronary artery

Tunneled epicardial coronary artery (myocardial bridge)

Congenital absence, atresia, or hypoplasia of a coronary artery[†]

*Usually causes fatal or nonfatal myocardial ischemia or cardiac dysfunction.
†Only occasionally causes fatal or nonfatal myocardial ischemia or cardiac dysfunction.

Figure 3-17.

Congenital coronary arterial anomalies unassociated with other major anomalies of the heart or great arteries. AA—ascending aorta; CS—crista supraventricularis; LADCA—left anterior descending coronary artery; LCCA—left circumflex coronary artery; LMCA—left main coronary artery; PT—pulmonary trunk; RCA right coronary artery; RV—right ventricle.

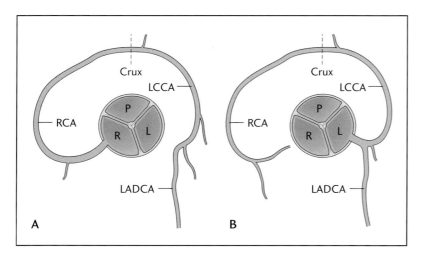

Figure 3-18.
The two most common varieties of single coronary ostium are shown. **A,** The single ostium arises in the right (R) aortic sinus (IVA1). **B,** The single ostium arises in the left (L) aortic sinus (type IVB1). When the single coronary artery arises from the right aortic ostium, the right coronary artery crosses the crux to continue as the left circumflex coronary artery (LCCA), which in turn continues as the left anterior descending coronary artery (LADCA) (IVA1). When the single ostium is located in the left aortic sinus, the LMCA gives rise to the LADCA and the LCCA, and the LCCA crosses the crux to continue as the right coronary artery (IVB). (*Adapted from* Roberts [1].)

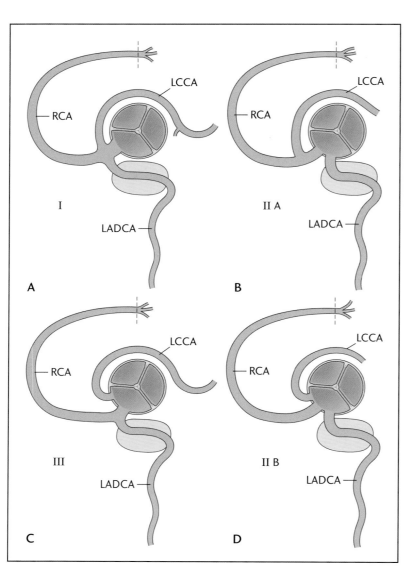

Figure 3-19.
The four types of retroaortic epicardial left circumflex coronary arteries (LCCAs) and anteroaortic intramyocardial left anterior descending coronary arteries (LADCAs) showing the possible origins of the LCCA and LADCA from either the aorta or the right coronary artery (RCA). **A,** In type I, only a single coronary artery arises from the aorta, and both the LCCA and the LADCA arise from the right (type IVA4b). **B** and **C,** In type II, there are two coronary ostia in the right sinus of Valvsalva of the aorta: the RCA and either the LADCA (type IIa) or the LCCA (type IIb). No reports are available describing the type IIb variety. **D,** In type III, there are three coronary ostia in the aorta: LCCA, RCA, and LADCA. (*Adapted from* Dollar and Roberts [19].)

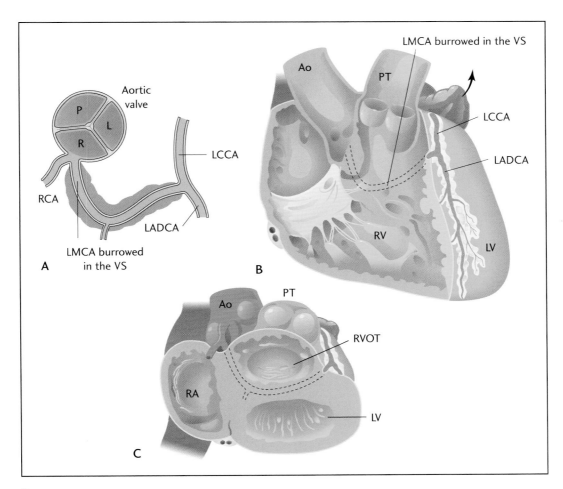

Figure 3-20.

A heart in which the left main coronary artery (LMCA) arose from the right aortic sinus and then coursed behind the right ventricular outflow tract (RVOT) and within the crista supraventricularis (CS) before entering the epicardium just anterior to the ventricular septum (IVA2b). The LMCA then divided into the left anterior descending coronary artery (LADCA) and left circumflex coronary artery (LCCA). This coronary artery causes no cardiac dysfunction despite the fact that the LMCA may have a length of approximately 5 cm within the myocardium. Ao—aorta; VS—ventricular septum. (*Adapted from* Roberts and coworkers [29].)

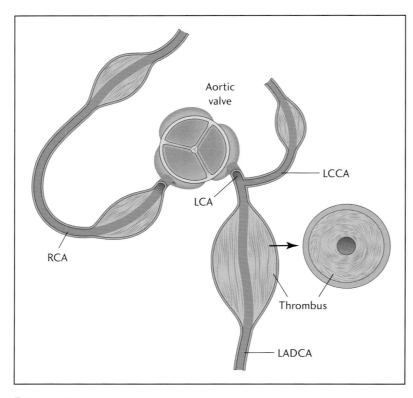

Figure 3-21.
Dilatation of epicardial coronary arteries can be diffuse or localized.
Very elderly individuals often have dilated coronary arteries, as do
younger individuals with huge hearts (most commonly from chronic
aortic regurgitation or hypertrophic cardiomyopathy). Patients with
supravalvular aortic stenosis have hugely dilated coronary arteries

because these vessels fill mainly in ventricular systole rather than in
diastole in this condition. Patients with severe cyanotic congenital
heart disease who survive well into adulthood also usually have very
large coronary arteries that dilate in response to the severe systemic
arterial desaturation. An occasional adult has considerable diffuse
dilatation of one coronary artery unassociated with any of the afore-
mentioned conditions. Localized dilatation of one portion of one or
more epicardial coronary arteries, in contrast to diffuse dilatation, is
rare. Probably its most common cause is that occurring as a part of
the mucocutaneous lymph node syndrome (*ie*, Kawasaki disease).
Atherosclerosis is most likely the next most common cause. Other
extremely rare causes include infection, particularly as a part of a septic
embolus; trauma; and congenital causes. The atherosclerotic coronary
aneurysms are seen only in older individuals, they nearly always
contain intra-aneurysmal thrombus that may narrow or completely
obstruct the lumen, and they are associated with extensive atherosclerosis in the portions of coronary artery that are not aneurysmal. In
contrast, the congenital aneurysms are mainly present in younger individuals, they are not associated with atherosclerotic plaquing in the
aneurysmal or nonaneurysmal portions of the coronary arteries, and
they usually do not contain intra-aneurysmal thrombus.

Shown here are multiple coronary arterial aneurysms in a 30-
month-old boy who was known to have coronary aneurysms at least
since age 6 months. He died suddenly at age 30 months and had been
asymptomatic before that time. At necropsy, the anterior wall of the
left ventricle was scarred, and all coronary aneurysms contained
thrombus. The child had other features consistent with the mucocutaneous lymph node syndrome. LADCA—left anterior descending
coronary artery; LCCA—left circumflex coronary artery. (*Adapted
from* Roberts [30].)

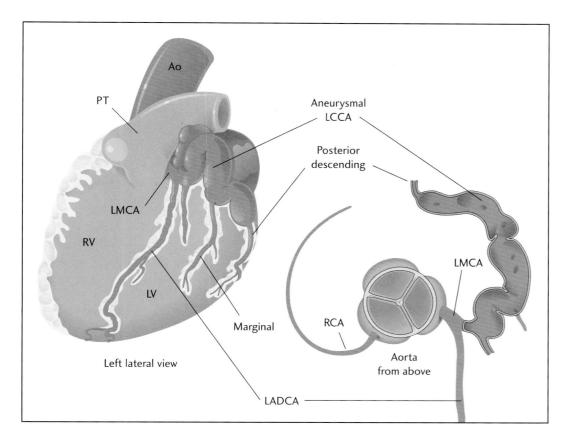

Figure 3-22.

A congenital coronary aneurysm unassociated with a fistula in a 70-year-old man who died from a head injury. The coronary aneurysm was an unexpected finding at necropsy. There were never signs or symptoms of cardiac dysfunction. The aneurysm was devoid of thrombus, and few atherosclerotic plaques were present in any of the epicardial coronary arteries. The right coronary artery was hypoplastic. LADCA—left anterior descending coronary artery; LCCA—left circumflex coronary artery; LMCA—left main coronary artery; PT—pulmonary artery. (*Adapted from* Roberts [30]).

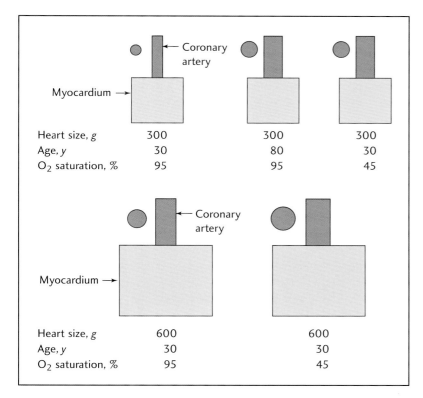

Figure 3-23.

The relationship between the sizes of the coronary arteries and the arterial oxygen saturation. In each of the *upper diagrams*, the heart weighs 300 g. At age 30 years, the coronary artery supplying that heart muscle is not dilated. The arterial oxygen saturation is normal (95%). In the *upper central diagram*, the arterial oxygen saturation is normal, but the patient is 80 years old; therefore, it is shown that the coronary arteries may dilate with age. In the *upper right diagram*, the patient is only 30 years old, but the arterial oxygen saturation is 45%; in this situation, the coronary arteries may dilate considerably. In the *lower diagrams*, the heart muscle quantity is twice that in the *upper diagrams*. The size of the coronary artery is roughly proportional to the amount of myocardium it needs to supply with blood; therefore, the coronary arteries are dilated with increased mass. In addition, if arterial oxygen desaturation is present, as shown in the *bottom right diagram*, the coronary arterial dilatation is much greater. (*Adapted from* Roberts [30].)

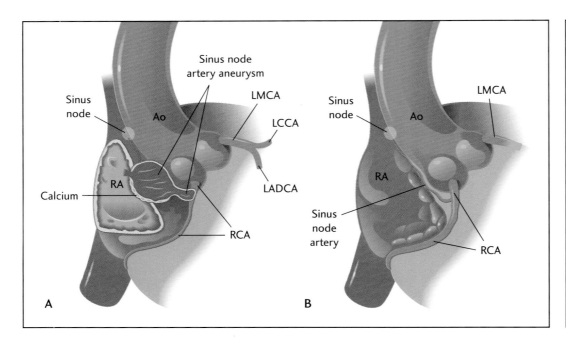
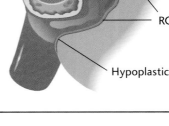

Figure 3-24.
Coronary artery fistula unassociated with a cardiac valve anomaly, such as pulmonic valve atresia or aortic valve atresia, is rare. It is estimated that about 350 cases have been reported since coronary artery fistula was first described in 1965. The fistulae involve the right coronary artery (RCA) or one or more of its branches in about 60% of the patients, and either the left anterior descending coronary artery (LADCA) or left circumflex coronary artery (LCCA) or one of their branches in the other 40%. Rarely, more than one coronary artery is part of the fistula, or a fistula may involve a single or an accessory coronary artery. The site of termination of the fistula in 90% of patients is the right side of the heart or vessels attached to it, most commonly the right ventricle (RV) followed by right atrium (RA) and pulmonary trunk. The other 10% terminate in either the left atrium or left ventricle. The connection between the coronary artery fistula and the site of termination may be a single opening or multiple openings. Some of those with multiple openings may have telangiectatic-type connections. The coronary artery that is part of the anomalous communication with the cardiac chamber or attached cardiac vein or artery nearly always is dilated, the dilatation being both transverse and longitudinal. The latter is manifest by tortuosity. The enlarged coronary artery often has focal outpouching (saccular aneurysms superimposed on the fusiform aneurysm), and its wall may contain focal calcific deposits. Symptoms appear to be determined mainly by the magnitude of the shunt via the coronary artery fistula. If the shunt is large, congestive heart failure or signs and symptoms of myocardial ischemia may result. The myocardial ischemia appears to result from the coronary steal effect, whereby blood intended to be used to perfuse myocardium is stolen by the cardiac chamber or vessel proximal to its intended myocardial termination. Some individuals with coronary artery fistula are asymptomatic, and attention is called to the presence of a coronary artery fistula by a continuous precordial murmur. Symptoms may appear in infancy or not until older adulthood.

A, Shown is an aneurysmal sinus node artery arising from the RCA and terminating in the RA. The wall of the fistula contains calcific deposits. B, The normal heart for comparison. Ao—aorta; R—right. (*Adapted from* Roberts [30].)

Figure 3-25.
A thrombosed sinus node artery that had served as a fistula between the right coronary artery (RCA) and the right atrium is shown in a 14-year-old girl who died of complications of regional ileitis. During life, she had no evidence of cardiac disease. The RCA was hypoplastic. Ao—aorta; LADCA—left anterior descending coronary artery; LCCA—left circumflex coronary artery; LMCA—left main coronary artery; R—right. (*Adapted from* Roberts [30].)

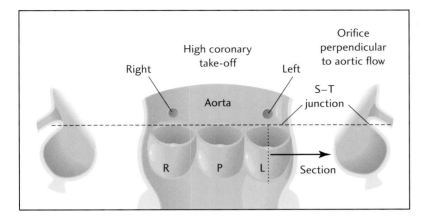

Figure 3-26.
High take-off coronary artery (VII). Normally, both coronary arterial ostia are located just caudal to an imaginary line separating the sinuses of Valsalva from that portion of aorta just above the sinuses, commonly referred to as the "tubular" portion of aorta. Occasionally, one, and rarely both, coronary arteries arise just cephalad to the sinotubular junction, and their origin may be called "high take-off." High take-off of a coronary artery is usually of no functional significance. When only one coronary artery is of high take-off, it is nearly always the right one. That artery may arise on occasion 1 to 2 cm above the sinotubular junction. Shown in this diagram are ostia of both the right coronary artery and left main coronary artery, each of which arise cephalad to the sinotubular (S–T) junction. (*Adapted from* Roberts [30].)

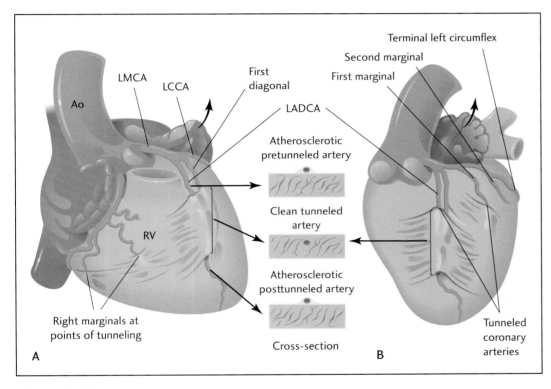

tunneling is of clinical significance (*ie*, causing symptomatic or even fatal myocardial ischemia), the author is not convinced that tunneling is of any clinical significance. In patients with considerable coronary atherosclerosis, the tunneled portion of a coronary artery is nearly always devoid of atherosclerotic plaques. It appears likely that the blood is "squeezed out" of the tunneled portion of the coronary artery by the adjacent contracting myocardium and that these contractions prevent the deposition of atherosclerotic plaques. Of course, the coronary arteries fill primarily during ventricular diastole; therefore, any narrowing during ventricular systole would not appear to be of functional significance.

Shown in this drawing is the heart from a 71-year-old man in whom several coronary arteries coursing over the left ventricle tunneled into myocardium for varying lengths. The nontunneled portions of the coronary arteries contained atherosclerotic plaques distributed diffusely, but the tunneled portions of the same coronary arteries were devoid of atherosclerotic plaques. This patient died of colon cancer and was severely cachectic, hence the near absence of subepicardial adipose tissue, which often "hides" coronary tunneling. The heart weighed only 260 g. Ao—aorta; RV—right ventricle. (*Adapted from* Roberts [30].)

Figure 3-27.
Tunneled major coronary arteries (myocardial bridge) (type VIII). Much has been written about tunneling of a major epicardial coronary artery. Any epicardial coronary artery can burrow into myocardium for variable distances and then reappear in the epicardium. Myocardial tunneling most commonly involves the left anterior descending coronary artery (LADCA), left diagonal, and left obtuse marginal. In about 20% of hearts, one or more of these arteries have tunneled in left ventricular myocardium. Far less commonly, a portion of the right coronary artery (RCA) or left circumflex coronary artery (LCCA) burrows into atrial myocardium. Although there are reports suggesting that myocardial

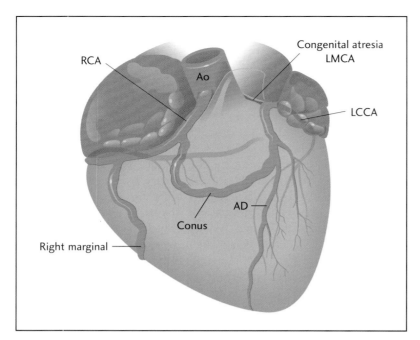

Figure 3-28.

Congenital absence, atresia, or hypoplasia of a coronary artery (IX). These are very rare occurrences. The author has seen atresia of the left circumflex coronary artery (LCCA) in an older man and atresia of the left main coronary artery (LMCA). The latter is similar to single right coronary artery (RCA) as long as the RCA is large. Hypoplasia of the LCCA is common with a dominant right circulation, and hypoplasia of the RCA is common with a dominant left circulation. Hypoplasia of the left anterior descending coronary artery (LADCA) has not been described except when there is a single coronary artery that arises from the right aortic sinus and courses in the atrioventricular sulcus to continue into the LCCA and then into the LADCA. On occasion, the artery is quite small by the time it gets to the anterior wall.

Shown are the epicardial coronary arteries in a 61-year-old man who died suddenly because of severe coronary narrowing by atherosclerotic plaques. The LMCA was congenitally atretic. This anomaly is equivalent to single coronary ostium with the single ostium in the right side of Valsava. R—right. (*Adapted from* Fortuin and Roberts [31].)

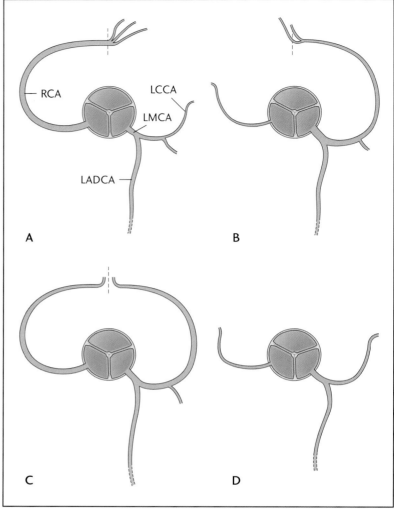

Figure 3-29.

Congenital absence, atresia, or hypoplasia of a coronary artery (type IX). Shown are graphic definitions of dominance and hypoplasia. **A,** When the right coronary artery (RCA) is dominant, the left circumflex coronary artery (LCCA) is usually hypoplastic. **B,** When the LCCA is dominant, the RCA is usually hypoplastic. **C,** Occasionally, both the RCA and the LCCA are dominant. **D,** On extremely rare occasions, both the RCA and the LCCA are hyoplastic. The latter is not a benign circumstance because perfusion of the posterior wall of the left ventricle in this circumstance may be inadequate. Sudden death, often during strenuous exertion, may be the consequence. (*Adapted from* Roberts and Glick [32].)

REFERENCES

1. Roberts WC: Anomalous origin of both coronary arteries from the pulmonary artery. *Am J Cardiol* 1962, 10:595–600.

2. Abbott ME: Anomalous origin from the pulmonary arteries. In *Osler's Modern Medicine, Its Theories and Practice,* vol 4. Edited by Osler W. Philadelphia: Lea and Febiger; 1980:420.

3. Bland EF, White PD, Garland J: Congenital anomalies of coronary arteries: report of an unusual case associated with cardiac hypertrophy. *Am Heart J* 1933, 8:787–801.

4. Edwards JE: Anomalous coronary arteries with special reference to arteriovenous-like communications. *Circulation* 1958, 17:1001–1006.

5. Edwards JE: The direction of blood flow in coronary arteries arising from the pulmonary trunk. *Circulation* 1964, 29:163–166.

6. Sabiston DC Jr, Floyd WL, McIntosh HD: Anomalous origin of the left coronary artery from the pulmonary artery in adults: surgical management. *Arch Surg* 1968, 97:963–968.

7. Fontana RS, Edwards JE: *Congenital Cardiac Disease: A Review of 357 Cases Studied Pathologically.* Philadelphia: WB Saunders; 1962:291.

8. Ogden JA: Congenital anomalies of the coronary arteries. *Am J Cardiol* 1970, 25:474–479.

9. Tingelstad JB, Lower RR, Eldredge WJ: Anomalous origin of the right coronary artery from the main pulmonary artery. *Am J Cardiol* 1972, 30:670–673.

10. Lerberg DB, Odgen JA, Zuberbuhler JR, Bahnson HT: Anomalous origin of the right coronary artery from the pulmonary artery. *Ann Thorac Surg* 1979, 27:87–94.

11. Roberts WC, Robinowitz M: Anomalous origin of the left anterior descending coronary artery from the pulmonary trunk with origin of the right and left circumflex coronary arteries from the aorta. *Am J Cardiol* 1984, 54:1381–1383.

12. Roberts WC: Major anomalies of coronary arterial origin seen in adulthood. *Am Heart J* 1986, 111:941–963.

13. Roberts WC, Siegel RJ, Zipes DP: Origin of the right coronary artery from the left sinus of Valsalva and its functional consequences: analysis of 10 necropsy patients. *Am J Cardiol* 1982, 49:863–868.

14. Kragel AH, Roberts WC: Anomalous origin of either the right or left main coronary artery from the aorta with subsequent coursing between aorta and pulmonary trunk: analysis of 32 necropsy cases. *Am J Cardiol* 1988, 62:771–777.

15. Barth CW III, Bray M, Roberts WC: Sudden death in infancy associated with origin of both left main and right coronary arteries from a common ostium above the left sinus of Valsalva [brief report]. *Am J Cardiol* 1986, 57:365–366.

16. Barth CW III, Roberts WC: Left main coronary artery originating from the right sinus of Valsalva and coursing between the aorta and pulmonary trunk. *J Am Coll Cardiol* 1986, 7:366–373.

17. White NK, Edwards JE: Anomalies of the coronary arteries: report of 4 cases. *Arch Pathol* 1948, 45:766–771.

18. Roberts WC, Waller BF, Roberts CS: Fatal atherosclerotic narrowing of the right main coronary artery: origin of the left anterior descending or left circumflex coronary artery from the right (the true "left-main equivalent"). *Am Heart J* 1982, 104:638–641.

19. Dollar AL, Roberts WC: Retroaortic epicardial course of the left circumflex artery and anteroaortic intramyocardial (ventricular septum) course of the left anterior descending coronary artery: an unusual coronary anomaly and a proposed classification based on the number of coronary ostia in the aorta. *Am J Cardiol* 1989, 64:828–829.

20. Roberts WC, Kragel AH: Anomalous origin of either the right or left main coronary artery from the aorta without coursing of the anomalistically arising artery between aorta and pulmonary trunk. *Am J Cardiol* 1988, 62:1263–1267.

21. Odgen JA: Anomalous aortic origin: circumflex, anterior descending or left main coronary arteries. *Arch Pathol* 1969, 88:323.

22. Zumbo O, Fani K, Jarmdyeh J, Daoud AS: Coronary atherosclerosis and myocardial infarction in hearts with anomalous coronary arteries. *Lab Invest* 1965, 14:571.

23. Dicicco BS, McManus BM, Waller BF, Roberts WC: Separate aortic ostium of the left anterior descending and left circumflex coronary arteries from the left aortic sinus of Valsalva (absent left main coronary artery). *Am Heart J* 1982, 104:153–154.

24. Shirani J, Roberts WC: Solitary coronary ostium in the aorta in the absence of other major congenital cardiovascular anomalies. *J Am Coll Cardiol* 1993, 21:137–143.

25. Hyrtl J: Einige in chirurgischer Hinsicht wichtige Gefässvarietäten. *Med Jahrb Österr Staats* 1841, 33:17–38.

26. Smith C: Review of single coronary artery with report of 2 cases. *Circulation* 1950, 1:1168–1175.

27. Odgen JA, Goodyer AVN: Pattern of distribution of the single coronary artery. *Yale J Biol Med* 1970, 43:11–21.

28. Lipton MJ, Barry WH, Obrez I, *et al.*: Isolated single coronary artery: diagnosis, angiographic classification and clinical significance. *Radiology* 1979, 130:39–47.

29. Roberts WC, Dicicco BS, Waller BF, *et al.*: Origin of the left main from the right coronary artery or from the right aortic sinus with intramyocardial tunneling to the left side of the heart via the ventricular septum: the case against clinical significance of myocardial bridge or coronary tunnel. *Am Heart J* 1982, 104:303–305.

30. Roberts WC: Congenital coronary arterial anomalies unassociated with major anomalies of the heart or great vessels. In *Adult Congenital Heart Disease*. Edited by Roberts WC. Philadelphia: FA Davis; 1987:583–629.

31. Fortuin NJ, Roberts WC: Congenital atresia of the left main coronary artery. *Am J Med* 1971, 50:385–389.

32. Roberts WC, Glick BN: Congenital hypoplasia of both right and left circumflex coronary arteries. *Am J Cardiol* 1992, 70:121–123.

Atherosclerosis

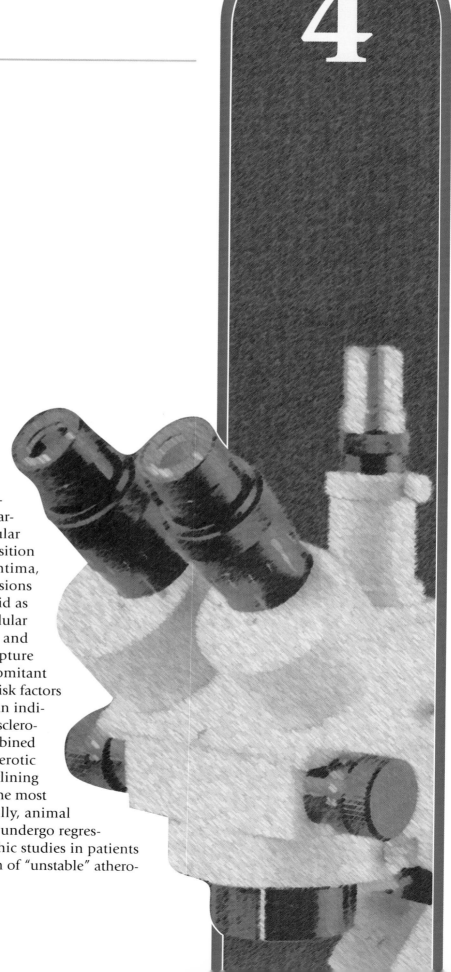

4

Peter G. Anderson
James B. Atkinson

Atherosclerosis and the myriad conditions that it engenders constitute the leading cause of death among middle-aged men and women older than 60 years of age. Although the clinical sequelae of atherosclerosis usually occur in middle-aged and older adults, the disease originates in childhood and progresses over the course of decades to culminate in myocardial infarction, cerebral infarction, or peripheral vascular disease. Atherosclerosis in childhood begins with deposition of cholesterol and cholesterol esters in the arterial intima, forming fatty streaks. Fatty streaks evolve into raised lesions in young adulthood by continued accumulation of lipid as well as proliferation of cells and production of extracellular matrix. In middle age, raised lesions increase in size and may become susceptible to complications, such as rupture and thrombosis, leading to ischemic injury with concomitant morbidity and mortality. From epidemiologic studies, risk factors have been identified that predict the probability that an individual will develop the clinical manifestations of atherosclerosis. Recognition of these cardiovascular risk factors, combined with advances in detection and treatment of atherosclerotic coronary artery disease, has been associated with a declining incidence of death from ischemic heart disease, one of the most dramatic manifestations of atherosclerosis. Additionally, animal studies have demonstrated that atherosclerotic lesions undergo regression with cholesterol-lowering therapy, and angiographic studies in patients indicate that regression is associated with transformation of "unstable" atherosclerotic plaques to "stable" lesions.

Atherosclerosis is a disease of the arterial intima. It does not occur randomly but has a predilection for "lesion-prone" sites in the arterial system. Whereas some arteries, such as the internal mammary artery, are resistant to atherosclerosis, others, such as the coronary arteries, are highly susceptible. Moreover, in any individual the extent and severity of atherosclerosis may vary in the coronary, cerebral, carotid, and femoral arteries and aorta. Atherosclerosis is also a focal disease that is characterized by the accumulation of molecules (*eg*, lipids, collagen, and proteoglycans) in the intima as well as recruitment and proliferation of inflammatory cells, smooth muscle cells, and fibroblasts. Although atherosclerosis is focal, it still can be associated with generalized abnormalities in the arterial system, such as increased vascular responsiveness, that can exacerbate the ischemic effects of arterial occlusion (*eg*, coronary spasm). Atherosclerosis begins as an intimal disease, but this chronic inflammatory process within the vessel wall progresses to eventually destroy the normal elastic and muscular components of the entire arterial wall, leading to replacement by connective tissue, lipid, and calcium. Indeed, atherosclerosis appears to be a chronic inflammatory condition rather than an inevitable consequence of aging. It is a dynamic process, not just the passive accumulation of amorphous debris in the artery. Two hypotheses from the 19th century laid the groundwork for the currently popular "response-to-injury" theory for the pathogenesis of atherosclerosis: the "incrustation" hypothesis of von Rokitansky, which proposed that intimal thickening was the result of fibrin deposition followed by secondary lipid accumulation, and the "lipid" hypothesis of Virchow, which suggested that transduction of lipid into the arterial wall exceeded its ability for removal. Although the precise events that initiate and promote the development and progression of atherosclerosis are still unclear, it appears that the disease begins with an "injury," or abnormality, of the endothelium, probably resulting from multiple interactions among various stimuli, which then evokes a series of molecular and cellular events that result in the chronic inflammatory and reparative processes.

This chapter focuses on the macroscopic and histologic features that define atherosclerosis and its complications. Recent pathobiologic studies have allowed a classification of atherosclerotic lesions beginning from those seen in children to advanced lesions in adults, and this classification has already begun to enhance an understanding of the development of lesions and the role of risk factors in their progression. Although a detailed discussion of the pathogenesis of atherosclerosis is beyond the scope of this chapter, a brief survey will be presented that emphasizes specific areas that have recently been elucidated as being potentially important in the initiation and progression of lesions. Such emphasis does not imply a lesser role for other mechanisms that are important in atherogenesis. The pathology of complications and interventions to treat atherosclerotic vascular disease are also presented.

PATHOLOGY OF ATHEROSCLEROSIS

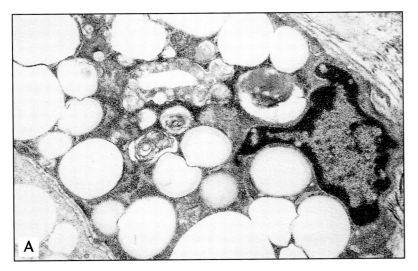

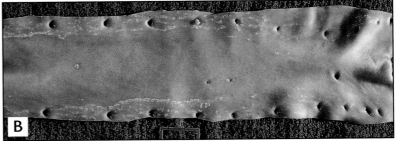

Figure 4-1.

Type I and type II lesions. **A,** Electron micrograph showing a macrophage foam cell in the intima of a macroscopically normal aorta from a 5-year-old child. Type I, or initial, lesions are the first microscopically and chemically detectable deposits of lipid in the intima. They may not be grossly apparent, or they may appear as small yellow streaks or dots. Type I lesions are composed of isolated or small groups of macrophage foam cells that may occur in areas of adaptive intimal thickening or in atherosclerosis-prone areas. Similar lesions are found as an initial abnormality in experimental animals with induced hypercholesterolemia.

Type II lesions are fatty streaks that macroscopically appear as yellow streaks, patches, or spots on the intimal surface. **B,** Fatty streaks in lesion-prone areas of the thoracic aorta from a 19-year-old woman.

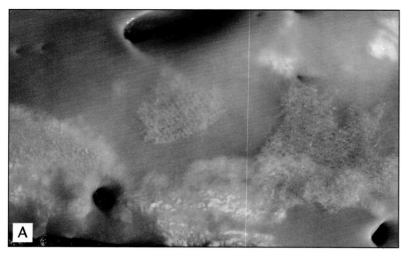

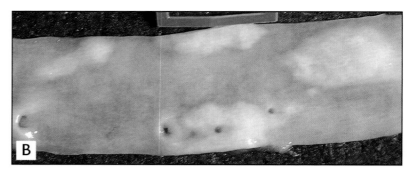

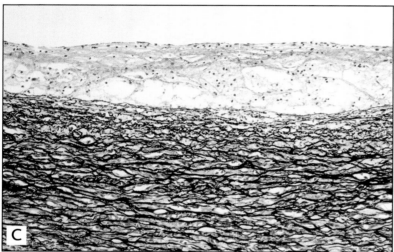

Figure 4-2.

Type III (intermediate, transition) lesions. Type III lesions are the transition between type II lesions (fatty streaks) and advanced raised lesions (atheromas). They are also called intermediate lesions or preatheromas. Type III lesions usually occur in lesion-prone areas, as in the thoracic aorta from an 18-year-old man (*panel A*) and the right coronary artery from a 23-year-old woman (*panel B*). However, they cannot be reliably distinguished from type II lesions macroscopically. Their identification rests on light microscopic features that include extracellular lipid in addition to lipid-containing foam cells (*panel C*; Movat's pentachrome stain). This extracellular lipid, which is both membrane bound and free by electron microscopy, forms small pools that replace extracellular matrix and moves cells apart but does not cause any other type of arterial deformity and does not form a lipid core that characterizes the atheroma (type IV lesion). Type III lesions have biochemical characteristics that are intermediate between type II lesions and atheromas, including more free cholesterol, fatty acid sphingomyelin, lysolecithin, and triglycerides than type II lesions, and a melting point of cholesterol ester that is between that of type II lesions and atheromas. The cells in type III lesions are similar to those found in type II lesions.

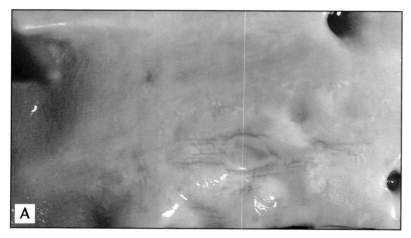

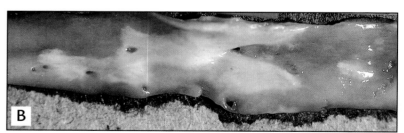

Figure 4-3.

Type IV lesions (atheromas). **A,** Intimal surface of abdominal aorta from a 28-year-old man. **B,** Intimal surface of right coronary artery from a 32-year-old man. Atherosclerotic lesions are advanced when the accumulation of lipid, cells, and matrix are associated with disorganization, repair, and thickening of the intima and deformity of the arterial wall. Type IV lesions, also called atheromas, are advanced lesions in which extracellular lipid

occupies a well-defined and extensive area in the intima, called the lipid core, that develops by coalescence of smaller isolated pools of extracellular lipid. When seen in younger people, atheromas occur in areas of previous adaptive intimal thickening. Although atheromas are raised lesions, they do not necessarily result in significant luminal occlusion. (*continued on next page*)

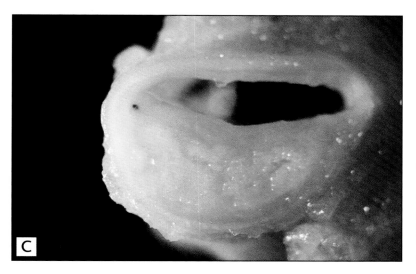

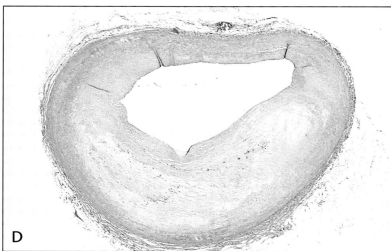

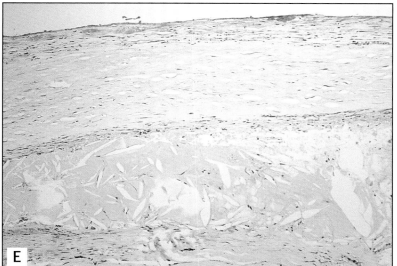

Figure 4-3. (*continued*)
Microscopically, the extracellular lipid in atheromas displaces and replaces smooth muscle cells and extracellular matrix. **C,** A cross-section of coronary artery that has significant luminal obstruction by an atheroma. A lipid-rich core can be seen in the center of the lesion that is also illustrated in the corresponding microscopic section in *panel D* (hematoxylin and eosin stain). Macrophages and small numbers of smooth muscle cells with and without lipid, lymphocytes, mast cells, proteoglycans, and extracellular matrix (collagen, proteoglycans) are located between the lipid core and the endothelial surface. Capillaries are at the lateral edge of the lipid core. The fibrous cap that overlies the lipid-rich core may vary in thickness. **E,** Although a relatively thick fibrous cap is present in this carotid artery atheroma (Movat's pentachrome stain), thin fibrous caps may be at risk for disruption ("rupture"), leading to thrombosis.

rests on histologic analysis. Type Vc (fibrotic) lesions are often found in arteries of the lower extremities. Whereas the production of fibrous connective tissue occurs as a reparative response in arteries with large amounts of extracellular lipid, calcification is a response to cell death. Fibroatheromas may also contain macrophages, foam cells, lymphocytes, and capillaries. In addition to intimal changes, there may be loss of the integrity of the internal elastic lamina and damage to adjacent smooth muscle, and macrophage foam cells and lymphocytes may be found in the media and even the adventitia. Increased mast cells have also been observed in adventitia of arteries with fibroatheromas.

Smooth muscle cells in the intima of advanced lesions are derived from preexisting intimal as well as medial smooth muscle cells and have the phenotype of "synthetic" smooth muscle, with abundant rough endoplasmic reticulum and fewer myofilaments than "contractile" smooth muscle cells. Macrophages in these lesions have ultrastructural evidence of cell injury. Advanced lesions contain T and B lymphocytes, and T cells have both T helper (CD4+) and T killer (CD8+) phenotypes. The extracellular lipid in advanced lesions is ultrastructurally heterogeneous in terms of its structure and particle size. Other noncellular components of advanced lesions are fibrinogen, proteoglycans (predominantly chondroitin sulfate-containing molecules [versican-like] as well as dermatan sulfate proteoglycans [decorin and biglycan]), fibrillar collagen type I, and elastin. Apatite (hydroxyapatite, carbonate apatite) is the predominant form of calcium in advanced lesions, and mineral deposits are often associated with elastic fibers.

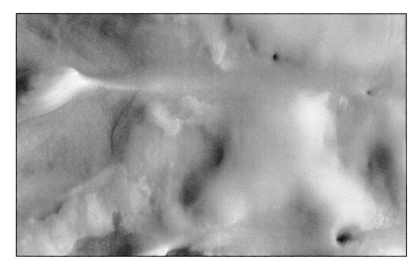

Figure 4-4.
Type V lesions (fibroatheromas). As fibrous tissue in atheromas increases, they evolve into type V lesions, or fibroatheromas. Atheromas and fibroatheromas are raised and may be indistinguishable macroscopically because the lipid core in type IV lesions is covered by an upper fibrous intimal layer. In the past, type IV and type V lesions have been collectively referred to as fibrous plaques. By careful examination of the intimal surface, fibroatheromas may appear whiter (*ie*, more "fibrotic") than atheromas (luminal surface of abdominal aorta), but precise classification

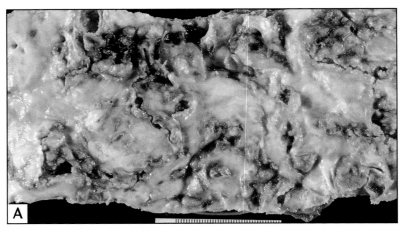

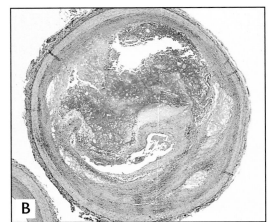

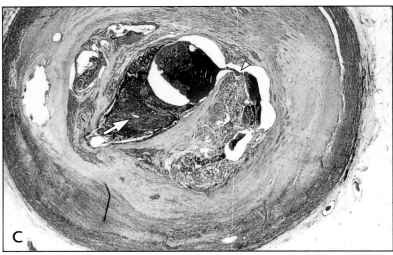

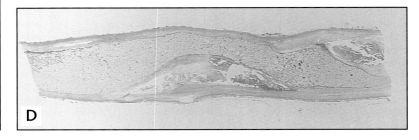

Figure 4-5.

Type VI lesions (complicated lesions). When the intimal surface of type IV and type V lesions becomes disrupted or has associated plaque hemorrhage or thrombosis, morbidity and mortality from atherosclerosis may become significant. Type VI, or complicated, lesions are type IV or V lesions with these complications. They can be subdivided into VIa (with disruption of the surface), VIb (with hematoma or hemorrhage), and VIc (with thrombosis). Features of all three subtypes can be seen in single lesions as well. Disruption of the surface may include fissures (with loss of the endothelial cell layer and usually visible only microscopically) and ulcerations (with exposure of the deep lipid core and often macroscopically visible). **A,** Ulceration in advanced atherosclerotic plaques in the abdominal aorta are seen macroscopically. **B,** Intraplaque hemorrhage in the histologic section of coronary artery (Movat's pentachrome stain) is defined as erythrocytes within an atheromatous plaque and is a common finding in patients with sudden cardiac death as well as those with noncardiac death. **C,** Plaque rupture (*arrowhead*) associated with intraplaque hemorrhage and thrombotic occlusion of the arterial lumen (*arrow*) is shown in the coronary artery (Movat's pentachrome stain). Thrombosis can contribute to the progression of atherosclerotic plaques. Evidence of thrombi can be seen in advanced lesions generally beginning in the fourth decade of life and may vary from microscopically to macroscopically visible deposits. Thrombi can have different ages and may contribute to lesion enlargement and gradual obstruction of the arterial lumen over the course of many years. Factors that promote thrombosis are disruption of the intimal surface by various triggers (discussed later), elevated fibrinogen or low-density lipoprotein or Lp (a) levels, decreased fibrinolytic activity (caused by increased levels of type 1 plasminogen activator inhibitor), and smoking.

Adaptive intimal thickening occurs in all people from birth, particularly at branch points. Type I and II lesions are early lesions that occur usually in infants and children but also occasionally in adults. Type III lesions, which are a bridge between early and advanced lesions, are usually seen soon after puberty. Type IV lesions are frequently found beginning at the third decade, and type V and VI lesions may become the predominant types of lesion in middle-aged and older people. Atherosclerotic lesions may vary in type along the extent of the artery and are generally classified according to the most advanced pathology. **D,** Although atherosclerotic lesions may extensively involve arteries, lesions are focal, as shown in the longitudinal section of a coronary artery here (hematoxylin and eosin stain; contrast pigment fills the arterial lumen).

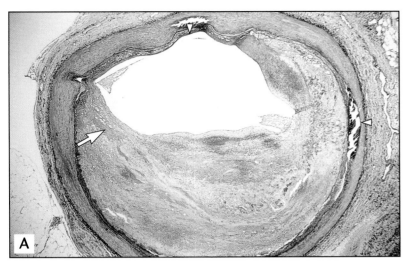 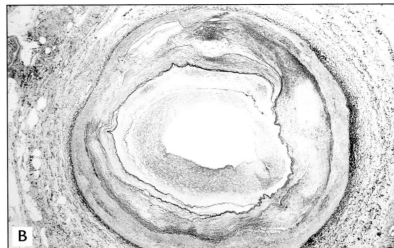

Figure 4-6.

Atherosclerosis in the extremities. Atherosclerosis is more frequent in the lower extremities than the upper extremities. Despite the clinical importance of peripheral vascular disease, little is known about the natural history or progression of atherosclerosis in the extremities or the ways the various risk factors relate to atherogenesis. Although the severity of atherosclerosis in the lower extremities generally correlates with that in the aorta and coronary arteries, the incidence of clinically silent lower extremity atherosclerosis may be twice that of the coronary arteries, and the incidence is increased fivefold in patients with diabetes [1,2]. Whereas the distribution of disease in patients younger than the age of 40 years is aortoiliac, lesions are found more often in the femoropopliteal distribution in those older than 40 years of age [3]. Atherosclerosis in the lower extremities may develop in the setting of age-related arterial degeneration, such as Monckeberg's medial calcification. **A,** An eccentric fibroatheroma in the femoral artery from a patient with gangrene of the foot; occasional foam cells are in the shoulder region (*arrow*), and focal calcification around the internal elastic lamina is present (*arrowheads*; Movat's pentachrome stain). Peripheral vascular disease leading to ischemia and gangrene are well-known complications of atherosclerosis. Thrombosis is a frequent complication of lower extremity atherosclerosis, particularly in the femoropopliteal arteries. **B,** The concentric fibroatheroma that narrows the lumen of the femoral artery is further occlusive by concentric layers of cellular fibrous tissue that represents remote (organized) mural thrombosis (Movat's pentachrome stain).

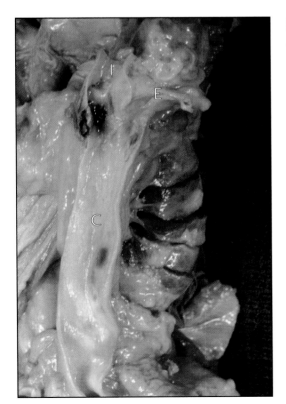

Figure 4-7.

Atherosclerosis in the carotid arteries. The unique anatomic and flow characteristics of the carotid artery bifurcation make this a high-risk area for plaque formation. It is especially important to understand the topography and morphology of arteriosclerosis in carotid arteries as more invasive procedures are being used in the carotid arteries. Angioplasty and stent placement have revolutionized the treatment modalities available for carotid disease [4,5]. The usual topographic localization of atherosclerotic plaque formation is demonstrated in this autopsy specimen of the carotid artery. Although there is little atherosclerotic plaque along the length of the common carotid artery (C), significant plaque has formed at the bifurcation of the internal (I) and external (E) carotid arteries.

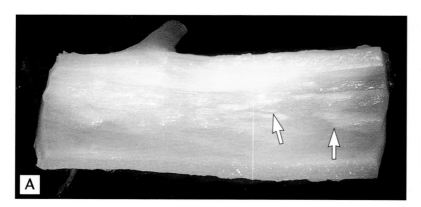

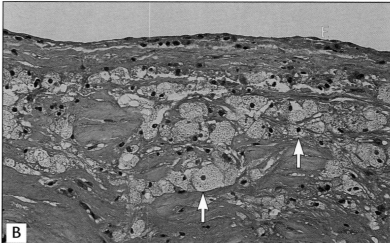

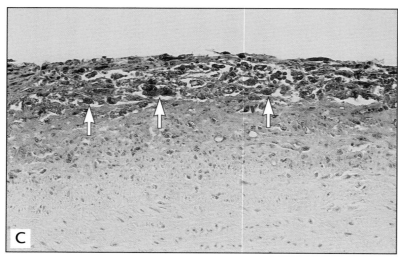

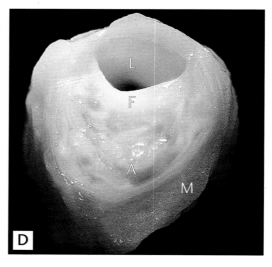

Figure 4-8.

Nitrotyrosine in early and advanced atherosclerotic lesions. Because peroxynitrite plays an integral role in the development of atherosclerosis [6], the stable marker of peroxynitrite activation, nitrotyrosine, should be present in atherosclerotic tissues. **A,** Gross photograph of a section of coronary artery that has been opened lengthwise demonstrating early fatty streak lesions on the endothelial surface (*arrows*). These are early lesions in this 31-year-old woman who died acutely from a ruptured berry aneurysm. **B,** Photomicrograph of a plastic embedded specimen from the vessel in *panel A* demonstrating the histologic appearance of these early fatty streak lesions. The endothelial layer (E) is intact, and there are lipid-laden macrophages in the intima (*arrows*). In this early lesion, the lipid is primarily intracellular. **C,** Immunohisto-chemical staining was performed on paraffin-embedded sections

from this same coronary artery using a primary antibody specific for nitrotyrosine. Because nitrotyrosine is formed by the reaction of peroxynitrite with tyrosine residues in tissues, nitrotyrosine serves as a stable marker for the reaction of peroxynitrite on tissues. In this immunoperoxidase-stained reaction, the presence of nitrotyrosine is indicated by the intense brown coloration of the lipid-laden macrophages in these early fatty streak lesions (*arrows*). **D,** Nitrotyrosine is also present in the late stages of atherosclerosis. This gross photograph of a cross-section of a coronary artery demonstrates advanced atherosclerosis. The vessel lumen (L) is compromised by the large eccentric atheroma (A) that is covered by a fibrous cap (F). The media (M) is still visible, and serves to demarcate the original vessel diameter.

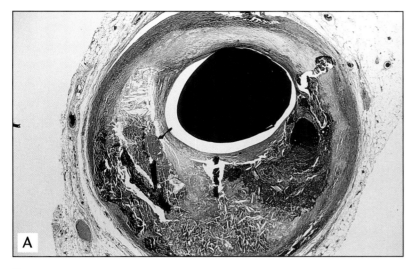

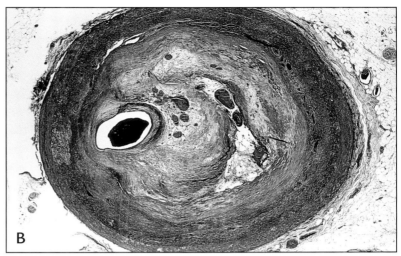

Figure 4-9.

Types of atherosclerotic plaques and complications. Athero-sclerotic plaques that are associated with acute or unstable coro-nary syndromes are usually small and nonocclusive, but they are lipid-rich lesions with thin fibrous caps. If the fibrous cap ruptures, thrombogenic material in the atheromatous core is exposed to flowing blood that can induce thrombosis. **A,** The coronary artery in this unstable (vulnerable) lesion has a large lipid-rich core, plaque hemorrhage, and a thin fibrous cap; contrast media is in the lumen (Movat's pentachrome stain). Atherosclerotic plaques in coronary arteries that are associated with chronic stable angina and silent occlusion tend to be severely stenotic and fibrotic lesions. **B,** An example of a "stable" plaque, with a thick fibrous

cap and a lipid-rich core that is smaller than that seen in *panel A*; several small vascular channels within the lesion may indicate neo-vascularization (contrast dye is in the lumen; Movat's pentachrome stain). Although stenotic lesions can progress to total thrombotic occlusion, these lesions do not produce acute myocardial infarction as often as unstable lesions because of the development of collat-eral vessels. Fibrous tissue stabilizes plaques, protecting them against disruption. Less occlusive atheromatous (lipid-rich) plaques, however, are at increased risk for disruption and subse-quent thrombotic complications. After thrombus formation, the thrombus may lyse and recanalize, or it may organize and eventu-ally produce total luminal occlusion.

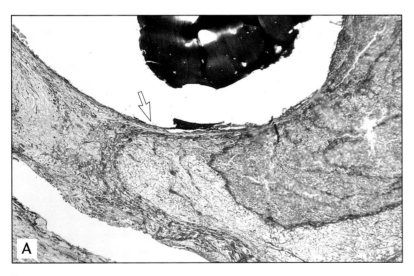

Figure 4-10.

Morphologic features of unstable lesions. The morphologic deter-minants that characterize unstable atherosclerotic plaques are 1) the size and composition of the atheromatous core, 2) thickness

and collagen content of the fibrous cap that overlies the core, and 3) the extent and location of inflammation in the plaque [7]. This substrate is modified by hemodynamic influences on the plaque as well as various "triggers" listed previously. Stability of individual lesions depends on the size of the atheromatous core [7]. There is a direct relationship for both the coronary arteries and the aorta between atheromatous core size and plaque disruption; plaques that have a lipid core of more than 40% of the lesion are at the greatest risk for rupture and thrombosis [8]. In an analysis of the relationship between plaque composition and vulnerability to rupture, Davies *et al.* [8] evaluated the composition of three types of aortic plaques: stable, vulnerable, and ruptured.

Lipid-lowering therapies may be important in depleting plaque lipid, resulting in more fibrotic but less vulnerable lesions. The thickness of the fibrous cap in advanced lesions varies widely. **A,** Photomicrograph illustrating that fibrous caps are often the thinnest at the shoulder region (*arrow*); this is where disruption frequently occurs (Movat's pentachrome stain). Fibrous caps in ruptured plaques contain fewer smooth muscle cells and less colla-gen than intact fibrous caps. (*continued on next page*)

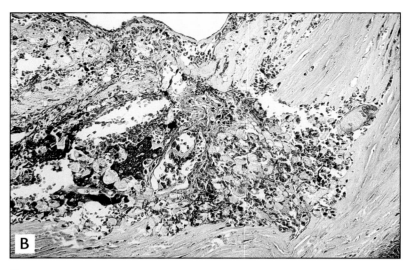

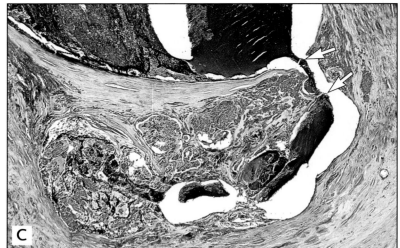

Figure 4-10. (*continued*)

B, Fibrous caps in unstable lesions are also usually infiltrated with macrophage foam cells, particularly at the vulnerable shoulder region (the junction of the fibrous cap with the more normal intima), as illustrated in this photomicrograph, which shows large numbers of macrophage foam cells in a hemorrhagic complicated plaque (Movat's pentachrome stain). These macrophages are activated and capable of degrading extracellular matrix by proteolytic enzymes such as plasminogen activators and matrix metalloproteinases (collagenases, gelatinases, and stromelysins), all of which could weaken the fibrous cap to make it vulnerable to rupture

[8,9]. Activated mast cells may also be found in the shoulder region of vulnerable plaques, and mast cells secrete proteolytic enzymes (*eg*, tryptase and chymase) and can activate matrix metalloproteinases secreted by macrophages [9,10]. **C,** In addition to these morphologic substrates for plaque disruption, the highest tensile circumferential stress from hemodynamic forces is at the lateral edge of large lipid cores, at the weakened shoulder region [10], and this is a frequent site of plaque disruption, shown here (*arrows*) (Movat's pentachrome stain).

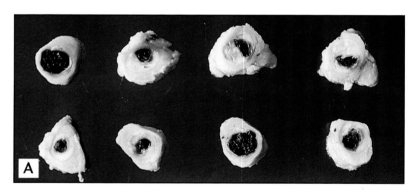

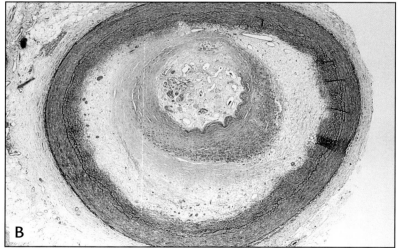

Figure 4-11.

Consequences of plaque rupture. After disruption of an atherosclerotic plaque in the coronary arteries, plaque hemorrhage or luminal thrombosis can lead to myocardial ischemia and trigger ventricular fibrillation and sudden death, acute myocardial infarction, or acute coronary syndromes [10]. **A,** Cross-sections of the right coronary artery in which plaque rupture resulted in acute occlusion and acute myocardial infarction. The thrombotic response to plaque disruption is influenced by the extent of plaque disruption and content of the exposed plaque components. Thrombosis may also be related to risk factors such as smoking [11]. Loss of only the endothelial cell surface may result in a limited response, with formation of a mural thrombus that

contributes to growth of the lesion. If there is a plaque fissure, transient thrombotic occlusion may occur, resulting in repetitive episodes of ischemia. Evidence of recurrent thrombosis causing gradual occlusion can be seen in layered thrombi overlying ruptured lesions in some coronary arteries. **B,** Photomicrograph of a coronary artery that is totally occluded by remote (organized) thrombosis, in which several layers can be seen, with recanalization in the center (Movat's pentachrome stain). If the disruption is deep, exposure of the lipid core, collagen, tissue factor, and other thrombotic elements may produce a persistent thrombus that results in acute myocardial infarction.

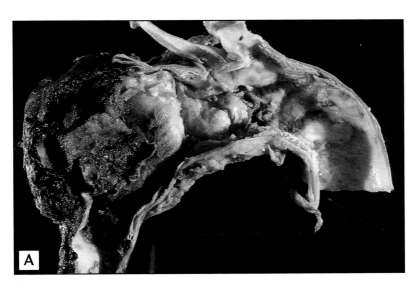

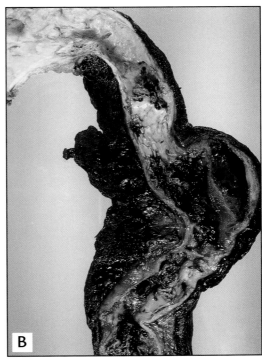

Figure 4-12.

Atheromas, fibroatheromas, and complicated lesions (type IV, V, and VI) may cause localized dilatations of the underlying arterial wall. Aneurysms, defined as an increase in arterial diameter of more than 1.5 times its normal diameter [12], are most often found in the abdominal aorta in association with complicated atherosclerotic lesions. Although atherosclerosis may not directly cause aneurysms, the association between aneurysms and atherosclerosis is high, and their development probably requires the combination of arterial wall damage with systemic and local pathophysiologic factors that serve as initiators and promoters of aneurysm development. Risk factors for aneurysms include hypertension, and there is evidence for genetic susceptibility [13]. Lesion progression may be accompanied by an enlargement of the artery as a compensatory mechanism to maintain perfusion. This enlargement, combined with the degenerative changes associated with atherosclerosis, results in disruption of the underlying media. Aortic aneurysms characteristically have atrophy of the media and loss of normal lamellar architecture with loss of elastic tissue. Some have proposed that if there is regression of the plaque late in the development of the disease, insufficient tensile support is maintained and aneurysm formation occurs [14]. Aneurysms have an associated inflammatory infiltrate that is usually more severe than that seen in accompanying atherosclerosis. T lymphocytes are abundant in aneurysmal artery segments, and they may interact with macrophages to induce release of proteinases (elastase and collagenase), plasminogen activators (that can initiate a cascade of other enzymes such as procollagenase and plasminogen), and matrix metalloproteinases [14,15]. Protease activity may promote degradation of elastin and collagen, resulting in an arterial wall that cannot bear the usual hemodynamic load, leading to progressive dilatation. These influences may be modified by genetic predisposition or degenerative changes associated with aging [14,15].

A, An atherosclerotic aneurysm in the thoracic aorta of a 74-year-old-man. The intimal surface proximal to the aneurysm has raised, advanced atherosclerosis (on the *right*), and the aneurysm contains a large amount of organizing and recent thrombus. Although most atherosclerotic aneurysms are fusiform and located in the abdominal aorta, some may be saccular, as seen here, and located in the thoracic aorta. **B,** The fusiform aneurysm shown located in the distal thoracic portion of a severely atherosclerotic aorta demonstrates features of a false aneurysm, with mural disruption that allows a hematoma to form from extravasated blood but is confined by the perivascular tissues, producing a tamponade effect locally. Survival and prognosis depend on the size of the aneurysm at the time of presentation and the rapidity of enlargement. Aortic aneurysms that are at a high risk for rupture are those with a diameter of greater than 6 cm, or that increase in diameter more than 1 cm per year. (*continued on next page*)

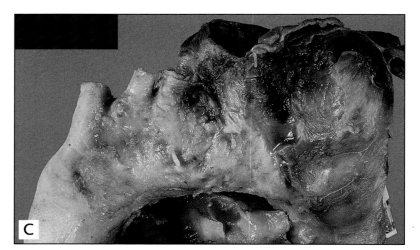

Figure 4-12. (*continued*)

C, Rupture usually occurs through a tear at the site of maximum width, as seen in the ruptured aortic arch aneurysm shown here. Ruptures are caused by a combination of progressively increased wall tension caused by the law of Laplace and weakness of the arterial wall.

In addition to the aorta, atherosclerotic aneurysms can also occur in the popliteal, splenic, axillary, renal, iliac, femoral, and coronary arteries.

PERCUTANEOUS TRANSLUMINAL CORONARY ANGIOPLASTY

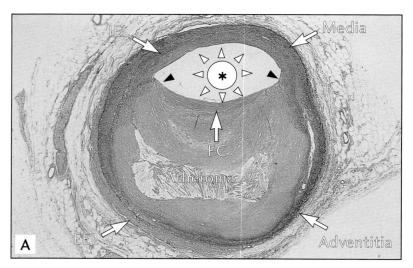

Figure 4-13.

Mechanisms of percutaneous transluminal coronary angioplasty (PTCA). Interventional techniques to treat patients with clinically significant atherosclerosis have been extremely successful, with over 300,000 procedures being performed each year in the United States alone. Recent studies have demonstrated that PTCA has the same 5-year survival as saphenous vein bypass grafting [16,17]. Considering the extensive pathologic changes associated with atherosclerosis, it is hard to imagine that an angioplasty balloon would be able to open a stenotic vessel. Intravascular ultrasound examination has shown that there is very little compression of atherosclerotic material at the site of PTCA and there is minimal redistribution of atherosclerotic material proximal or distal to the point of balloon inflation. However, a successful PTCA leads to a significant increase in lumenal cross sectional area. So how does the lumenal area increase? **A,** A trichrome-stained histology section of a typical atherosclerotic vessel. **B,** A vessel before and after PTCA. If an angioplasty balloon is inflated inside the lumen of this vessel, pressure will be exerted on the plaque, resulting in of the plaque at the shoulder regions. A dissection plane (*arrowheads*) usually forms and extends circumferentially between the plaque and the media along the plane of the internal elastic lamina (IEL) or between the media and the adventitia along the plane of the external elastic membrane (EEL). In either case the laceration of the plaque and the development of the dissection allow the angioplasty balloon to stretch the media and the adventitia and leads to an increased luminal area [18].

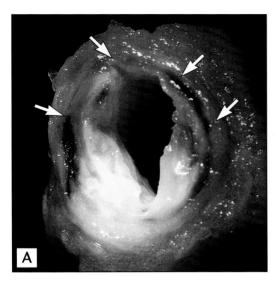

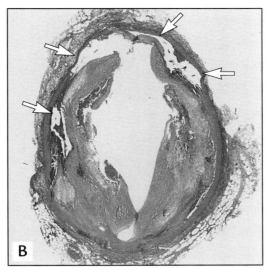

amount of injury. Postmortem samples of atherosclerotic coronary arteries after PTCA often demonstrate the damage caused by the PTCA; however, despite the visible injury, these vessels did not thrombose and they were not the cause of death of these patients (as is the case with many of the specimens shown in this chapter). **A,** A high-power view of an atherosclerotic vessel 24 hours after angioplasty. Note the hemorrhage in the adventitia and the thrombotic material in the dissection plane between the plaque and the media (*arrows*). **B,** The histologic section of this same vessel segment also demonstrates the dissection plane (*arrows*) and the thrombotic material trapped in this space. Also note the way the media has been stretched and it is very thin at the top of the image. This dissection, medial stretching, and adventitial stretching leads to the increase in vessel lumen area after PTCA.

Figure 4-14

Acute percutaneous transluminal coronary angioplasty (PTCA) injury. In order to obtain a beneficial PTCA outcome, significant vessel injury must occur. Obviously, the goal of the interventionalist is to obtain the best possible hemodynamic result while producing the least

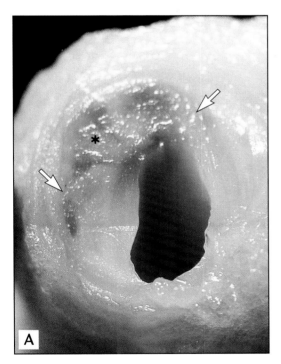

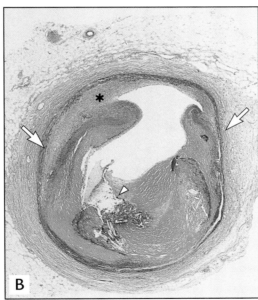

angioplasty injury. These processes activate smooth muscle cells and lead to modulation from the contractile phenotype of normal medial smooth muscle cells to a synthetic phenotype. The synthetic smooth muscle cells play a role in the wound healing process. Stretching of the adventitia and initiation of the inflammatory response lead to activation of adventitial fibroblasts such that they transform into the myofibroblasts commonly seen in granulation tissue. Endothelial cells are also stimulated to divide and migrate over the area denuded by PTCA. This normal healing process is demonstrated in sections of coronary artery taken 1 month after PTCA. **A** and **B,** The typical morphology of PTCA is noted with a dissection plane (*arrows*) between the plaque and the media. In this case, there is still some residual thrombus that can be seen trapped in this dissection plane (*panel A*). The *asterisk* denotes the neointimal tissue that has formed. Note how this tissue has filled in the defects produced by the PTCA injury and has stabilized the dissection flaps. Also note the fissure in this section (*arrowhead*).

Figure 4-15.

Subacute percutaneous transluminal coronary angioplasty (PTCA) injury. After PTCA, the vessel must go through a normal healing process. As with all injury and wound healing, there is initiation of an inflammatory response and activation of growth factors. In the vasculature, there is also release of growth factors from the platelets that attach at the site of

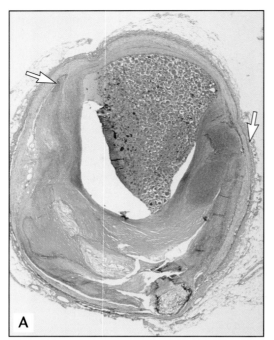

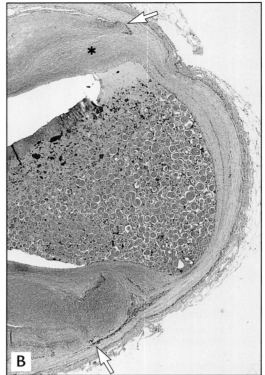

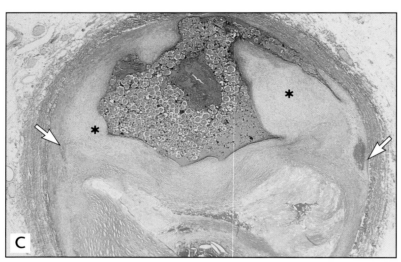

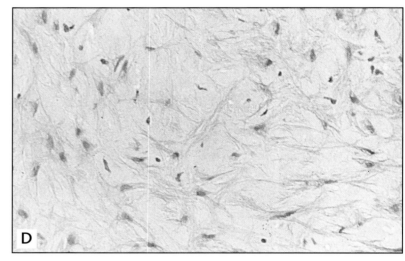

Figure 4-16.

Late percutaneous transluminal coronary angioplasty (PTCA) changes and restenosis. Healing of the vessel after PTCA injury is a natural and necessary process. However, approximately 35% of patients who undergo successful PTCA develop clinically significant restenosis within 6 months of the original procedure. As we have seen, initiation of the healing response is necessary to stabilize the vessel segment that has been injured by the PTCA procedure. **A** and **B,** Four months after PTCA, the dissection plane (*arrows*) is still visible and an area of residual thrombus can also be seen (*panel B*; *bottom arrow*). The dissection flaps are closely abutted against that outer vessel wall and the "bulging" of lumen produced by the PTCA procedure is evident. Also present are areas of neointima (*asterisk*). In approximately 65% of patients who undergo PTCA, the neointimal response heals the injured vessel segment and then stops. Also evident in these specimens is the lack of a robust adventitial reaction. Often after PTCA injury, the adventitia produces significant amounts of fibrous connective tissue. As with any scar, this

tissue contracts as the scar matures, and this contraction of the adventitial tissue leads to constriction of the vessel [19,20]. This vessel was infused with a barium gelatin mixture at the time of autopsy to distend the vessels and allow for postmortem radiographs. **C** and **D,** A vessel 3 months after PTCA. In this case, there is a more fulminate neointimal proliferative response (*asterisk*), and this neointima decreases the lumen area. The dissection plane is visible (*arrows*), and an area of thrombus is still present within the dissection plane. A high-power photomicrograph of the neointimal tissue (*panel D*) demonstrates the stellate appearance of these secretory smooth muscle cells and the abundant extracellular matrix material. The restenosis process is a combination of neointimal proliferation and extracellular matrix production as well as adventitial remodeling. The combination of these processes as well as the progression of the underlying atherosclerosis can lead to clinically significant restenosis.

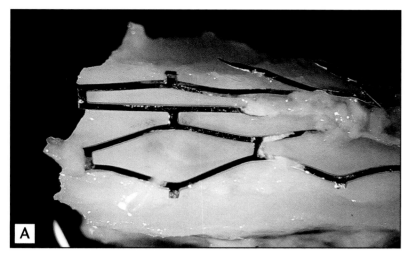

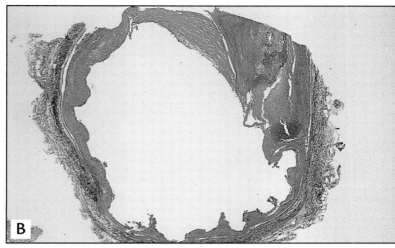

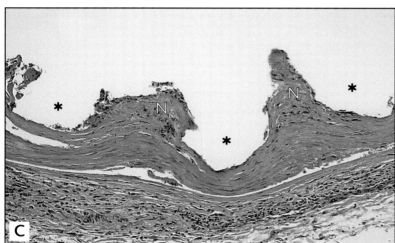

Figure 4-17.

Acute stent implantation. Coronary stents have been used for "bail out" when a suboptimal percutaneous transluminal coronary angioplasty (PTCA) jeopardizes the well-being of a patient. Stents have also been used in order to achieve and maintain the greatest vessel luminal area. Specimens for pathologic evaluation have been obtained at autopsy from surgically removed saphenous vein graft and from hearts at the time of cardiac transplantation. **A,** Five days after a Palmaz-Schatz biliary stent (Johnson & Johnson Interventional Systems, NJ) stent was placed in the ostium of the left main coronary artery, the patient died and was autopsied. Note that there is no thrombus associated with this stent. The glistening white material associated with the stent is the neointimal tissue that has begun to cover the stent wires. **B,** On histologic examination, the vessel is widely patent and the indentations produced by the stent wires can be seen in the media. **C,** At higher magnification, the indentations (*asterisks*) and the neointimal tissue (N) that is beginning to cover the stent wires are evident.

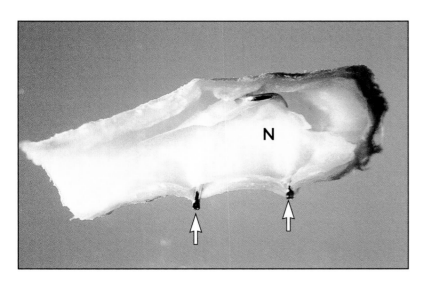

Figure 4-18.

Subacute stent implantation. After percutaneous transluminal coronary angioplasty (PTCA), a Gianturco-Roubin stent (Cook, Inc., Bloomington, IN) was placed in the left anterior descending coronary artery of a 71-year-old diabetic man with three-vessel coronary disease. The patient died 14 days after stent placement because of pneumonia and a lateral wall infarct. The stented vessel segment was patent and there was no evidence of thrombus in the stented region. A portion of the stented vessel was opened longitudinally to view the luminal surface. The stent wires (*arrows*) and the thin covering of neointima (N) are visible in this photograph.

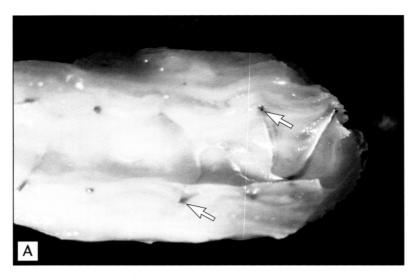

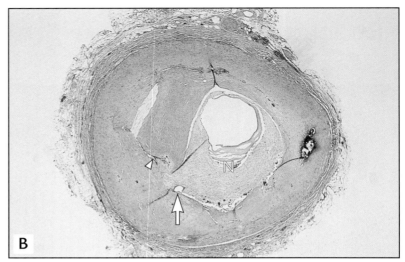

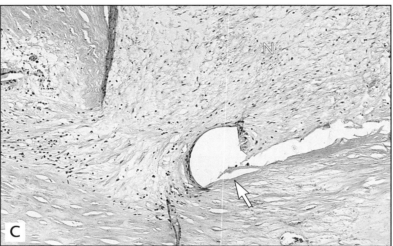

Figure 4-19.

Chronic stent implantation and restenosis. A common question regarding stents is the long-term effects that stents may have on coronary vessels. Because stents are fairly rigid foreign material placed inside a rhythmically pulsating vessel, chronic changes may

have deleterious effects on the coronary artery. Although few careful pathologic studies have been performed on human tissues, we have observed several vessels after chronic stent implantation [21,22]. Five months after implantation of a Gianturco-Roubin stent (Cook, Inc., Bloomington, IN), the patient represented here underwent cardiac transplantation for end-stage ischemic cardiomyopathy. **A,** A portion of the stented left circumflex coronary artery was opened longitudinally to expose the luminal surface. The stent wires (*arrows*) are covered by a layer of neointima (N). The stent on the *right* is covered by a thin layer of neointima; however, as one goes distally down the vessel (*left*), the thickness of the neointima increases. The wire was carefully removed and this section was processed for histologic evaluation. **B,** In this histology section, the hole where the stent wire was removed is visible (*arrow*), and the neointimal tissue can be seen partially filling in the vessel lumen. An area of old dissection can be seen in this section (*arrowhead*). **C,** A high-power photomicrograph of the hole left after removal of the stent. Note that even after 5 months, a very minimal inflammatory response surrounding the stent wire is present. The histologic character of the neointima is similar to that seen in restenotic tissue after PTCA.

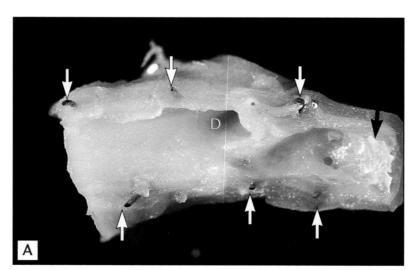

Figure 4-20.

Chronic stent implantation. Complications or restenosis after stent implantation may require additional interventions inside stented artery segments. In the case demonstrated here, this patient had a stent placed across the branch point of the first diagonal branch of the left anterior descending coronary artery (LAD) after a suboptimal percutaneous transluminal coronary angioplasty (PTCA). Five months later, the patient developed unstable angina; angiograms revealed restenosis of the stented segment. A repeat balloon angioplasty was performed inside the stented vessel segment, including the diagonal branch. This produced a good angiographic result; however, the patient again presented with unstable angina 5 months later. At this time, the patient elected to undergo coronary artery bypass grafting, but she died during the operative procedure. **A,** A portion of the artery was opened longitudinally to expose the luminal surface. The stent wires are visible along the cut edge of the vessel wall (*white arrows*), but the stents are not visible through the neointima, suggesting a thick neointimal covering. The letter *D* indicates the branch point for the diagonal artery. Also note that in the distal LAD, there is an area of recanalized thrombus (*black arrow*). (*continued on next page*)

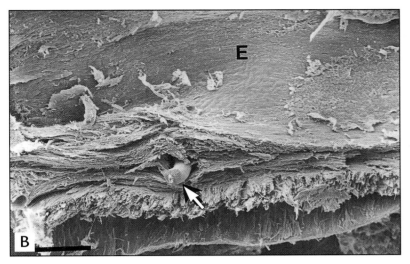

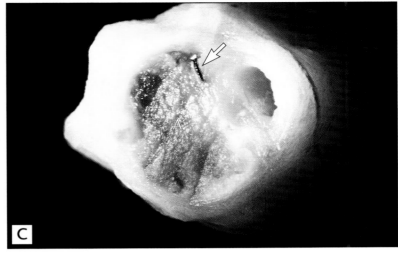

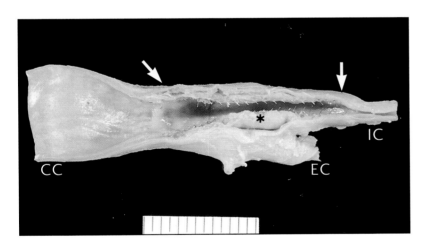

Figure 4-20. (*continued*)
B, Using scanning electron microscopy, the thickness of the neointima over the stent wire (*arrow*) and the endothelial cells (E) lining the lumen were seen (the *bar* indicates 500 μm). **C,** Another segment of this stented vessel was transversely sectioned. In this section, there is a large eccentric atheromatous plaque (A), and the stent wire is visible (*arrow*), abutted against the fibrous cap. There is white glistening neointima overlying the stent wire and impinging on the lumen. **D,** The histologic section of the vessel shows the large atheromatous plaque (A) with areas of mineralization (*blue material*). The *arrow* points to the hole where the stent was removed. The neointimal tissue (N) is visible overlying the stent. (*From* Waller and Anderson [21]; with permission.)

Figure 4-21.
Carotid artery stents. Recent studies by investigators at the University of Alabama at Birmingham have demonstrated that carotid artery percutaneous transluminal coronary angioplasty (PTCA) and stenting may be an alternative to carotid endarterectomy surgery. Yadav *et al.* [4,5] have shown that PTCA and stenting can be used effectively to treat atherosclerotic carotid artery disease. In one patient from this series who died of non-neurologic causes, the stented carotid artery was available for evaluation 6 months after stenting. The vessel was opened longitudinally to show that the stent extended from the common carotid artery (CC) across the bifurcation of the internal (IC) and external carotid (EC) arteries and extended distally into the internal carotid artery. The wires of this Wallstent (Schneider, Inc., Plymouth, MN) are visible along the length of the stented segment (*white arrows*). There is a large atheromatous plaque (*asterisk*) visible under the stent wires at the carotid bulb.

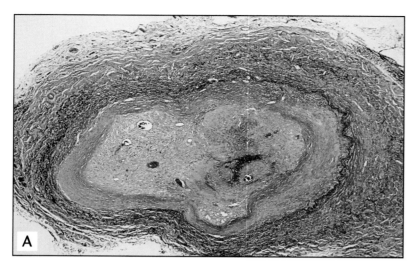

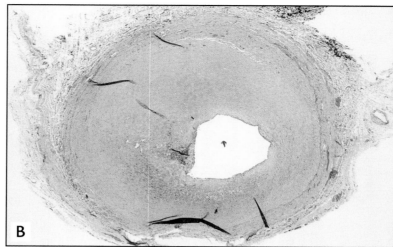

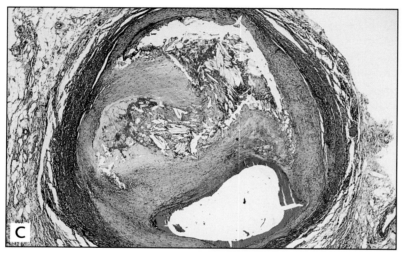

Figure 4-22.

Saphenous vein bypass grafts. Coronary artery bypass surgery has been widely used for more than 25 years as an important treatment of coronary artery disease. Despite well-defined indications and low operative mortality, long-term survival of saphenous veins when used as coronary artery conduits is still limited, thus encouraging use of the internal mammary artery as a bypass vessel.

The pathology of saphenous vein bypass grafts is related to early and late complications and consists of three changes: thrombosis, fibrointimal proliferation, and atherosclerosis. Early vein graft occlusion (within 1 month after surgery) is usually caused by thrombosis [23,24]. **A,** The thrombus organizes and causes total graft occlusion by fibrotic tissue (note several small recanalized vascular channels [Movat's pentachrome stain]). Virtually all vein bypass grafts have some degree of intimal thickening that can be seen as early as 1 month after surgery. This fibrointimal proliferation consists of smooth muscle cells in an extracellular matrix (collagen and proteoglycans). **B,** It may progress to near total graft occlusion (Movat's pentachrome stain). The pathogenesis of fibrointimal proliferation in vein grafts is not known but probably relates to reparative processes after vein ischemia or hemodynamic stresses that can cause endothelial damage, and it may be accelerated by systemic hypertension [23]. More importantly, fibrointimal proliferation provides the foundation for graft atherosclerosis. Some vein grafts, usually those that have been in place longer than 3 years, may develop atherosclerosis similar to that seen in native arteries, with advanced and complicated plaques composed of foam cells and a lipid core, fibrous caps, and calcification. **C,** Plaque hemorrhage and rupture with luminal occlusion by thrombosis may also occur in atherosclerotic vein grafts (Movat's pentachrome stain). Atherosclerosis is diffuse and rapidly progressive in vein grafts and may be promoted by smoking and hyperlipidemia [23,25].

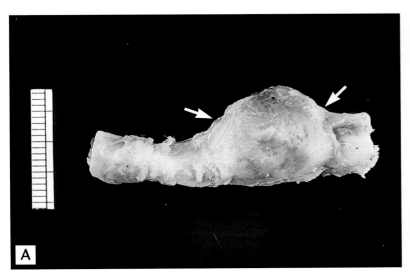

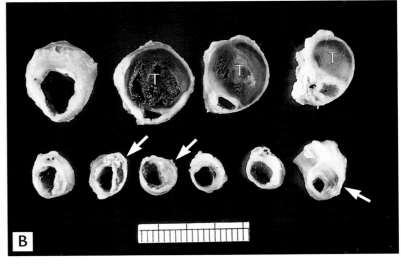

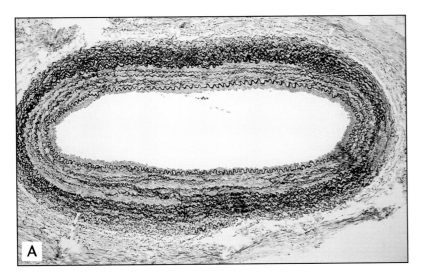

Figure 4-23.

Percutaneous transluminal coronary angioplasty (PTCA) and stents in saphenous vein bypass grafts. The technique of PTCA in saphe-

nous vein grafts is similar to that in native coronary arteries. Despite the diffuse nature of the lesions seen in saphenous vein bypass grafts and the problems this causes the interventional cardiologist, published success rates are good and complication rates are acceptable [26]. One complication of PTCA within vein grafts is the formation of aneurysmal dilatation (*panels A and B*). As seen in this case, a large aneurysmal dilatation occurred at the site of the PTCA (*arrows in panel A*). This was an incidental finding at autopsy 1 year after the PTCA. Serial sections of this vein graft show a large eccentric atheromatous plaque (*arrows in panel B*). In this case, the aneurysm is filled with thrombus (T) and the lumen of the vein graft is patent. Stents are also used extensively in saphenous vein grafts. As with native coronary arteries, stents act as a scaffold to hold open the saphenous vein graft and produce the maximal luminal area after an intervention. In this case, a Palmaz-Schatz biliary stent (Johnson & Johnson Interventional Systems, NJ) was used after PTCA 2 months before death. The stented saphenous vein was opened longitudinally (*panel C*) to demonstrate the smooth, glistening luminal surface and the stent wires (*arrows*) embedded into the wall of the vein graft.

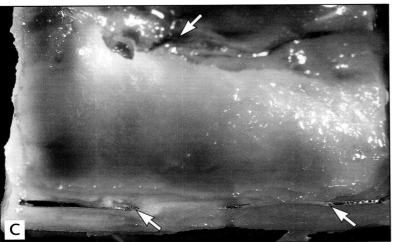

Figure 4-24.

Internal mammary artery (IMA) as an aortocoronary bypass graft. The IMA used as a bypass vessel for the coronary arteries has been one of the most important advances to account for improved survival and long-term graft patency [24]. Although the IMA delivers a smaller blood flow compared with saphenous veins, it can adapt and enlarge to some extent, and long-term patency is better than for vein grafts. **A,** A normal IMA used for aortocoronary bypass (Movat's pentachrome stain). Graft failure with the IMA usually occurs early and is caused by thrombosis secondary to technical problems. (*continued on next page*)

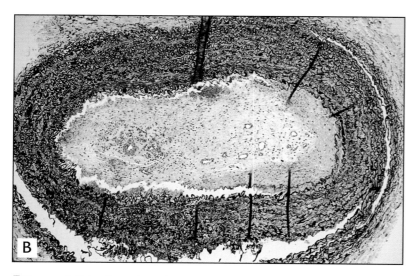

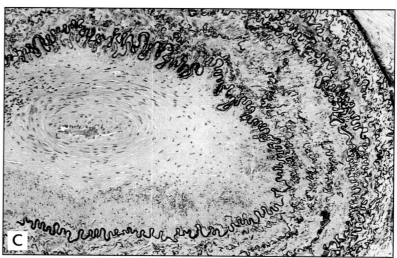

Figure 4-24. (*continued*)
B, A remote (organized) thrombus in an IMA bypass graft (Movat's pentachrome stain). The intima of the IMA changes little over the course of time, and the most common finding is subendothelial intimal proliferation, probably related to trauma of mobilizing the artery. **C,** Although fibrointimal proliferation in the IMA is usually mild, it can occasionally result in significant occlusion (Movat's pentachrome stain). In contrast to vein grafts, atherosclerosis in IMA grafts is exceedingly rare [26].

REFERENCES

1. Insull W: Peripheral vascular disease: a clinician's view. In *Syndromes of Atherosclerosis*. Edited by Fuster V. Armonk, NY: Futura Publishing Company; 1996:261–267.

2. Kannel WB, McGee DL: Diabetes and cardiovascular disease: the Framingham Study. *JAMA* 1979, 241:2035–2038.

3. McDaniel MD, Cronenwitt JL: Basic data relative to the natural history of intermittent claudication. *Ann Vasc Surg* 1989, 3:273–277.

4. Yadav JS, Roubin GS, King P, *et al.*: Angioplasty and stenting for restenosis after carotid endarterectomy: initial experience. *Stroke* 1996, 27:2075–2079.

5. Yadav JS, Roubin GS, Iyer S, *et al.*: Elective stenting of the extracranial carotid arteries [see comments]. *Circulation* 1997, 95:376–381.

6. Beckman JS, Ye YZ, Anderson PG, *et al.*: Extensive nitration of protein tyrosines in human atherosclerosis detected by immunohistochemistry. *Biol Chem Hoppe Seyler* 1994, 375:81–88.

7. Falk E, Shah PK, Fuster V: Coronary plaque disruption. *Circulation* 1995, 92:657–671.

8. Davies MJ, Richardson PD, Woolf N, *et al.*: Risk of thrombosis in human atherosclerotic plaques: role of extracellular lipid, macrophage, and smooth muscle cell content. *Br Heart J* 1993, 69:377–381.

9. Matrisian LM: The matrix degrading metalloproteinases. *Bioessays* 1992, 14:455–463.

10. Atkinson JB: Pathobiology of sudden death: coronary causes. *Cardiovasc Pathol* 1994, 3:105–115.

11. Burke AP, Farb A, Malcom GT, *et al.*: Coronary risk factors and plaque morphology in men with coronary disease who died suddenly. *N Engl J Med* 1997, 336:1276–1282.

12. Johnston KW, Rutherford RB, Tilson MD, *et al.*: Suggested standards for reporting on arterial aneurysms. *J Vasc Surg* 1991, 13:453–458.

13. Majumder PP, St. Jean PL, Ferrell RE, *et al.*: On the inheritance of abdominal aortic aneurysm. *Am J Hum Genet* 1991, 48:164–170.

14. Patel MI, Hardman DTA, Fisher CM: Current views on the pathogenesis of abdominal aortic aneurysms. *J Am Coll Surg* 1995, 181:371–382.

15. MacSweeney STR, Powell JT, Greenhalgh RM: Pathogenesis of abdominal aortic aneurysm. *Br J Surg* 1994, 81:935–941.

16. Chaitman BR, Rosen AD, Williams DO, *et al.*: Myocardial infarction and cardiac mortality in the Bypass Angioplasty Revascularization Investigation (BARI) randomized trial [see comments]. *Circulation* 1997, 96:2162–2170.

17. Narins CR, Holmes DR Jr, Topol EJ: A call for provisional stenting: the balloon is back. *Circulation* 1998, 97:1298–1305.

18. Farb A, Virmani R, Atkinson JB, Anderson PG: Long-term histologic patency after percutaneous transluminal coronary angioplasty is predicted by the creation of a greater lumen area. *J Am Coll Cardiol* 1994, 24:1229–1235.

19. Andersen HR, Maeng M, Thorwest M, Falk E: Remodeling rather than neointimal formation explains luminal narrowing after deep vessel wall injury: insights from a porcine coronary (re)stenosis model. *Circulation* 1996, 93:1716–1724.

20. Shi Y, Pieniek M, Fard A, *et al.*: Adventitial remodeling after coronary arterial injury. *Circulation* 1996, 93:340–348.

21. Waller BF, Anderson PG: The pathology of interventional coronary artery techniques and devices. In *Textbook of Interventional Cardiology*. Edited by Topol EJ. Philadelphia: WB Saunders, 1999.

22. Anderson PG, Bajaj RK, Baxley WA, Roubin GS: Vascular pathology of balloon-expandable flexible coil stents in humans. *J Am Coll Cardiol* 1992, 19:372–381.

23. Atkinson JB, Forman MB, Vaughn WK, *et al.*: Morphologic changes in long-term saphenous vein bypass grafts. *Chest* 1985, 88:341–348.

24. Virmani R, Atkinson JB, Forman MB: Aortocoronary bypass grafts and extracardiac conduits. In *Cardiovascular Pathology*. Edited by Silver MD. New York: Churchill Livingstone; 1991:1607–1647.

25. Motwani JG, Topol EJ: Aortocoronary saphenous vein graft disease: pathogenesis, predisposition, and prevention. *Circulation* 1998, 97:916–931.

26. Shelton ME, Forman MB, Virmani R, *et al.*: A comparison of morphologic and angiographic findings in long-term internal mammary artery and saphenous vein bypass grafts. *J Am Coll Cardiol* 1988, 11:297–307.

Topography of Coronary and Aortic Atherosclerosis

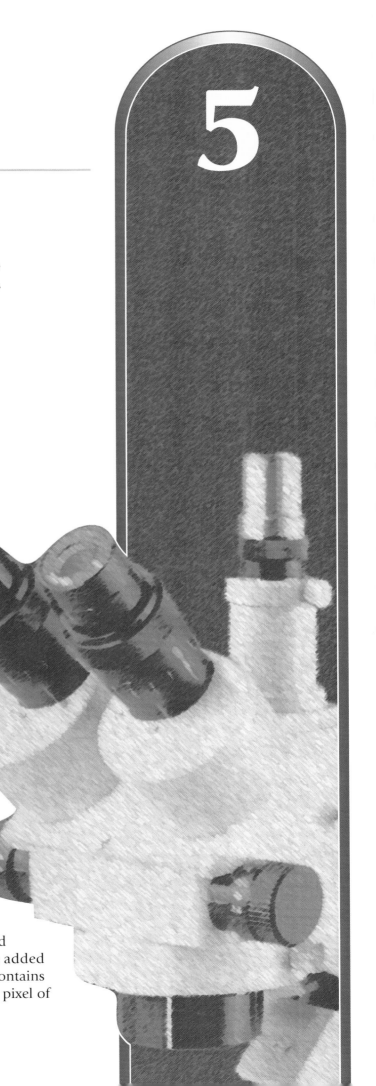

J. Fredrick Cornhill
Edward E. Herderick

The study of the topography of aortic and coronary atherosclerosis has benefited from dramatic advances in imaging techniques, computer hardware, and related technologies. Early studies of the distribution of atherosclerosis required experts' visual estimation of disease in a small number of regions; the resulting data were plotted manually [1]. These techniques yielded important information about the general distribution of disease but lacked the spatial precision required to study the pattern of the disease. Using high-resolution scanning equipment, high-capacity disk drives, and advanced imaging techniques, the topographic distribution of atherosclerosis can now be studied [2,3].

The probability-of-occurrence map is one result of such studies. To construct a probability-of-occurrence map, a large number of images of a vessel, such as the abdominal aorta, are scanned and stored on computer disks. Fiducial points, such as the origin of ostia and other landmarks common to all individuals, are placed on each image. A standard template, which is the average of anatomic data from all the individuals, is calculated. Each individual image is spatially transformed to the standardized shape to remove anatomic variation. Each transformed image is segmented into a binary image, with each pixel assigned either a value of one (disease, *ie*, sudanophilic lesion) or a value of zero (no disease, *ie*, normal). The transformed and segmented images for a particular group, *eg*, those aged 15 to 19 years, may be added together to create a summed image. Each pixel in this summed image contains the number of cases for which there was a one (disease). Dividing each pixel of the summed image by the number of cases and storing the resultant image yields the probability-of-occurrence map. This image is displayed in banded isopleths. Probability-of-occurrence maps may be created for different types of lesions (*eg*, fatty streaks or raised atherosclerotic plaques) and for various risk factors (*eg*, cholesterol level, smoking). Because each map is the same size, the relationship of the risk factors of interest to the incidence of disease is readily apparent.

A multicenter cooperative study entitled Pathobiological Determinants of Atherosclerosis in Youth (PDAY) collected the aortas, coronary arteries, and related data from approximately 2800 victims of traumatic death who were aged 15 to 34 years [4]. The probability-of-occurrence maps from the first 1378 (examples of which are presented in this chapter) show that whereas the early fatty streaks and raised lesions in the abdominal aorta and right coronary artery occur in very specific (*ie*, lesion-prone) regions of the vessel, other regions are relatively spared (*ie*, lesion-resistant). In addition, the pattern of disease appears to be similar regardless of the risk factors involved. Such risk factors act to increase or decrease the incidence of disease in lesion-prone areas but do not change the location of these areas.

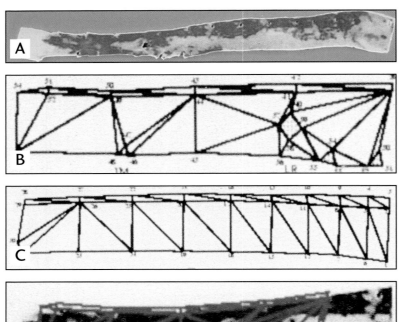
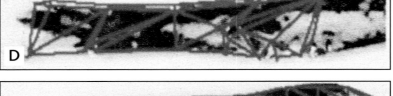
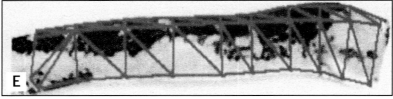
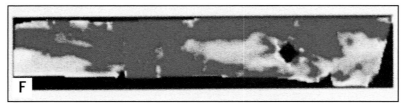
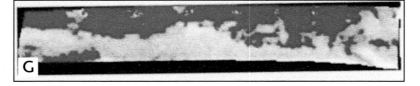

Figure 5-1.

Creation of probability-of-occurrence maps for the human aorta. It has been shown that lesions occur symmetrically in the aorta around the ventral midline [3]. Therefore, to fully use all tissue, each aorta was divided in half. One half was used to study topography; the other half was divided into several sections and used for histologic and chemical analyses. **A,** A half of a human aorta stained with Sudan IV to highlight fatty lesions. Sudan-positive areas stain a bright red; normal tissue is white. **B** and **C,** The standard template (*ie*, the average anatomy for the population of vessels under study) for the abdominal aorta and thoracic aorta, respectively. In the abdominal aorta, the celiac (C), the superior mesenteric (SM), left renal (LR), and inferior mesenteric (IM) arteries are shaded *gray*.

D and **E,** Digital scans of the abdominal and thoracic aortas through a green filter to enhance the contrast between sudanophilic lesions (*red* in *panel A*) and normal tissue (*white* in *panel A*).

F and **G,** Each image is transformed to the standard template in *panel B* and *panel C* and thresholded into a binary image (*ie*, disease is given a value of one [*dark areas*]; normal tissue is given a value of zero [*white areas*]) using a computer thresholding algorithm [2,3]. (*continued on next page*)

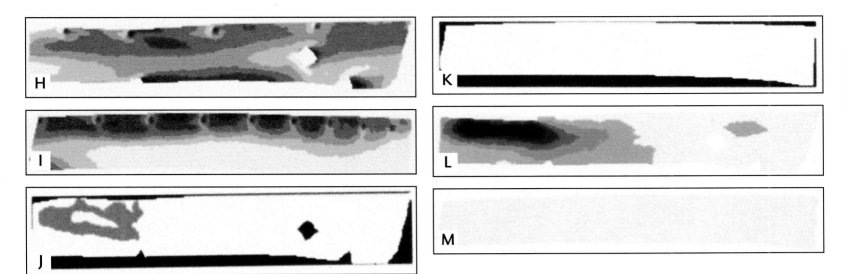

Figure 5-1. (*continued*)

H and **I,** Probability-of-occurrence map for sudan-positive lesions constructed from 1378 cases [4]. The map is displayed in 10% isopleths to highlight areas of high and low probability.

J and **K,** A panel of pathologists examined each vessel and identified those with raised atherosclerotic plaques. Black-and-white photographs of the abdominal and thoracic aortas were provided with these lesions manually identified (not shown). These manually

thresholded photographs were scanned, transformed, and segmented in a manner similar to that in sudanophilic lesions (*panels D to G*).

L and **M,** Probability-of-occurrence maps for raised atherosclerotic lesions for the same 1378 cases shown in *panels H* and *I*. Note that the map is displayed in 2% isopleths because of the lower incidence of such lesions in this young (15- to 34-year-old) age group. Raised lesions are prevalent in the abdominal aorta but are rarely present in the thoracic aorta in this population.

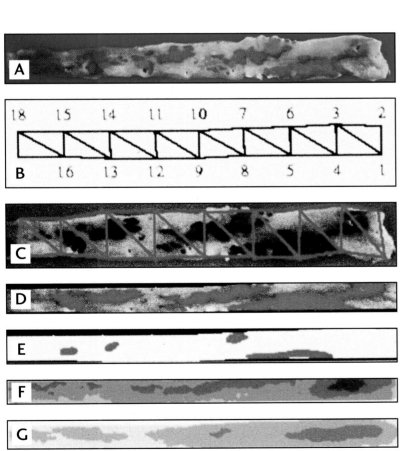

Figure 5-2.

Creation of probability-of-occurrence maps for the human right coronary artery (RCA). There are few stable landmarks in the right coronary artery; therefore, 1-cm marks were used as fiducial points [4]. In addition, the lengths of the RCAs varied greatly, with some vessels 1 cm in length and others up to 20 cm. After reviewing the distribution of lengths, it was decided to use only the first 8-cm portion for probability-of-occurrence maps. If a vessel was shorter than 8 cm, only the available portion was added into the map. **A,** A human RCA stained with Sudan IV to highlight fatty lesions. Sudan-positive areas stain a bright red; normal tissue is white. **B,** The standard template (*ie,* the average anatomy for the population of vessels under study). **C,** Digital scans of the RCA through a green filter to enhance the contrast between sudanophilic lesions (*red in panel A*) and normal tissue (*white in panel A*). The 1-cm fiducial marks have been placed on this image. **D,** Each image is transformed to the standard template shown in *panel B* and thresholded into a binary image (*ie,* disease is given a value of one [*dark*]; normal tissue is given a value of zero [*white*]) using a computer thresholding algorithm [2,3]. **E,** A panel of pathologists examined each vessel and identified those with raised atherosclerotic plaques. Black-and-white photographs of the RCA were provided with these lesions identified (not shown). These photographs were scanned, transformed, and segmented in a manner similar to that in sudanophilic lesions (*panel D*). **F,** Probability-of-occurrence map for sudan-positive lesions as constructed from 1378 cases. The map is displayed in 2% isopleths rather than 10% isopleths (as used for the aorta) because the incidence of fatty streaks in the RCAs of this young population is much lower than that in the aorta. **G,** Probability-of-occurrence maps for raised atherosclerotic lesions for the same 1378 cases. Note that the map is displayed in 2% isopleths based on the lower incidence of such lesions in this young population.

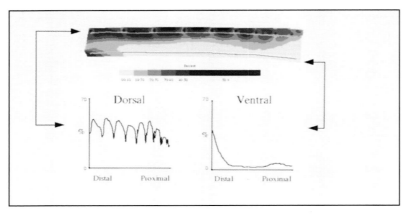

Figure 5-3.

Dorsal and ventral profiles of the incidence of sudanophilic lesions in the thoracic aorta constructed from 1378 cases [4]. *Top,* Thoracic probability-of-occurrence map with dorsal and ventral profiles. *Bottom left,* In the dorsal region, the areas of highest probability of lesions occur midway between the origins of the intercostal ostia, with relative sparing of the regions immediately distal to the ostia. *Bottom right,* In the ventral region, virtually no lesions are present until the region just proximal to the origin of the celiac artery.

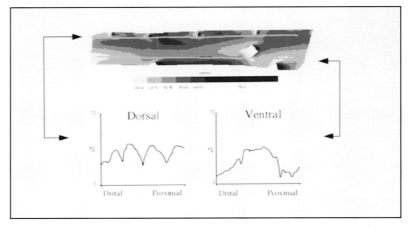

Figure 5-4.

Dorsal and ventral profiles of the incidence of sudanophilic lesions in the abdominal aorta constructed from 1378 cases. *Top,* Abdominal probability-of-occurrence map with dorsal and ventral profiles. *Bottom left,* The dorsal distribution of sudanophilic lesions observed in the thoracic aorta continues distally. *Bottom right,* In the ventral region, an area of high probability occurs from the level of the renal arteries to the origin of the inferior mesenteric artery, with relative sparing of the region distal to the inferior mesenteric artery.

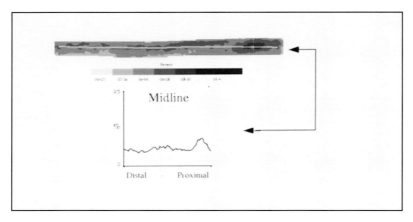

Figure 5-5.

Midline profile of the incidence of sudanophilic lesions in the right coronary artery (RCA). *Top,* RCA probability-of-occurrence map with dorsal and ventral profiles. *Bottom,* Midline profile graph. The areas of highest probability occur in the first 2 cm immediately distal to the origin of the RCA from the aorta. The highest probability of fatty streaks observed in the RCA was approximately one fifth those observed in the thoracic and abdominal aortas. This decreased probability reflects the later onset of the development of such lesions in the coronary arteries compared with in the aorta. Note that the incidence isopleth scale has been expanded from that used for the sudanophilic lesions in the thoracic and abdominal aorta. The maximum incidence displayed is 10% as opposed to 50% in the thoracic and abdominal aorta.

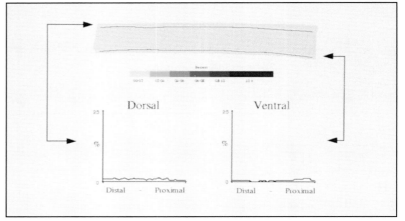

Figure 5-6.

Dorsal and ventral profiles of the incidence of raised atherosclerotic lesions in the thoracic aorta generated from 1378 cases [4]. *Top,* Thoracic aorta probability-of-occurrence map with dorsal and ventral profiles. *Bottom left,* Dorsal profile graph of the thoracic aorta showing a raised lesion. *Bottom right,* Ventral profile graph of the thoracic aorta showing a raised lesion. No region has a probability in excess of 2% for the development of raised lesions. Note that the incidence isopleth scale is expanded from that used in the sudanophilic map with the maximum value being 10%.

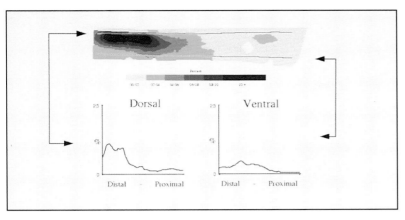

Figure 5-7.
Dorsal and ventral profiles of the incidence of raised atherosclerotic lesions in the abdominal aorta generated from 1378 cases [4]. *Top*, Abdominal aorta probability-of-occurrence map with dorsal and ventral profiles. *Bottom left*, Dorsal profile graph of the abdominal aorta showing a raised lesion. *Bottom right*, Ventral profile graph of the abdominal aorta showing a raised lesion. One significant region of high probability exists; this region exists on the dorsal-lateral surface of the abdominal aorta just distal to the origin of the inferior mesenteric ostia and proximal to the aorto-iliac bifurcation.

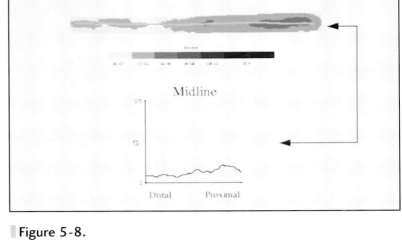

Figure 5-8.
Midline profile of the incidence of raised atherosclerotic lesions in the right coronary artery (RCA) generated from 1378 cases [4]. *Top*, RCA probability-of-occurrence map with dorsal and ventral profiles. *Bottom*, Midline profile graph of the RCA showing a raised lesion. The distribution of raised atherosclerotic lesions closely parallels the distribution of sudanophilic lesions, with the region of highest probability occurring in the first 2 cm of the vessel.

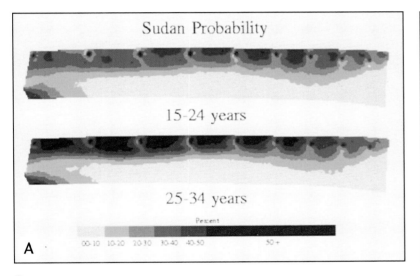

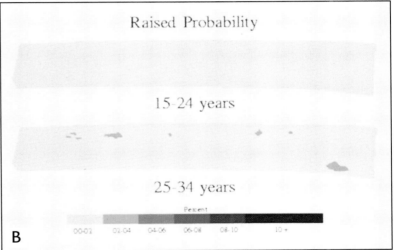

Figure 5-9.
Probability-of-occurrence maps by age for the thoracic aorta. The maps were constructed from individuals aged 15 to 24 years (*n* = 675) and 25 to 34 years (*n* = 703) [4]. **A,** The distribution of sudanophilic lesions is the same, with age acting to increase the incidence of lesions. The areas of highest probability, between the ostia, are approximately 30% to 40% in the younger age group; the same areas in the older age group increase to more than 50%. **B,** The distribution of raised atherosclerotic lesions is less than 2% in both age groups.

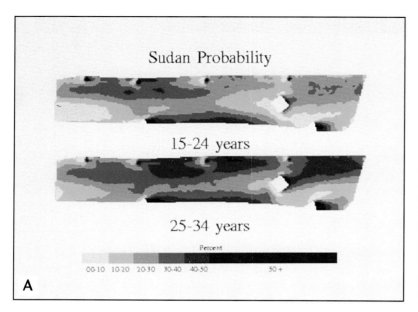

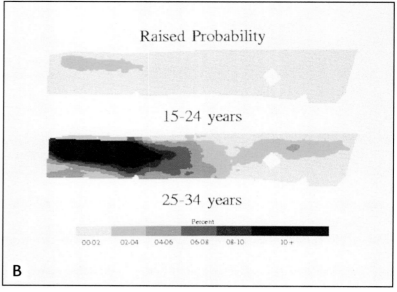

Figure 5-10.

Probability-of-occurrence maps by age for the abdominal aorta. The maps were constructed from individuals aged 15 to 24 years (*n* = 675) and 25 to 34 years (*n* = 703) [4]. **A,** The distribution of sudanophilic lesions is the same, with age acting to increase the incidence of lesions. The region just proximal to the flow divider on the dorsal side of the aorta does not show an increase in the incidence of sudanophilic lesions. This is caused by the increase in raised atherosclerotic lesions in this region. These raised lesions have a fibrous cap that no longer stains positive for sudan. **B,** Raised atherosclerotic lesions are just beginning to appear in the younger age group (*top*) with the highest incidence of lesions just under 4%. In the older age group (*bottom*), raised lesions appear in significant numbers; the highest incidence of lesions is well over 10%.

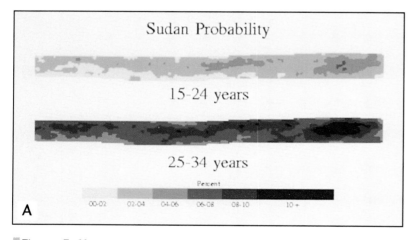

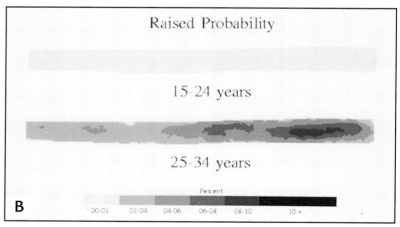

Figure 5-11.

Probability-of-occurrence maps by age for the right coronary artery. The maps were constructed from individuals aged 15 to 24 years (*n* = 675) and 25 to 34 years (*n* = 703) [4]. **A,** The distribution of sudanophilic lesions is the same, with age acting to increase the incidence of lesions. The areas of highest incidence in the younger age group is approximately 2% to 4% with the incidence increasing fivefold to 10% in the same region of the older year age group. **B,** Raised atherosclerotic lesions do not appear in significant numbers in the younger age group with no region having an incidence of greater than 2%. In the older age group, lesions begin to appear, with the regions of highest incidence at 6% to 8%.

REFERENCES

1. Strong P: Atherosclerotic lesions: natural history, risk factors, and topography. *Arch Pathol Lab Med* 1992, 116:1268–1275.

2. Cornhill JF, Barrett WA, Herderick EE, *et al.*: Topographic study of sudanophilic lesions in cholesterol-fed minipigs by image analysis. *Arteriosclerosis* 1985, 5:415–426.

3. Cornhill JF, Herderick EE, Stary HC: Topography of human aortic sudanophilic lesions. In *Monographs in Atherosclerosis.* 1990,15:13–19.

4. PDAY Research Group.: Natural history of aortic and coronary atherosclerotic lesions in youth: findings from the PDAY study. *Arterioscler Thromb* 1993, 13:1291–1298.

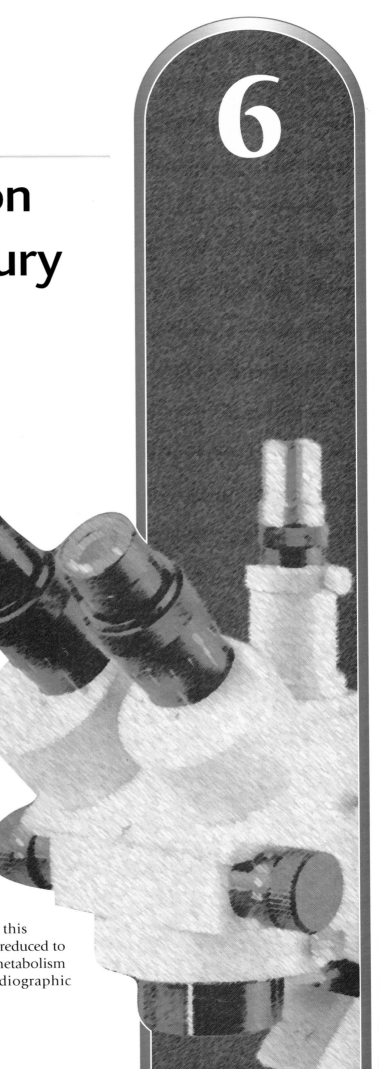

Myocardial Infarction and Reperfusion Injury

Robert B. Jennings
Keith A. Reimer

A myocardial infarct is a region of myocardial cell death restricted to the territory of a coronary artery that is, or temporarily was, obstructed sufficiently to allow little or no arterial flow to the infarcted tissue. In most instances, the involved artery is atherosclerotic and contains an acute thrombus that impedes or obstructs arterial flow. Often, the thrombus is located at the point of rupture of the fibrous cap of an atherosclerotic plaque (atheroma), but in other instances, the thrombus forms on an apparently intact atheroma. Other causes of obstruction of flow through a single coronary artery include severe spasm, embolization, and arteritis. The incidence of spasm of sufficient severity and duration to cause infarction is unknown. Thromboembolization and arteritis occur but are uncommon causes of infarction. Myocardial infarction involving one or more coronary territories may occur because of prolonged hypoperfusion caused by hypotension, hypoxemia, or both, especially if superimposed in a circumstance of fixed coronary stenosis by atherosclerotic plaque. Circumferential subendocardial infarction may be seen in patients who survive transient global myocardial ischemia.

Myocardium is dependent on arterial flow to maintain contractile function and viability. When a coronary artery is obstructed suddenly, arterial flow to the myocardium supplied by that vessel is reduced or eliminated; the myocardium supplied by this vessel is ischemic. Acute ischemia is present when the arterial flow is reduced to the point that the myocardium converts from aerobic to anaerobic metabolism and functional defects such as contractile failure and electrocardiographic changes appear [1,2]. If the ischemia is both severe and unrelieved, much of the ischemic myocardium becomes infarcted.

Myocardium can tolerate episodes of severe or total ischemia of brief duration without dying. Reperfusion of such tissue with arterial blood prevents myocyte death; the surviving myocytes are reversibly injured [3]. However, although alive, this tissue does not return to its initial condition. Monuments to the injury persist in the reperfused myocardium for seconds, minutes, hours and, in some cases, days. For example, electrocardiographic changes disappear after only a few minutes of reperfusion while, for a period of hours or days, this same myocardium will not contract as efficiently as it did prior to the episode of ischemia [4]. This contractile deficit is termed *stunning*. In addition, for about 1 to 2 hours, this tissue is more resistant to subsequent periods of sustained ischemia. This myocardial protection is termed *ischemic preconditioning* [5,6].

If severe ischemia is allowed to persist for 25 to 30 minutes, scattered myocytes exhibit electron microscopic evidence of necrosis [3]. As the period of ischemia is extended, more and more myocytes become necrotic. Although all myocytes destined to die in a zone of severe ischemia in the canine heart are dead after 6 hours of ischemia have passed [7,8], the presence of necrosis still cannot be detected by routine techniques of light microscopy. Although normal by light microscopy [9], these myocytes are irreversibly injured, *ie*, they cannot be salvaged by removing the cause of the injury via reperfusion of the tissue with arterial blood.

If severely ischemic myocardium is reperfused successfully after lethal injury first has developed, the dead myocytes undergo a disruptive form of necrosis termed *contraction-band necrosis* (CBN) [10,11]. CBN develops in the same myocytes that showed electron microscopic changes of necrosis prior to reperfusion. Other myocytes in an area of reperfusion, particularly those on the subepicardial border of the ischemic focus, often survive.

Processes initiated by reperfusion may damage the heart. These changes comprise reperfusion injury [12]. Stunning is the best established manifestation of reperfusion injury, in that much of the stunning effect clearly is due to deleterious effects of oxygen-derived free radicals formed in the myocardium at the onset of reperfusion [4]. It is less clear that reperfusion causes significant additional myocyte death through any mechanism [13], although possible ongoing myocyte apoptosis is under active investigation. In any event, reperfusion with arterial blood is the only therapy known to salvage myocytes damaged by ischemia.

Most of our knowledge of the pathobiology of acute ischemic injury has been established in studies of ischemia in experimental animals with permanent or transient occlusions of a coronary artery. Virtually all mammalian hearts exhibit similar changes following ischemia and reperfusion, and it seems certain that identical changes occur in the human heart [14]. Differences between species are qualitative and are caused by differences in heart rate, the presence or absence of collateral blood flow, and so on.

Once acute myocardial infarction is fully developed, acute inflammatory cells begin to appear at the periphery of zones of infarction. In the absence of reperfusion, the first such cells appear as early as 4 hours [15], but are most numerous at 2 to 4 days. Phagocytic activity usually is evident by 4 to 5 days, and the initiation of repair (in-growth of new capillaries and fibroblasts to replace the dead myocardium by scar), is evident after about 1 week. Reperfusion accelerates the time course of both inflammation and repair [15,16].

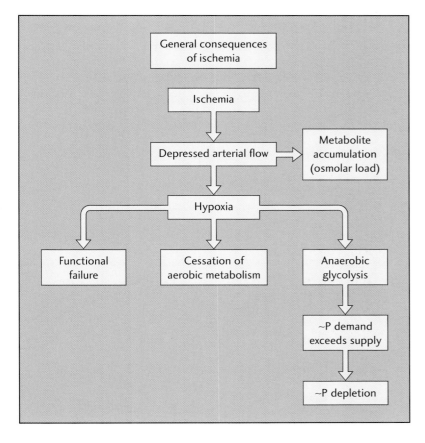

Figure 6-1.

General metabolic consequences of ischemia. Sudden obstruction of a coronary artery results in depressed or absent arterial flow. If the flow is reduced to the point that the supply of O_2 is inadequate to maintain aerobic metabolism, only seconds are required for the tissue to become hypoxic and to utilize much of the reserve creatine phosphate (CP); simultaneously, anaerobic glycolysis (AG) becomes active. Within a few seconds of the onset of low or absent flow, alterations in function appear; the myocardium ceases contracting and electrocardiographic changes develop. Once AG and the utilization of reserve ~P (high energy phosphate) has begun, lactate, H^+ ion, inorganic phosphate (Pi), and other metabolites accumulate in the intracellular space. This results in an intracellular osmotic load [1]. In severe or total ischemia, this causes an increase in myocyte intracellular H_2O and a decrease in extracellular H_2O. However, myocyte swelling is limited by the small amount of extracellular H_2O available to support swelling. Because the demand of the tissue for ~P to run ion pumps, to attempt to contract, and to fuel the mitochondrial ATPase [17] exceeds the supply available from AG and reserve ~P, the level of ~P decreases to virtually zero in less than an hour at 37°C in vivo. The failure of ~P supplies to meet the demand for ~P by the ischemic myocytes results in destruction of the adenine nucleotide pool. (*Adapted from* Jennings and coworkers [1].)

DEVELOPMENT OF NECROSIS IN ISCHEMIA

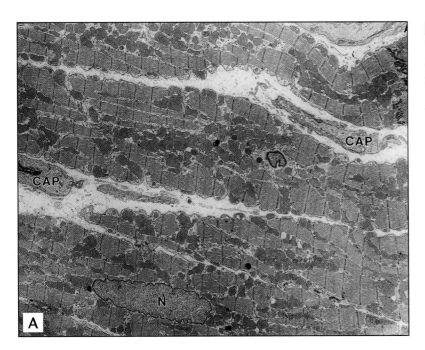

Figure 6-2.

Ultrastructure of control (nonischemic) left ventricular myocardium of the dog. **A,** Several myocytes. Note that the chromatin of the nuclei (N) is distributed evenly. Several capillaries (CAP) are present in the interstitial space. Abundant mitochondria with tightly packed cristae are present between the myofibrils. (Magnification, × 17,000). (*continued on next page*)

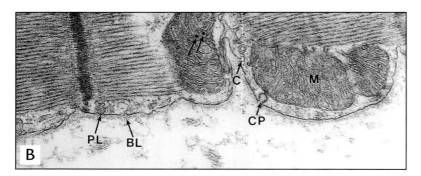

B

Figure 6-2. (*continued*)

B, A high-power view of the sarcolemma. The basal lamina (BL) or glycocalyx and the plasmalemma (PL) are both intact. An early phase of invagination of a pinocytotic vesicle is indicated at *C*. A coated pit is at *CP*. Note the tightly packed cristae of the mitochondria (M). Occasional matrix granules (*arrows*) are present. These granules disappear very early in ischemia. Junctional sarcoplasmic reticulum is present adjacent to the mitochondrion with the labeled matrix granules. (Magnification, × 51,000.) This and all subsequent electron micrographs in this chapter are of tissue fixed in glutaraldehyde with postosmication except where indicated otherwise. Thin sections were stained with uranyl acetate and lead citrate. No en bloc staining was used [19]. (*From* Jennings and coworkers [20]; with permission.)

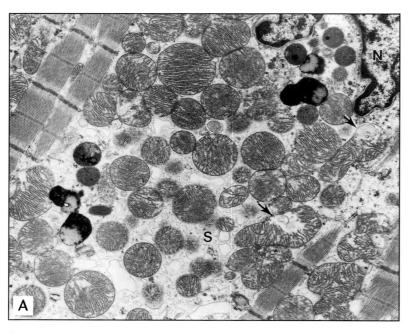

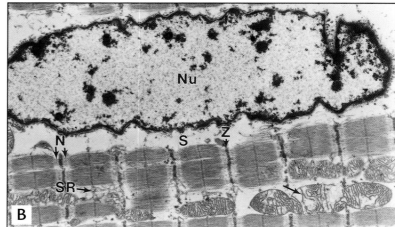

Figure 6-3.

Reversible ischemic injury. **A,** Reversible injury induced by 15 minutes of ischemia in canine heart. The structural changes typical of the late phase of reversible injury in the subendocardial myocardium are shown in this panel and should be contrasted to representative control tissue in Figure 6-2. Note that the chromatin of the nucleus (N) is aggregated peripherally. Also, the sarcoplasm (S) of the damaged myocyte is clearer than control due to cellular edema and partial loss of glycogen. There is increased matrix space in some mitochondria, as well as focal swelling (*arrows*). The normal matrix granules have disappeared. Although not illustrated here, the sarcolemma was indistinguishable from control at this time.

(Magnification, × 15,750). **B,** The most marked ultrastructural changes observed after 15 minutes of severe low-flow ischemia. The chromatin of the nucleus (Nu) is markedly aggregated peripherally. The sarcoplasm (S) is clear and contains very little glycogen. The myofibrils are relaxed and contain N bands (N) in the prominent I-band region on either side of the Z line (Z). The I band is wide because the myofibrils are acontractile (they stretch rather than shorten during systole). The sarcoplasmic reticulum (SR) is intact. The matrix space is increased in virtually all mitochondria, and the cristae are occasionally disorganized (*arrow*). (Magnification, × 12,500). (*From* Jennings and coworkers [1]; with permission.)

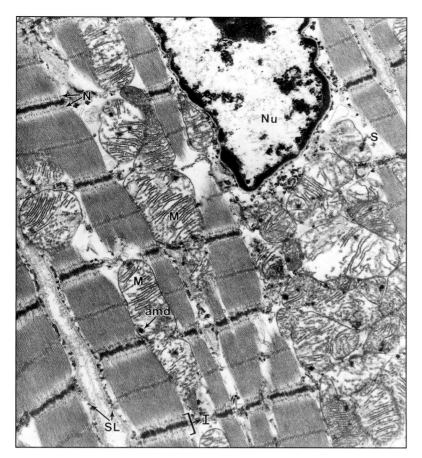

Figure 6-4.

Early irreversible injury induced by 40 minutes of low-flow ischemia in the canine heart. The chromatin of the nucleus (Nu) is aggregated peripherally. Note the clarity of the sarcoplasmic space (S) and the generalized mitochondrial (M) swelling. Prominent amorphous matrix densities (amd) are present in virtually every mitochondrial profile and the matrix granules have disappeared. The myofibrils are relaxed. The I bands (I) are prominent due to stretching and now exhibit an N line (N). (Magnification, × 17,500.) SL—sarcolemma. (*From* Basuk and coworkers [21]; with permission.)

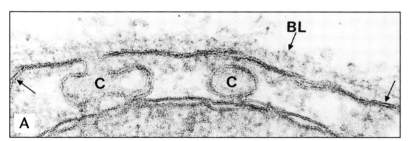

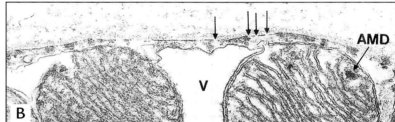

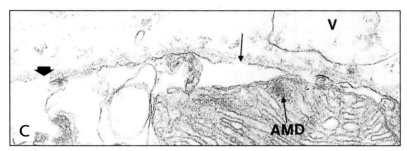

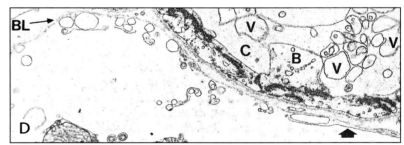

Figure 6-5.

Sarcolemmal disruption in irreversible injury. **A,** The typical architecture of the sarcolemma of control nonischemic tissue. The trilaminar structure of the plasmalemma is shown clearly (*arrows*), but where it tilts away from the perpendicular, it appears less distinct. A fuzzy coat (BL), the basal lamina or glycocalyx (15 to 35 mm thick) covers the unit membrane. Two caveolae (C) are present. **B,** A myocyte irreversibly injured by 30 minutes of ischemia. At this early time interval, only a few ischemic myocytes exhibit the ultrastructural changes of irreversible injury. Note that there are numerous tiny defects in the plasmalemma (*arrows*), vacuoles (V) in the sarcoplasm, and that the mitochondria are enlarged and exhibit a clear matrix that contains prominent amorphous matrix densities (AMD). **C,** The changes in the sarcolemma caused by 40 minutes of ischemia in vivo. There is one small (60 nm) gap in the plasmalemma and a larger region where the glycocalyx is generally intact but the plas-

malemma is not identifiable (*thick arrowhead*). The vesicle (V) in the interstitium is typical of fully developed ischemic injury. A large matrix density (AMD) is present in the enlarged mitochondria. **D,** A view of a subsarcolemmal bleb adjacent to a capillary (C) after 3 hours of severe ischemia in vivo without reflow. The capillary shows blebs (B) of endothelium extending into the lumen and vesicles of swollen endothelium within the lumen. Much of the basal lamina of both the capillary and myocyte is intact. However, the plasmalemma of the sarcolemma is broken up and can be identified as circular profiles under the basal lamina. Intact plasmalemma is present (*thick arrowhead*). The most marked damage to the plasmalemma occurs in localized areas of cell swelling. Magnification in each panel is as follows: **A,** × 108,000; **B,** × 70,000; **C,** × 60,000; **D,** × 15,000 (the magnification is reduced by 85%.) (*From* Jennings and coworkers [22]; with permission.)

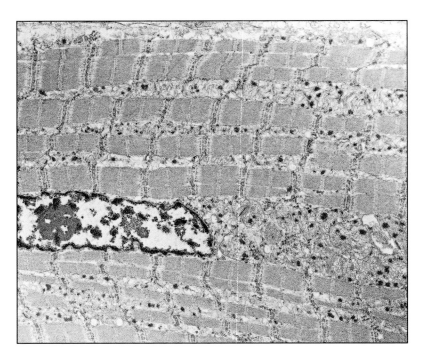

Figure 6-6.
Fully developed acute myocardial infarct after 24 hours of ischemia. This electron micrograph of a myocyte exhibits fully developed coagulation necrosis induced by 24 hours of severe ischemia in the canine heart. The changes are qualitatively similar to those found in myocytes irreversibly injured by 40 minutes of severe ischemia. The amorphous matrix densities in the mitochondria are larger and more abundant. However, the mitochondria still are intact. The myofibrils are superstretched, but generally have remained in register. The sarcolemma is disrupted totally. No attachment complexes between the sarcolemma and the Z bands are present. The nuclear chromatin is peripherally aggregated. Note that all of the electron microscopic changes noted in fully developed coagulation necrosis are present in irreversibly injured myocytes after only 40 minutes of ischemia. (Magnification, × 12,500). (*From* Jennings and Hawkins [23]; with permission.)

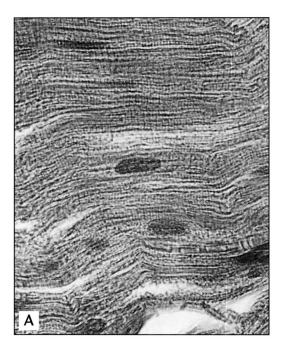 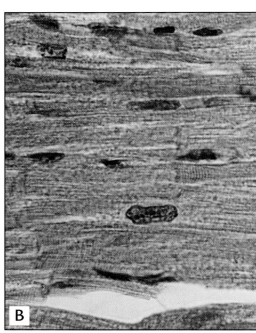

Figure 6-7.
Light microscopic view of early irreversible injury. Control myocytes and myocytes irreversibly injured by 60 minutes of ischemia are indistinguishable by routine light microscopy. **A,** The irreversibly injured tissue. **B,** Control tissue is in the right panel. (Hematoxylin and eosin, × 1000). (*From* Jennings and coworkers [24]; with permission.)

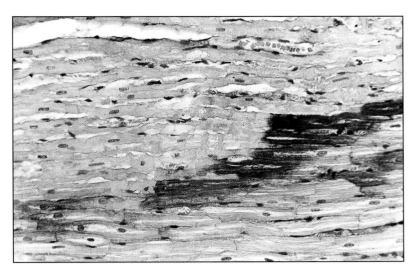

Figure 6-8.

View of an acute myocardial infarct, 4 hours old, stained for glycogen with the periodic acid–Schiff technique. This longitudinal section of canine heart was obtained 4 hours after occlusion of the circumflex branch of the left coronary artery. On the left is the ischemic tissue of the infarct. These myocytes contain no stainable glycogen, whereas

viable myocytes just outside the border of the infarct show increased stainable glycogen. In addition, dead myocytes at the border show contraction bands. Longitudinal sections are required to detect this narrow (1 to 3 cells thick) zone of contraction band necrosis. Finally, the myofibers of the infarct itself are stretched and appear both more wavy (termed *wavy fiber change*) and narrower than control myocytes. Although this change clearly is present early in acute myocardial infarction [25], it is not a good "objective" sign of early irreversible injury. That the dead myocytes are superstretched by ultrastructural criteria was illustrated in Figure 6-4. Note that the nuclei of the wavy fibers in the infarct are indistinguishable at 4 hours from the nuclei of nonischemic control myocytes.

The contraction-band necrosis first is detectable 60 to 90 minutes after the onset of ischemia. The explanation for the enhanced glycogen staining just beyond the infarct border is unknown. There may be increased glycogen synthesis in the myocytes immediately adjacent to the zone of ischemia. An alternate hypothesis involves solubility. Glycogen is slightly soluble in the formalin used to fix the tissue shown in this figure. Perhaps glycogen in the myocytes with enhanced staining has been altered to a less soluble form of glycogen than exists in the better perfused myocytes of the normal left ventricle. (Periodic acid–Schiff, × 309.)

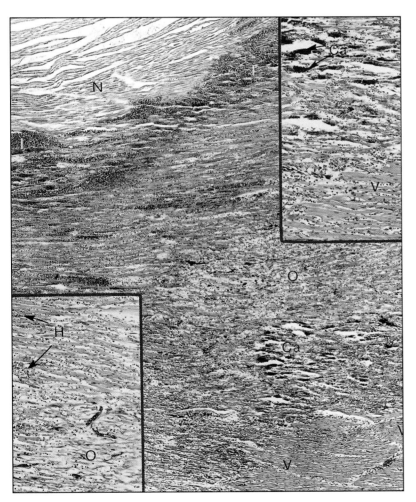

Figure 6-9.

View of a fully developed acute myocardial infarct after 4 days of ischemia. This figure shows the characteristic histologic zones of inflammation and repair in an infarct induced by ligation of the left circumflex coronary artery in the dog heart. This view is from the center of the circumflex bed and incorporates much of the transmural wall from the subendocardial region (*top*) to the subepicardial region (*bottom*). There is a subendocardial central core of coagulation necrosis (N), with separation of fibers due to interstitial and cellular edema but with relatively little cellular infiltration. This zone is surrounded by a zone with hemorrhage (H) and an intense acute inflammatory response (I). In the peripheral zone, organization (O) has begun and is characterized by macrophages, which have removed some of the necrotic cells, and ingrowth of fibroblasts and capillaries. This is better seen in the *lower inset*. Some heavily calcified cells (Ca) also are present in the peripheral zone. Some viable muscle (V) survived in the subepicardial region seen at the *lower right*. This region, between the organizing zone of the infarct and viable myocardium, is shown at higher power in the *upper inset*. (Hematoxylin and eosin, × 55; insets, × 120.) (*From* Reimer and Jennings [19]; with permission.)

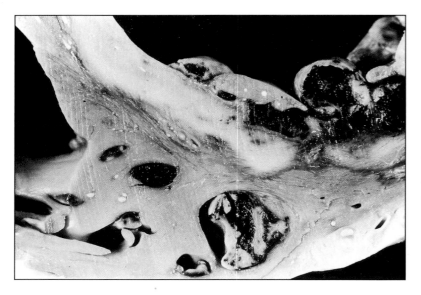

Figure 6-10.

Gross appearance of a fully developed acute myocardial infarct in a human heart. This image is a cross-section of the anterior wall of the right and left ventricles and anterior interventricular septum of a human heart containing an organizing infarct. The section is viewed from the base, with the anterior wall toward the bottom. An acute infarct is present in the subendocardial zone of the anteroseptal region of the left ventricle (anterior descending artery territory). This infarct occurred about 10 days before the patient's death and is characterized by a central core of necrotic muscle that was yellow-gray, surrounded by a rim of granulation tissue that was dark red. The slightly darker color of this peripheral rim is caused by erythrocytes within the proliferating capillaries. The dark tissue separating muscular trabeculae in the cardiac chamber is mural thrombus, a further complication of myocardial infarction that may result in systemic embolization. Some vessels in this cross-section contain a barium gelatin mixture (*white*) that was injected postmortem to demonstrate the vascular tree on radiography. (*From* Jennings and Reimer [1]; with permission.)

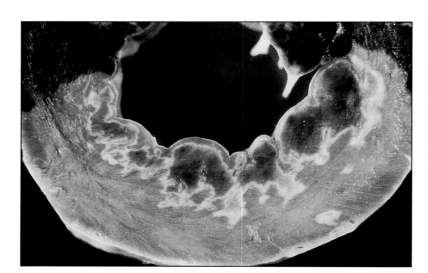

Figure 6-11.

Identification of myocardial infarcts grossly with dehydrogenase staining. This subendocardial myocardial infarct in a dog heart is delineated by dehydrogenase staining using triphenyl tetrazolium chloride (TTC). The illustration includes part of a cross-sectional slice of a dog left ventricle, viewed from the apex. Before sectioning, the ischemic and nonischemic vascular regions were identified by postmortem coronary perfusion with blue dye (nonischemic; dark regions at *top*) and TTC (ischemic region). In viable subepicardial areas, TTC was reduced by tissue dehydrogenases from its colorless oxidized state to a brick red color. The lighter subendocardial areas demarcate the edge of an infarct caused by 40 minutes of circumflex coronary occlusion followed by 4 days of reperfusion. The lack of TTC staining in the infarct is caused by the loss of tissue dehydrogenase reactions. Although myocardial dehydrogenase enzymes eventually are destroyed following 3 to 6 hours of ischemia, the loss of TTC staining in dead myocytes occurs much more quickly if the tissue has been reperfused, because soluble cofactors and enzymes required for dehydrogenase activity leak to the extracellular space and are flushed from the area [27]. The *dark areas* within the confines of the infarct are caused by hemorrhage. Note that whereas the subepicardial half of the ischemic region was spared by reperfusion, lateral boundaries of viable myocardium within the previously ischemic vascular bed were narrow. (*From* Reimer and Jennings [28]; with permission.)

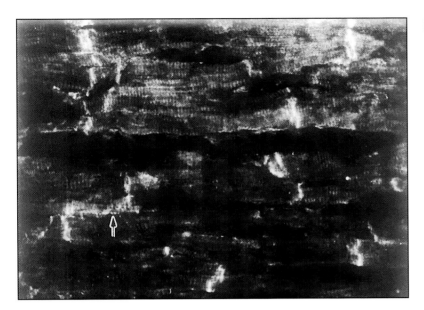

Figure 6-12.

Cytoskeletal changes in irreversibly injured myocytes. This fluorescence photomicrograph shows damage to the myocyte cytoskeleton, indicated by marked loss of vinculin immunofluorescence staining along the lateral margins of cells observed in canine myocardium injured by 180 minutes of total ischemia in vitro. In healthy myocardium, vinculin is localized at each attachment complex of the sarcolemma and in the intercalated disks. An example of persistent vinculin in typical costameric staining is shown at the *arrowhead*. The intercalated disk staining is unaffected by this period of ischemia. Disappearance of vinculin, a cytoskeletal component, coincides with the appearance of subsarcolemmal blebs and breaks in the plasma membranes of the affected cells. (*From* Steenbergen and coworkers [29]; with permission.)

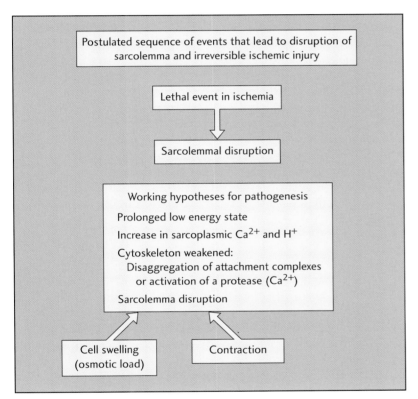

Figure 6-13.

Postulated sequence of events that lead to disruption of the sarcolemma and irreversible ischemic injury. The metabolic and structural changes induced by severe ischemia become more marked as the myocyte injury progresses from the reversible to the irreversible phase. Two distinctive ultrastructural features of irreversibility are the development of amorphous matrix densities in the mitochondria and disruption of the sarcolemma. The sarcolemmal disruption is considered to be the lethal event. It is associated with disaggregation of the attachment complexes between the myofibrils and the sarcolemma. This disaggregation permits the formation of subsarcolemmal blebs of edema fluid (see Fig. 6-5 *panels C and D*). The detached sarcolemma is stretched over these blebs, and such stretch, together with the continued contraction of adjacent myocardium, is thought to cause sarcolemmal ruptures. Attempts to demonstrate activation of a protease specific for vinculin or some other protein component of the attachment complex have not been successful. It is an attractive but unproved hypothesis that a protease is activated by a slight increase in Ca^{2+} late in the phase of reversible injury. (*Adapted from* Steenbergen and coworkers [30]; with permission.)

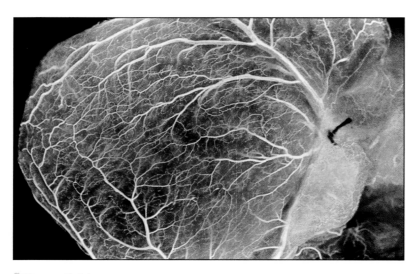

Figure 6-14.

Subepicardial collateral connections in a normal dog heart. In this photograph of the anterior surface of a normal dog heart, the vascular tree has been injected with a latex mixture. After the injection was complete, the myocardium was digested away to leave a cast of the anterior descending and circumflex branches of the left coronary artery and their branches. In most canine hearts, there are subepicardial connections between small branches of the coronary arteries. These collateral connections between major coronary territories range from 20 to 200 μm in diameter. When these connections are large, occlusion of one arterial bed is partially miti-

gated by passage of collateral arterial flow from the nonoccluded to the occluded arterial bed.

The response to slow occlusion of the proximal circumflex artery over a period of 1 week in the canine heart results in enough collateral growth to prevent myocyte death when the occlusion is complete [31]. Moreover, the collateral enlargement induced by the slow occlusion is long-lasting. If the occlusion is removed and flow is restored through the proximal circumflex artery, sudden reocclusion of this vessel 6 months or more later will be followed by restoration of collateral flow from the left anterior descending artery and with preservation of the myocytes that were destined to die if collaterals had not been allowed to develop and enlarge during the phase of slowly progressive occlusion [31].

The initial stimulus to collateral growth clearly is stenosis of a coronary artery. However, it is unlikely that collateral growth results from stress-induced hemodynamic changes, per se. Rather, biochemical transmitters, especially mitogenic peptides released as a consequence of reduced flow, are a much more likely cause [32]. The underlying hypothesis is that the growth of a tissue as complex as a blood vessel requires a genetic blueprint. Evidence supporting this hypothesis is provided by the observation that growth factors such as β-endothelial cell growth factor (βECGF) and acidic and basic fibroblast growth factors have been isolated from tissue undergoing enlargement and growth of collaterals. Alternatively, an inhibitor, or inhibitors, of these growth factors that is active in normal vessels might be inactivated when a vessel becomes stenosed. In any event, the cause of the angiogenesis (vessel growth) in ischemia remains unknown. (*From* Schaper [33]; with permission.)

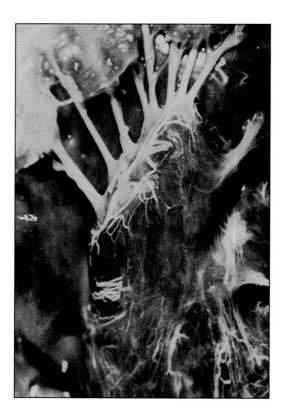

Figure 6-15.

Arterial collateral connections in the healthy pig heart. This view shows well-developed collateral connections in the subendocardium of the pig heart. In normal pig hearts, injection of a barium gelatin mixture reveals very few collateral connections. Those that are detectable are 15 to 20 μm in diameter and are located primarily in the subendocardial zone of the heart.

However, as shown in this figure, from Schaper's studies [33] of collateral formation in the pig, gradual occlusion of the anterior descending branch of the left coronary artery caused formation of collateral vessels of sufficient size to be easily detectable in gross coronary injection studies. (*From* Schaper [33]; with permission.)

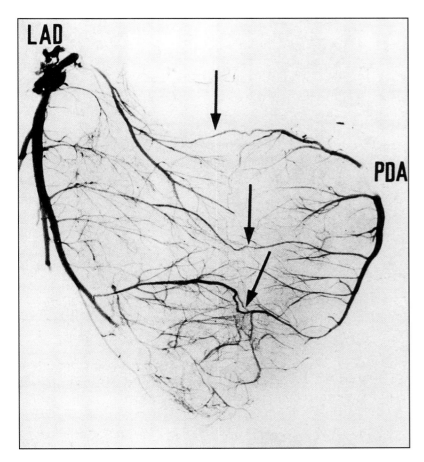

Figure 6-16.

Intramural collateral connections in the pig heart. This radiograph shows the coronary arterial tree of the pig 4 weeks after slow proximal occlusion of the left anterior descending coronary artery (LAD) with an ameroid constrictor. The constrictor is beneath the letters LAD. Moderate-sized septal intramural connections between the posterior descending coronary artery (PDA) and the LAD are shown at the arrows. No such connections are seen in control pig hearts. Because these hearts also showed some infarction, either these vessels carried insufficient flow or did not develop quickly enough to prevent infarction.

The normal human heart is similar to the normal pig heart in that few or no collateral connections greater than 15 μm exist. However, extensive collateral connections usually develop in human hearts if a coronary artery develops significant stenosis due to atherosclerosis. These collateral connections are important because they can prevent or delay the death of some myocardium after occlusion of a coronary artery. The phenomenon of infarction at a distance is explained by interruption of collateral flow. Myocardium may have survived occlusion of one coronary artery if collateral flow was provided from another coronary artery. A second coronary occlusion might then cause infarction both in the territory of the newly occluded artery and in the territory of the previously occluded artery because of the loss of both antegrade and collateral flow.

The importance of collateral flow for limiting myocardial infarct size has been studied in the greatest detail in the canine heart. Like the hearts of humans with extensive atherosclerosis, the normal dog heart exhibits variable-sized connections between the epicardial branches of the left coronary artery (see Fig. 6-14). Flow through these vessels affects the amount of cell death that results from sudden occlusion of a coronary artery. (*From* Reimer and Jennings [7]; with permission.)

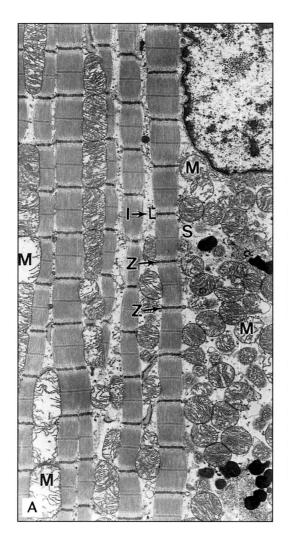

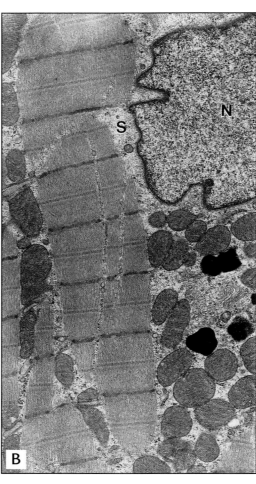

Figure 6-17.

Effect of reperfusion on tissue late in the phase of reversible injury. Canine myocytes reversibly injured by 15 minutes of ischemia exhibit the changes shown in Figure 6-3. Three minutes of reperfusion (*panel A*) is adequate to restore oxygenation and aerobic metabolism. (Magnification, × 7750.) **B,** Nonischemic myocardium from the same heart illustrated in *panel A*. All of the mitochondria (M) in the reperfused, reversibly injured tissue are swollen to a greater extent than they were when they were ischemic (compare with Figure 6-3), and in some, the swelling is very marked. Note that the chromatin of the nucleus still is aggregated peripherally. Compared to nonischemic myocardium from the same heart (*panel B*), the sarcoplasm (S) is less dense and contains much less glycogen. Also, the myofibrils are relaxed and demonstrate large I bands (I) that are not seen in myocytes of the control tissue. (Magnification, × 10,075.) N—nucleus; S—sarcoplasm. (*From* Jennings and coworkers [1]; with permission.)

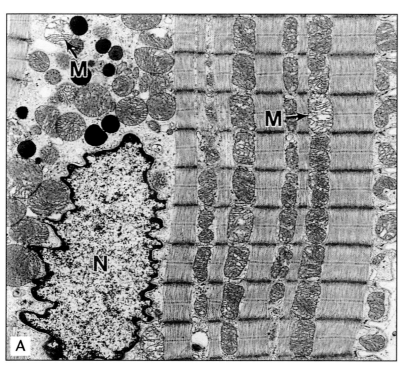

Figure 6-18.

Effect of 20 minutes of reperfusion with arterial blood on ultrastructure of myocardium reversibly injured by 15 minutes of ischemia. **A,** The lower power view shows that the architecture of the reperfused myocytes is well preserved. Note that these myocytes are virtually indistinguishable from typical control myocytes shown in Figures 6-2 or 6-17. The nuclear chromatin (N) is distributed evenly. An occasional swollen mitochondrion (M) is detected. The myofibrils are contracted. (Magnification, × 7000.) (*continued on next page*)

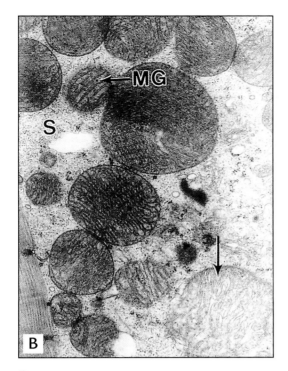

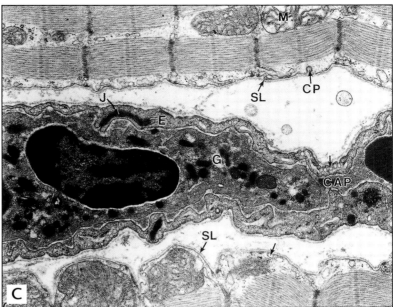

Figure 6-18. (*continued*)

B, Higher power view of typical mitochondria. Except for one swollen mitochondrion (*arrow*), they are indistinguishable from control mitochondria. Note that glycogen is present in the sarcoplasm (S). Matrix granules (MG), which disappeared during the episode of ischemia, again are present, but tiny. (Magnification, × 13,000.) **C,** This micrograph shows a granulocyte (G) in the lumen of a capillary (CAP) located between two myocytes. Granulocytes were seen in occasional capillaries of reversibly injured damaged tissue after reperfusion but were uncommon. No granulocytes were seen in the interstitial space, nor was attachment of granulocytes to endothelial cells observed. The endothelium (E) of the capillary is intact. The *arrow* shows the typical pinocytic vesicles of healthy myocardial capillaries. A tight junction (J) between endothelial cells also is present in the field. The sarcolemma (SL) of the myocytes is intact and also shows pinocytotic activity at the arrow in the lower myocyte. A swollen mitochondrion (M) also is present. However, most mitochondria were similar to control. (Magnification, × 25,000.) CP—coated pit. (*From* Reimer and Jennings [15]; with permission.)

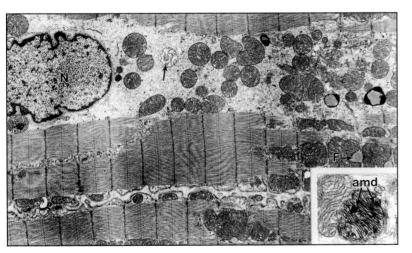

Figure 6-19.

Ultrastructure of myocytes reversibly injured by 15 minutes of ischemia and then reperfused for 24 hours. Except for an occasional badly swollen (*arrow*) or disrupted mitochondrion (*inset*), these myocytes are indistinguishable from control (Figs. 6-2 and 6-13*B*). The mitochondrion in the inset contains prominent amorphous matrix densities (amd). The chromatin of the nucleus (N) is distributed evenly. Glycogen is prominent. Occasional droplets of triglyceride (F) are detectable. However, it is unlikely that this fatty change is a true reflection of previous ischemic damage because control myocardium from the same dog also contained such fat droplets. (Magnification, × 10,750; inset magnification, × 22,000). (*From* Jennings and coworkers [1]; with permission.)

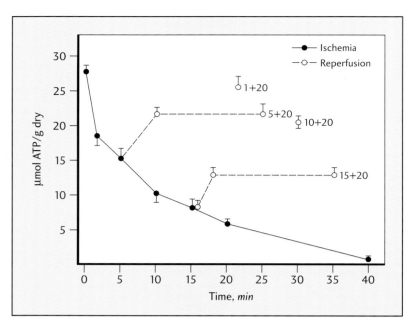

Figure 6-20.

Effect of reperfusion with arterial blood on the ATP of myocardium reversibly injured by 1, 5, 10, and 15 minutes of ischemia. During ischemia ATP is utilized at a rate that exceeds the supply available from anaerobic glycolysis, adenylate kinase, and reserves of ~P (high-energy phosphate). This results in the

changes in the adenine nucleotide pool in severely ischemic but viable canine myocardium; ATP declines early and the content of ADP and AMP increase. When reversibly injured myocytes are salvaged by reperfusion with arterial blood, aerobic metabolism resumes and the ADP and AMP that have accumulated in the ischemic tissue are converted to ATP. The quantity of ATP formed after reperfusion is limited by the quantity of ADP and AMP remaining in the tissue. As the period of ischemia is prolonged, AMP is degraded. The nucleosides and bases that have been formed during ischemia are flushed from the myocardium during reperfusion. ATP repletion is slow; therefore, depletion persists in the first hours after reperfusion.

The size of the total adenylate pool and the amount of ATP present after reperfusion is directly related to the amount of destruction of the pool. This figure shows that short periods of ischemia result in little depletion of ATP, whereas 15 minutes on ischemia reduces the amount of ATP in the tissue by 50%.

The speed of rephosphorylation of ADP and AMP to ATP in reversibly injured myocardium has not been measured. It is known to be complete after 3 minutes of reperfusion and it seems likely that it would be complete after 60 seconds of reperfusion. When it is complete, regardless of the size of the pool, the adenylate charge (AC), which reflects the degree of phosphorylation of the adenine nucleotides of the pool, is 0.89 to 0.91. *Bars* indicate ±SEM. (*Adapted from* Jennings and coworkers [18].)

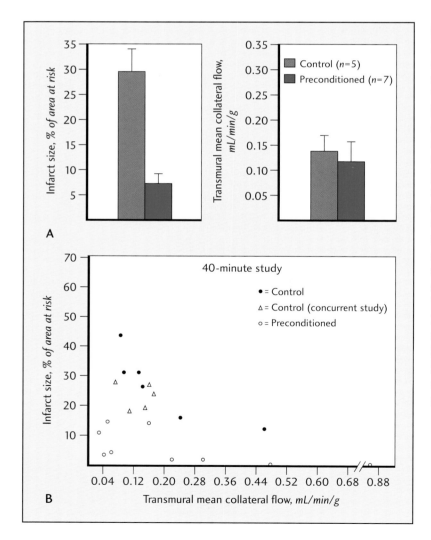

Figure 6-21.

Preconditioning with ischemia. A brief episode or several brief episodes of ischemia and reperfusion will delay the death of myocytes destined to die during an episode of severe ischemia. This beneficial effect is the strongest cardioprotective effect so far identified [5]. This figure shows the effect of preconditioning of myocardial infarct size in dogs. Dogs were preconditioned with four 5-minute occlusions of the proximal circumflex artery, each separated by 5 minutes of reperfusion. Then the tissue was subjected to a sustained 40-minute ischemic episode. Control animals received a single 40-minute circumflex occlusion. Infarcts were sized histologically after 4 days of reperfusion and related to anatomic area at risk and collateral blood flow (measured with radioactive microspheres midway through the sustained occlusion.) **A,** In control animals, infarct size averaged 29% of the area at risk. In preconditioned animals, infarct size was much smaller, averaging 7% of the area at risk. Collateral blood flow to the ischemic region was not significantly different between groups. **B,** Regression of infarct versus collateral blood flow. In control animals there was an inverse relation between infarct size and collateral blood flow (*ie,* low collateral flow was associated with large infarcts and vice versa). In preconditioned animals, infarcts were much smaller than controls at any level of collateral blood flow. (*Adapted from* Murry and coworkers [5].)

EFFECT OF REPERFUSION ON ACUTELY ISCHEMIC IRREVERSIBLY INJURED MYOCARDIUM

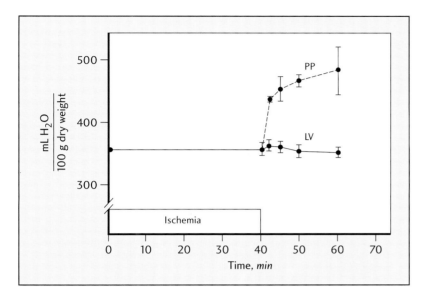

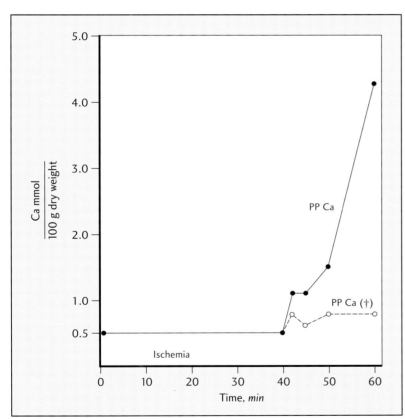

Figure 6-22.

Changes in total tissue water (TTW). Reperfusion of acutely ischemic myocardium with arterial blood early in the phase of irreversible injury produces dramatic changes in total tissue water (TTW), ions, and histology. In contrast to reversible injury, in which the myocytes remain intact following reperfusion (Figs. 6-17 to 6-19), the dead myocytes develop a distinctive form of necrosis termed *contraction band necrosis* (CBN) (Fig. 6-24). Accompanying CBN are the changes in TTW shown in this figure. The changes in TTW were measured in groups of hearts in which myocardium was irreversibly injured by 40 minutes of ischemia and then was reperfused for 2, 5, 10, and 20 minutes. The irreversibly injured myocytes swell enormously and very quickly. After only 2 minutes of arterial reflow, the TTW has increased by 16%. It slowly increases to 30% over the next 18 minutes of reflow [34]. *Bars* indicate ±SEM. (*Adapted from* Opie [34].)

Figure 6-23.

Changes in Ca^{2+}. The massive increase in total tissue water (TTW) shown in Figure 6-21 in irreversibly injured myocytes is accompanied by massive increases in tissue Na^+ and Cl^-, along with decreases in tissue Mg^{2+} and K^+ [34,35]. In contrast to reversibly injured reperfused tissue in which total tissue Ca^{2+} does not change, it increases markedly in irreversibly injured tissue during the first few minutes of reperfusion. In this figure, tissue calcium in mmol/100 g dry weight in the center of the zone of ischemia (posterior papillary muscle calcium [PP Ca]) is plotted as a function of minutes of reperfusion. The calcium level of severely ischemic tissue does not change during the first 40 minutes of permanent ischemia. However, it increases markedly after 2, 5, and 10 minutes of arterial reflow, and at 20 minutes there is eight to ten times more calcium in ischemic than in nonischemic control myocardium. The *dotted line* represents the theoretical Ca^{2+} content of the ischemic tissue PPCa(t), which would result from changes in the volume of extracellular fluid (ECF) in reperfused tissue if one assumes that the calcium content of ECF and plasma are essentially identical. To the extent that plasma Ca^{2+} is higher than ECF Ca^{2+}, the PPCa(t) would be lower than the curve plotted in this figure. Thus, much more Ca^{2+} is present than can be accounted for by tissue edema. Much of the difference between the two curves is due to mitochondrial accumulation of calcium phosphate. (*Adapted from* Whalen and coworkers [35].)

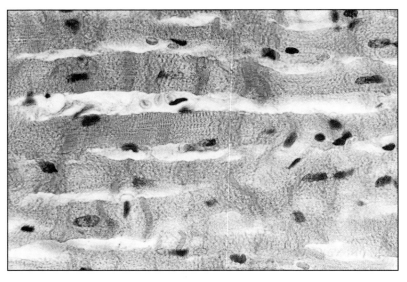

Figure 6-24.

Contraction band necrosis (CBN). This light micrograph shows CBN in canine myocardium irreversibly injured by 40 minutes of ischemia and reperfused for 20 minutes with arterial blood. The myocytes show striking bands of condensed myofibrils generally

separated by areas with much less dense cytoplasm in which the cross-striations often are out of register.

Contraction band necrosis appears after only 2 minutes of arterial reflow. The theoretical cause is entry of Ca^{2+} from the extracellular to the intracellular space where it induces massive contraction of the myofibrils [36–38]. CBN also appears in circumstances in which the tissue has not been subjected to ischemia. For example, CBN develops in experimental studies after toxic doses of catecholamines [39] or during the so-called calcium paradox [44]. In the latter condition, the lesion develops in isolated perfused hearts when calcium is added to the perfusate after a brief period of calcium-free perfusion. CBN develops as soon as the calcium is returned to the heart.

Contraction band necrosis also occurs following several types of cardiac injury in humans. For example, it may occur as a consequence of one or more aspects of cardiac arrest and resuscitation, including ischemia and reperfusion, or as a result of administration of catecholamines or as a consequence of injury from electrical defibrillation, calcium administration, or mechanical trauma.

Because reperfusion for days or weeks is followed by replacement of the dead myocytes with fibrous tissue [24], the lesion clearly represents a form of irreversible injury. (Magnification, × 1200.) (*From* Jennings and coworkers [24]; with permission.)

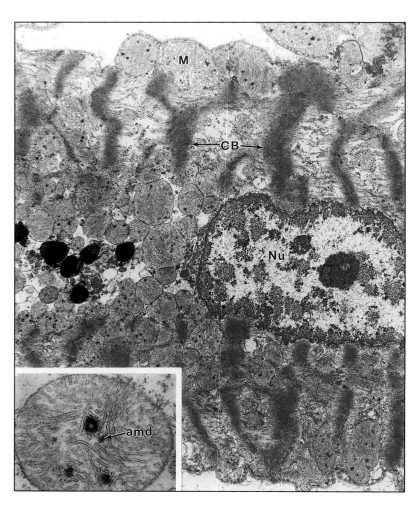

Figure 6-25.

Ultrastructural features of contraction band necrosis induced by 40 minutes of in vivo ischemia and 20 minutes of reperfusion are shown in this micrograph. Numerous dense contraction bands (CB) are obvious. Peripheral condensation of nuclear chromatin (Nu) also is apparent, and mitochondria (M) appear swollen and contain both amorphous and granular matrix densities. The inset on the lower left shows a higher power view of characteristic granular densities of calcium phosphate in mitochondria of these cells. Much of the excess Ca^{2+} found in CBN is presumed to be in mitochondrial calcium phosphate. Both amorphous (amd) and granular densities are present. The amds are known to develop prior to reperfusion (see Figs. 6-4 to 6-6). (Osmium fixation, × 14,000; inset magnification, × 45,000). (*From* Jennings and Hawkins [23]; with permission.)

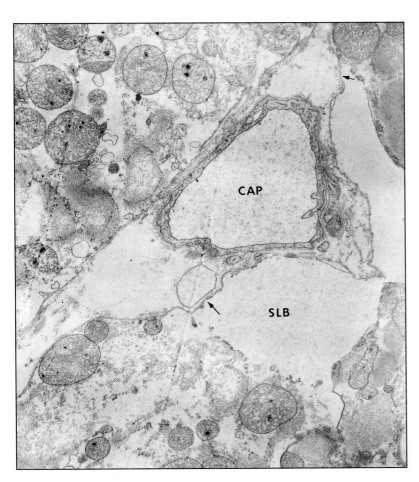

Figure 6-26.

Cross-sectional view of two myocytes exhibiting contraction band necrosis (CBN) caused by 40 minutes of ischemia and 20 minutes of reperfusion. This micrograph illustrates the extraordinary swelling of myocytes in CBN. Note the large subsarcolemmal bleb of edema fluid (SLB) covered by a focally disrupted sarcolemma (*arrows*). Note that the capillary (CAP) is compressed slightly by the myocyte swelling but is still patent; the endothelial cytoplasm does not appear to be swollen. Also, granular densities of calcium phosphate are prominent in most mitochondrial profiles. The myocytes in this micrograph were sectioned between contraction bands and show no organized myofibrils between the mitochondria. The contractile proteins have been condensed into the contraction bands that were present elsewhere in the myocytes, *ie*, out of the plane of this section. (Magnification, × 14,000.) (*From* Herdson and coworkers [10]; with permission.)

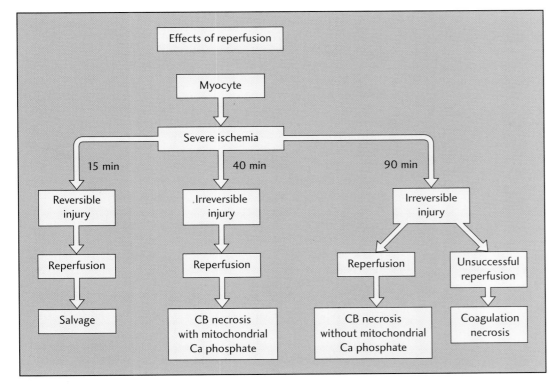

Figure 6-27.

Reperfusion after prolonged ischemia. The sequence of events observed when severely ischemic tissue is reperfused in the experimental animal heart are well established and are summarized in this figure. In the reversible and early irreversible phase, reperfusion is successful throughout the tissue even though edema (Fig. 6-21) may slow flow early in the irreversible phase. However, after 90 or more minutes of ischemia, reflow may be unsuccessful in severely ischemic areas in which severe vascular injury is present. This is termed the *no reflow* phenomenon [37]. This change occurs most often in the subendocardial center of an infarct where the most severe ischemia virtually always is present. If some flow reaches the area of vascular injury, the infarct may become markedly hemorrhagic.

One interesting feature of successful reperfusion after prolonged ischemia is the fact that mitochondrial Ca^{2+} accumulation does not occur. Mitochondrial accumulation of Ca^{2+} requires active metabolism that clearly can take place early but not late. (*Adapted from* Jennings and Reimer [41].)

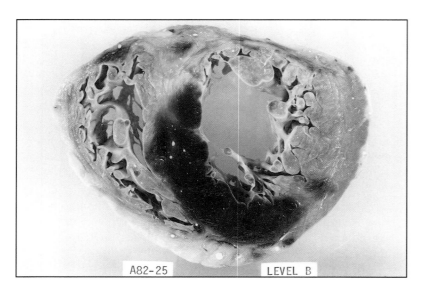

Figure 6-28.

Vascular injury in human infarction (hemorrhage after reperfusion). This is an example of hemorrhage occurring in a reperfused human infarct in a patient given streptokinase to lyse a clot in the anterior descending branch of the left coronary artery. This cross-section of the heart is viewed from the basal side (anterior wall at bottom of photograph). There is extensive hemorrhage within a nearly transmural anteroseptal infarct (*dark area*). A scar from a prior posteroseptal (inferior) myocardial infarct also is present. The hemorrhagic tissue exhibited classic contraction band necrosis by microscopic evaluation [10]. (*From* Kao and coworkers [42]; with permission.)

A82-25   LEVEL B

REFERENCES

1. Jennings RB, Reimer KA, Steenbergen C Jr.: Myocardial ischemia revisited: the osmolar load, membrane damage, and reperfusion [editorial]. *J Mol Cell Cardiol* 1986, 18:769–780.

2. Jennings RB, Reimer KA: The cell biology of acute myocardial ischemia. *Ann Rev Med* 1991, 42:225–246.

3. Jennings RB, Murry CE, Steenbergen C Jr, *et al.*: Development of cell injury in sustained acute ischemia. *Circulation* 1990, 82(suppl):II-2–II-12.

4. Bolli R, Marban E: Molecular and cellular mechanisms of myocardial stunning. *Physiol Rev* 1999, 79:609–634.

5. Murry CE, Jennings RB, Reimer KA: Preconditioning with ischemia: a delay of lethal cell injury in ischemic myocardium. *Circulation* 1986, 74:1124–1136.

6. Murry CE, Richard VJ, Reimer KA, *et al.*: Ischemic preconditioning slows energy metabolism and delays ultrastructural damage during sustained ischemia. *Circ Res* 1990, 66:913–931.

7. Reimer KA, Jennings RB: The "wavefront phenomenon" of myocardial ischemic cell death: II. Transmural progression of necrosis within the framework of ischemic bed size (myocardium at risk) and collateral flow. *Lab Invest* 1979, 40:633–644.

8. Reimer KA, Vander Heide RS, Richard VJ: Reperfusion in acute myocardial infarction: effect of timing and modulating factors in experimental models. *Am J Cardiol* 1993, 72:13G–21G.

9. Sommers HM, Jennings RB: Experimental acute myocardial infarction: histologic and histochemical studies of early myocardial infarcts induced by temporary or permanent occlusion of a coronary artery. *Lab Invest* 1964, 13:1491–1503.

10. Herdson PB, Sommers HM, Jennings RB: A comparative study of the fine structure of normal and ischemic dog myocardium with special reference to early changes following temporary occlusion of a coronary artery. *Am J Pathol* 1965, 46:367–386.

11. Ganote CE: Contraction band necrosis and irreversible myocardial injury. *J Mol Cell Cardiol* 1983, 15:67–73.

12. Jennings RB, Yellon DM: Reperfusion injury: definitions and historical background. In *Myocardial Protection: The Pathophysiology of Reperfusion and Reperfusion Injury*. Edited by Yellon D, Jennings RB. New York: Raven Press; 1992:1–11.

13. Reimer KA: Lethal reperfusion injury: does it exist and does it matter? *J Thromb Thrombolysis* 1997, 4:117–118.

14. Lee JT, Ideker RE, Reimer KA: Myocardial infarct size and location in relation to the coronary vascular bed at risk in man. *Circulation* 1981, 64:526–534.

15. Reimer KA, Jennings RB: Myocardial ischemia, hypoxia, and infarction. In *The Heart and Cardiovascular System*, vol 2, edn 2. Edited by Fozzard HA, Haber E, Jennings RB, *et al.* New York: Raven Press; 1991: 1875–1974.

16. Richard VJ, Murry CE, Reimer KA: Healing of myocardial infarcts in dogs: effects of late reperfusion. *Circulation* 1995, 92:1891–1901.

17. Vander Heide RS, Hill ML, Reimer KA, *et al.*: Effect of reversible ischemia on the activity of the mitochondrial ATPase: relationship to ischemic preconditioning. *J Mol Cell Cardiol* 1996, 28:103–112.

18. Jennings RB, Reimer KA, Steenbergen C, Jr, *et al.*: Energy metabolism in myocardial ischemia. In *Myocardial Ischemia*. Edited by Dhalla NS, Innes IR, Beamish RE. Boston: Martinus Nijhoff Publisher; 1987:185–198.

19. Reimer KA, Jennings RB: Myocardial ischemia, hypoxia, and infarction. In *The Heart and Cardiovascular System*. Edited by Fozzard HA, Jennings RB, Haber E, *et al.* New York: Raven Press; 1992:1874–1973.

20. Jennings RB, Reimer KA, Kinney RB, *et al.*: Sarcolemmal damage in ischemia. In *Proceedings of the Sixth Joint US-USSR Symposium on Myocardial Metabolism*. Edited by Smirnov VN, Katz AM. Switzerland: Harwood Publishers; 1987:120–154.

21. Basuk WL, Reimer KA, Jennings RB: Effect of repetitive brief episodes of ischemia on cell volume, electrolytes and ultrastructure. *J Am Coll Cardiol* 1986, 8(suppl):33A–41A.

22. Jennings RB, Steenbergen C, Jr, Kinney RB, *et al.*: Comparison of the effect of ischaemia and anoxia on the sarcolemma of the dog heart. *Eur Heart J* 1983, 4 (suppl):123–127.

23. Jennings RB, Hawkins HK: Ultrastructural changes of acute myocardial ischemia. In *Degradative Processes in Heart and Skeletal Muscle*. Edited by Wildenthal K. Amsterdam/New York: Elsevier; 1980:295–344.

24. Jennings RB, Sommers HM, Herdson PB, *et al.*: Ischemic injury of myocardium: part II. Cardiopathies and factors influencing myocardial degeneration. *Ann N Y Acad Sci* 1969, 156:61–78.

25. Bouchardy B, Majno G: Histopathology of early myocardial infarcts: a new approach. *Am J Pathol* 1974, 74:301–337.

26. Reimer KA, Jennings RB: The changing anatomic reference base of evolving myocardial infarction: underestimation of myocardial collateral blood flow and overestimation of experimental anatomic infarct size due to tissue edema, hemorrhage, and acute inflammation. *Circulation* 1979, 60:866–876.

27. Klein HH, Puschmann S, Schaper J, *et al.*: The mechanism of the tetrazolium reaction in identifying experimental myocardium infarction. *Virchows Arch (Pathol Anat Histopathol)* 1981, 393:287–297.

28. Reimer KA, Jennings RB: Effects of reperfusion on infarct size: experimental studies. *Eur Heart J* 1985, 6 (suppl E): 97–108.

29. Steenbergen C, Jr, Hill ML, Jennings RB: Cytoskeletal damage during myocardial ischemia: changes in vinculin immunofluorescence staining during total in vitro ischemia in canine heart. *Circ Res* 1987, 60:478–486.

30. Steenbergen C, Jr, Hill ML, Jennings RB: Volume regulation and plasma membrane injury in aerobic, anaerobic, and ischemic myocardium in vitro: effect of osmotic cell swelling on plasma membrane integrity. *Circ Res* 1985, 57:864–875.

31. Khouri EM, Gregg DE, McGranahan GM, Jr: Regression and reappearance of coronary collaterals. *Am J Physiol* 1971, 220:655–661.

32. Schaper W, Bernotat-Danielowski S, Nienaber D, *et al.*: Collateral circulation. In *The Heart and Cardiovascular System*. Edited by Fozzard HA, Haber E, Jennings RB, *et al.* New York: Raven Press; 1999:1427–1464.

33. Schaper W: The collateral circulation of the heart. In *Clinical Studies: A North-Holland Frontiers Series*. Edited by Black DAK. Manchester: North-Holland Publishing Company; 1971.

34. Opie LH: *Calcium-Antagonists and Cardiovascular Disease.* (ed.) New York: Raven Press; 1984.

35. Whalen DA, Jr, Hamilton DG, Ganote CE, *et al.*: Effect of a transient period of ischemia on mycardial cells: I. Effects on cell volume regulation. *Am J Pathol* 1974, 74:381–398.

36. Jennings RB, Baum JH, Herdson PB: Fine structural changes in myocardial ischemic injury. *Arch Pathol Lab Med* 1965, 79:135–143.

37. Kloner RA, Ganote CE, Jennings RB: The "no-reflow" phenomenon after temporary coronary occlusion in the dog. *J Clin Invest* 1974, 54:1496–1508.

38. Jennings RB, Ganote CE: Structural changes in myocardium during acute ischemia. *Circ Res* 1974, 35(suppl):III-156–III-172.

39. Rona G, Huttner I, Boutet M: Microcirculatory changes in myocardium with particular reference to catecholamine-induced cardiac muscle cell injury. In *Handbook der allgermeinen Pathologie III Mikrozirkulation/Microcirculation*. Edited by Meesen H. Berlin: Springer-Verlag; 1977:791–888.

40. Ganote CE, Nayler WG: Contracture and the calcium paradox [editorial review]. *J Mol Cell Cardiol* 1985, 17:733–745.

41. Jennings RB, Reimer KA: Lethal reperfusion injury: fact or fancy? In *Myocardial Response to Acute Injury*. Edited by Parratt JR. London: Macmillan Press; 1992:17–34.

42. Kao KJ, Hackel DB, Kong Y: Hemorrhagic myocardial infarction after streptokinase treatment for acute coronary thrombosis. *Arch Pathol Lab Med* 1984, 108:121–124.

Angiogenesis in Vascular and Myocardial Repair

Jeffrey M. Isner
Marianne Kearney

The full paradigm for angiogenesis has been suggested to begin with activation of endothelial cells (ECs) within a parent vessel followed by disruption of the basement membrane and subsequent migration of ECs into the interstitial space, possibly in the direction of an ischemic stimulus. Concomitant or subsequent EC proliferation, intracellular vacuolar lumen formation, pericyte "capping," and production of a basement membrane complete the developmental sequence.

More recently, it has been established that vasculogenesis—the formation of blood vessels from EC progenitors, or angioblasts—also contributes to postnatal neovascularization. Angiogenic cytokines responsible for natural as well as pathologic angiogenesis all share in common the ability to act as mitogens for ECs. The various growth factors that have been shown to promote angiogenesis include vascular endothelial growth factor (VEGF), basic fibroblast growth factor (bFGF), and acidic fibroblast growth factor (aFGF).

Examination of human atherosclerotic specimens obtained by directional atherectomy, obtained at necropsy, and studies performed in animal models have demonstrated expression of these growth factors in conjunction with neovascularization. These observations have established angiogenesis and vasculogenesis as key processes in a variety of cardiovascular pathologic states.

This chapter illustrates selected examples of native as well as therapeutic neovascularization in the cardiovascular system.

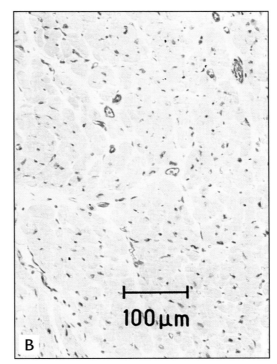

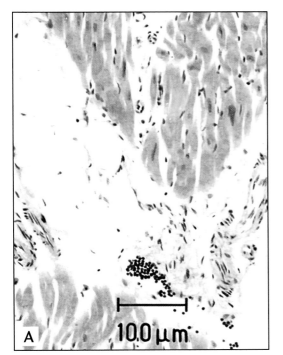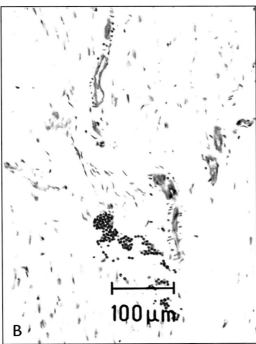

Figure 7-1.
Microvasculature typical of normal myocardium. Vessels are seen in interstitium among cardiomyocytes on hematoxylin and eosin–stained section (*panel A*) and more clearly on a section stained with an antibody to CD-31 (*panel B*).

Figure 7-2.
Neovascularity associated with myocardial infarction. These tissue specimens were harvested at necropsy from a patient with fatal myocardial infarction. The tissue was formalin fixed, paraffin embedded, and stained with hematoxylin and eosin for light microscopic examination. Additional immunohistochemical staining with CD31 was performed to identify endothelial cells as well as vascular endothelial growth factor (VEGF). **A**, Hematoxylin and eosin–stained section showing focus of myocardial fibrosis and lymphocytic infiltrate. **B**, Section stained with CD-31 explicitly identifies infarct-related vascularity. (*continued on next page*)

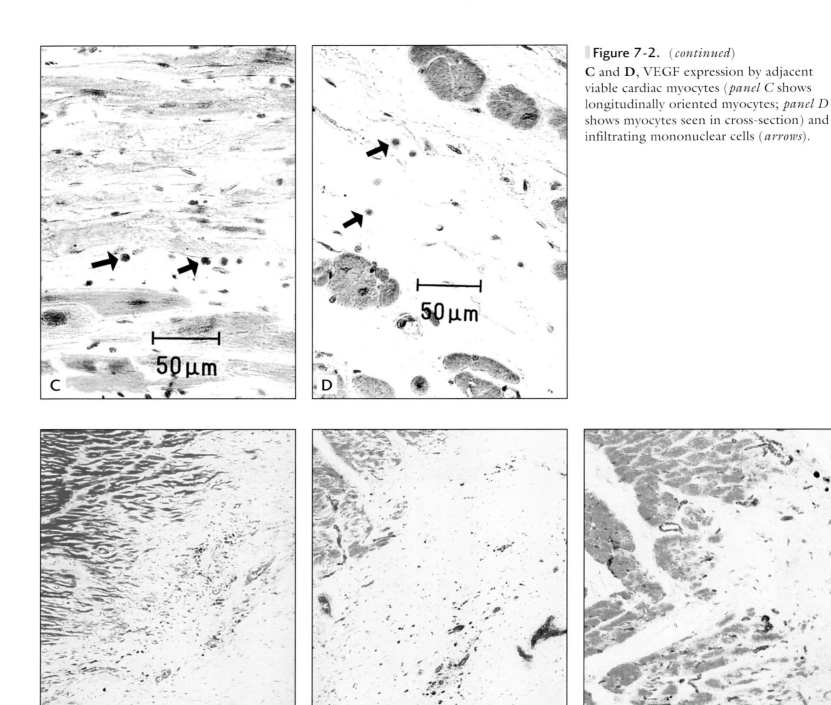

Figure 7-2. *(continued)*
C and **D**, VEGF expression by adjacent viable cardiac myocytes (*panel C* shows longitudinally oriented myocytes; *panel D* shows myocytes seen in cross-section) and infiltrating mononuclear cells (*arrows*).

Figure 7-3.

Vascularity associated with laser-induced myocardial wound in a dog. **A,** Multiple neovascular channels, as well as focal hemosiderin deposits, are observed at the site of the laser-induced myocardial fibrosis. **B** and **C,** The vascular channels seen on the hematoxylin and eosin–stained section are more easily identified on the section stained specifically for endothelial cells with an antibody (*reddish brown*). Smaller caliber vessels within the muscle fibers at the periphery of this fibrotic area, nearly undetectable on hematoxylin and eosin, are also identified with the antibody to factor VIII–related antigen (Ag). (*continued on next page*)

Figure 7-3. (*continued*)
D, Adjacent muscle fibers are expressing vascular endothelial growth factor protein detected by immunohistochemistry.

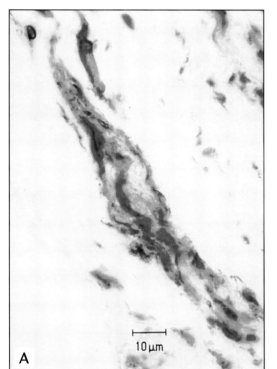

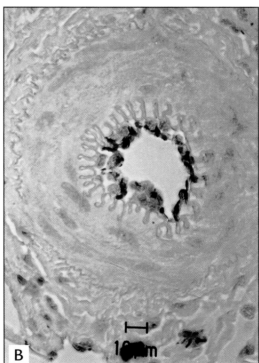

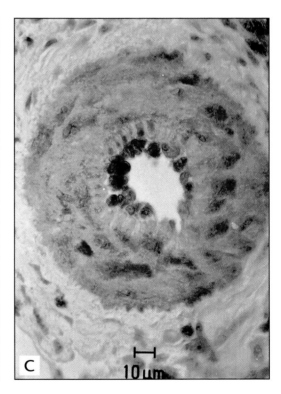

Figure 7-4.

Expression of the potent angiogenic cytokine, vascular endothelial growth factor (VEGF), by smooth muscle and endothelial cells in the artery wall. **A,** Double immunohistochemical staining for VEGF (*brown*) and smooth muscle α-actin (*red*) demonstrates smooth muscle cell production of VEGF in this specimen retrieved by directional atherectomy from a primary coronary atherosclerotic stenosis. **B** and **C,** Tissue specimen harvested from ischemic hind limbs of a C57 mouse. Immunohistochemical staining of adjacent sections illustrates that the intimal layer of endothelial cells (*B*) (*red/brown*; stained with CD31), medial layer of smooth muscle cells, and adventitia are producing VEGF (C) (*yellowish brown*). (Part A *from* Couffinhal and coworkers [1]; with permission.)

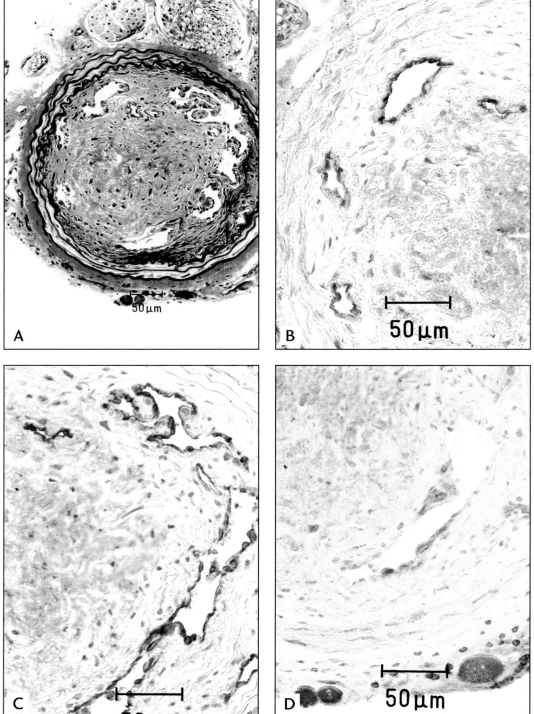

Figure 7-5.
Plaque neovascularization. Sections of
carotid artery from an ApoE[-/-]3 mouse
sacrificed 8 weeks after wire injury was performed. The histologic appearance suggests
that the artery has been totally occluded
but has now been partially recanalized.
A, Elastic tissue trichrome-stained section.
B and **C,** CD-31 immunostaining illustrates that these newly formed channels are
lined by endothelial cells. **D,** In addition,
immunostaining discloses an abundance of
vascular endothelial growth factor (VEGF).

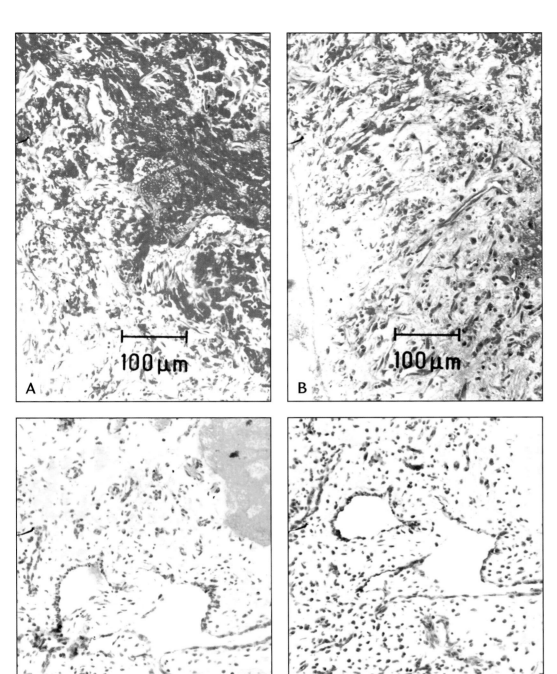

Figure 7-6.
Tissue retrieved by directional atherectomy from a primary coronary atherosclerotic lesion. **A** and **B**, Elastic tissue trichrome-stained sections. This tissue contains abundant neovasculature adjacent to an organizing thrombus. Endothelial cells were identified by immunohistochemical staining with both CD-31 (*panel C*) as well as CD-34 (*panel D*).

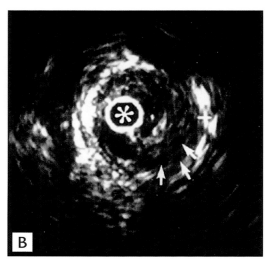

A

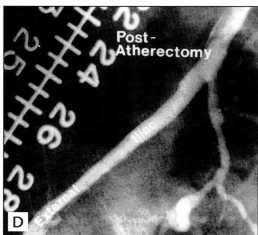

B

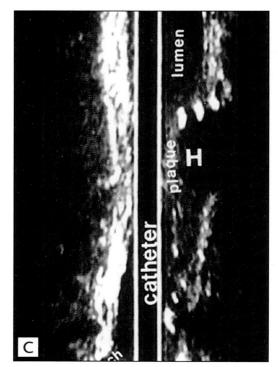

C

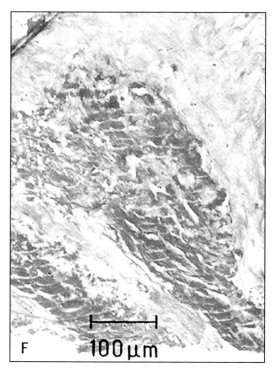

D

Figure 7-7.

Plaque rupture. Clinical and pathologic finding in a patient with crescendo claudication. **A,** Diagnostic arteriogram showing irregular, high-grade stenosis (*arrow*) in the right external iliac artery. **B,** Two-dimensional intravascular ultrasound (*asterisk* indicates the ultrasound transducer) obtained before atherectomy showing heterogeneous plaque with hypoechoic foci that are consistent with plaque hemorrhage (*arrows*). **C,** Three-dimensional reconstruction of intravascular ultrasound examination showing right external iliac artery narrowed by segmental stenosis that abuts the ultrasound catheter (hypoechoic foci of plaque hemorrhage [H] is now seen in longitudinal disposition). **D,** Angiogram obtained after atherectomy. In corroboration, the histologic findings in this case disclosed an apparent plaque rupture. **E,** Extensive foci of thrombus interspersed with fibrous tissue and hypocellular plaque tissue are present, which are consistent with plaque hemorrhage. **F,** The hemorrhagic fissures within the plaque extended to the edge of the specimen. **G,** As shown by the presence of medial elements (*black*) on this section, luminal thrombus adhered to the intimal surface of the specimen. (*From* Mecley and coworkers [2]; with permission.)

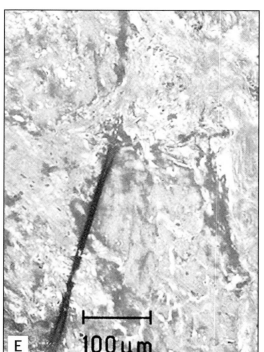

E   100 μm

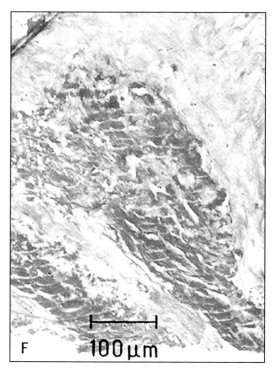

F   100 μm

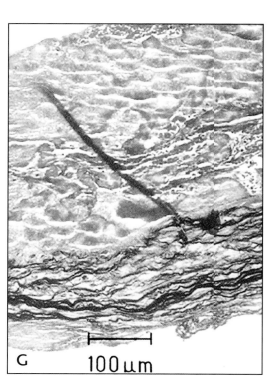

G   100 μm

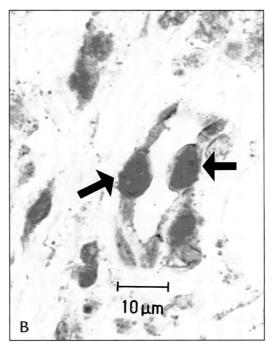

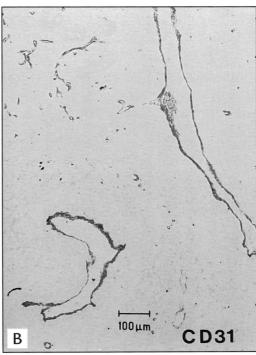

Figure 7-8.
Lower limb neovascularity associated with intramuscular vascular endothelial growth factor gene therapy. Shown is endothelial cell proliferation in two vessels (*panels A and B*) of tissue section harvested after below-the-knee amputation in a patient treated with intramuscular gene therapy. Double immunohistochemical staining with CD31 (*brown*), and Ki67 (*red*) illustrates proliferating endothelial cells (*arrows*). (*From* Baumgartner and coworkers [3]; with permission.)

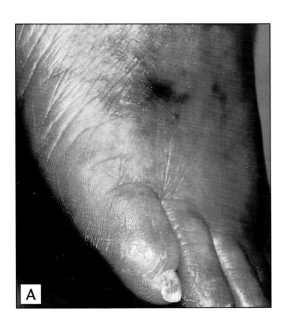

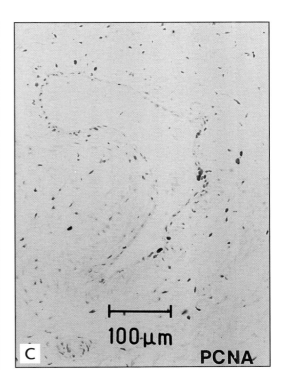

Figure 7-9.

Telangiectasia ("spider") developing in ischemic foot of a patient treated with intra-arterial vascular endothelial growth factor gene therapy. **A,** One of three spider angiomas that developed approximately 1 week after gene therapy in the distal portion of the ischemic limb. **B,** Tissue sections stained with antibody to endothelial antigen CD31 showing vascularity of lesion. **C,** Stain of adjacent section for proliferating cell nuclear antigen (PCNA) showing the extent of proliferative activity among endothelial cells in lesion. (*From* Isner and coworkers [4]; with permission.)

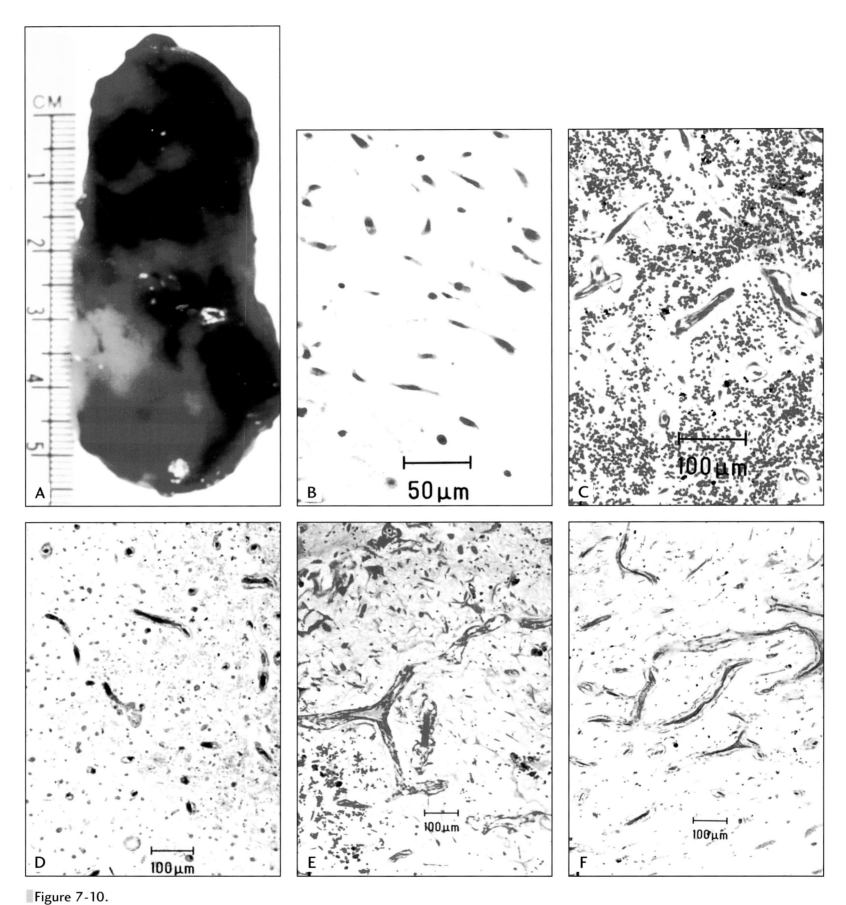

Figure 7-10.

Neovascularity and vascular endothelial growth factor (VEGF) expression in left atrial myxoma. **A,** Gross photograph taken of a surgically excised left atrial myxoma. **B** and **C,** Sections stained with hematoxylin and eosin illustrating classic myxoma cellularity seen singly or in small clusters within a rich extracellular matrix. Hemorrhage, evident in *panel* *A,* is also clearly seen in *panel C.* **D,** Microvasculature of myxoma demonstrates by anti–factor VIII immunostaining. **E,** Typical myxoma tube-like channels are composed of endothelial cells, demonstrated by CD-34 immunostaining in *panel F.* (*continued on next page*)

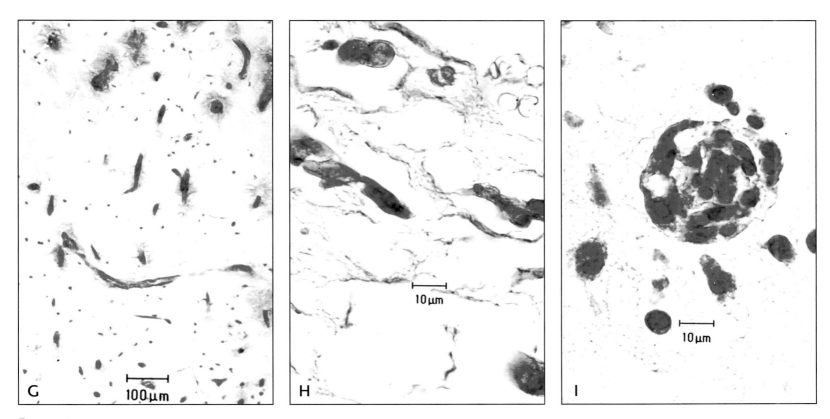

Figure 7-10. (*continued*)

G to **I**, Myxoma vascularity likely results from robust VEGF expression by myxoma cells, seen singly (*panel G*) or in clusters (*panels H* and *I*, both double immunostained for VEGF [*brown*] and CD-34 [*red*].)

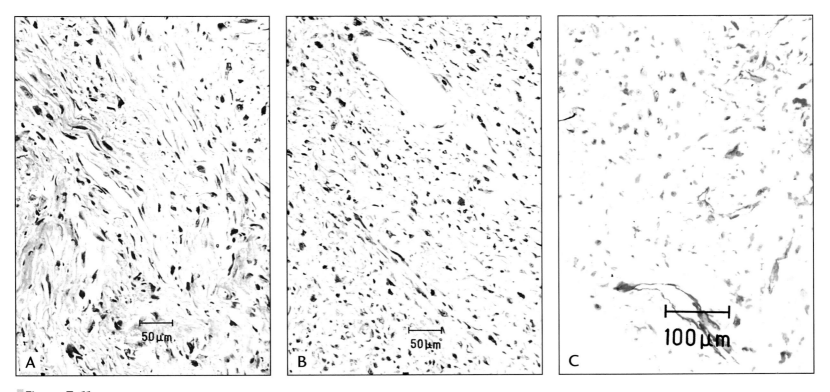

Figure 7-11.

Vascularity and vascular endothelial growth factor (VEGF) expression in angiosarcoma. Human angiosarcoma, hematoxylin and eosin–stained sections (*panels A and B*), as well as sections stained for CD31 (*panel C*), reveal many small blood vessels, including some dilated vessels. (*continued on next page*)

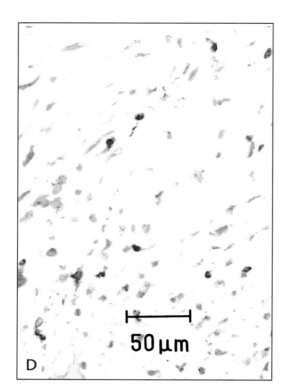

Figure 7-11. (*continued*)
VEGF protein, detected immunohistochemically (*panel D*), was expressed by multiple tumor cells.

REFERENCES

1. Couffinhal T, Kearney M, Witzenbichler B, *et al.*: Vascular endothelial growth factor/vascular permeability factor (VEGF/VPF) in normal and atherosclerotic human arteries. *Am J Pathol* 1997, 150:1673–1685.

2. Mecley M, Rosenfield K, Kaufman J, *et al.*: Atherosclerotic plaque hemorrhage and rupture associated with crescendo claudication. *Ann Intern Med* 1992, 117:663–666.

3. Baumgartner I, Pieczek A, Manor O, *et al.*: Constitutive expression of phVEGF165 after intramuscular gene transfer promotes collateral vessel development in patients with critical limb ischemia. *Circulation* 1998, 97:1114–1123.

4. Isner JM, Pieczek A, Schainfeld R, *et al.*: Clinical evidence of angiogenesis after arterial gene transfer of phVEGF165 in patient with ischaemic limb. *Lancet* 1996, 348:370–374.

Pulmonary Vascular Disease

John C. English

The pulmonary circulatory system contains many features that reflect its unique physiologic role. The lung is an organ with a dual circulation: pulmonary and bronchial. The pulmonary arterial circuit is responsible for directing the entire right ventricular output through a divergent system of vessels, ultimately forming an anastomosing capillary network where gas exchange takes place. The pulmonary circulation can respond to local alterations in alveolar hypoxia by shunting blood flow away from the hypoxic segment in an attempt to optimize perfusion with ventilation. The control of flow and pressure resides within intra-acinar vessels with diameters of 30 to 300 μm [1], the size range including vessels defined as small arteries and arterioles. Many humoral factors have been identified that operate in the normal regulation of vascular tone. Endothelium-derived nitric oxide is currently accepted as the prime pulmonary vascular vasodilator; the endothelium produces a variety of compounds, such as endothelin, angiotensin II, thromboxane A_2, and PGH_2 that are active in vasoconstriction [1]. Both vasodilatory and vasoconstrictive substances may also influence pulmonary vascular smooth muscle growth and vascular remodeling [2].

The morphology of the pulmonary vessels reflects their function. Because the circulation is one of low pressure and low resistance, the vessels, especially the arteries, have wider lumens and thinner medial layers than their systemic counterparts. This feature may hinder the distinction between artery and vein to those less familiar with microscopic pulmonary structure. The appearance of the pulmonary vasculature changes with respect to age; for example, in the fetus and neonate, the tunica media of the preacinar muscular arteries demonstrates increased thickness relative to the young adult. Remodeling toward the thinner adult structure proceeds rapidly in the postnatal period and at a slower pace during childhood [3], although often at rates that vary widely among individuals, especially in the first 3 months of life. Intra-acinar arteries, on the other hand, gradually acquire a smooth muscle coat that progressively extends toward the periphery of the respiratory unit [4]. Such development reaches mature levels by 7 years of age [3]. In older patients, intimal thickening, more fibrous than cellular in nature, is an accepted age-related change in both arteries and veins and does not necessarily indicate the presence of pulmonary hypertension.

The bronchial circulation supplies the nutritive component of the lung circulatory system, accounting for 1% of cardiac output; however, this may increase to as much as 30% in patients with cystic fibrosis and congenital heart disease [5]. Bronchial arteries are identified in close association with the conducting airways as far distal as the membranous bronchioles. The tunica media of the bronchiolar arteries is much thicker than that of the corresponding pulmonary arteries, and their dimensions are partially augmented by a layer of longitudinal smooth muscle internal to the typical circular smooth muscle layer. Anastomosis between the bronchial and pulmonary circulation occurs, and this communication contributes to the pathophysiology of hemorrhagic infarction after certain pulmonary thromboembolic events.

The pulmonary veins are readily recognizable within the loose fibrous tissue of the interlobular septae. The elastic arrangement of these thin-walled vessels differs from the structure of their arterial counterparts. Whereas the internal elastic lamina is easy to recognize, a prominent external layer is absent or at least difficult to distinguish. The true disposition of intra-acinar venules is only evident when confluence with an obvious vein is verified.

Proper preparation of lung specimens is necessary if critical assessment of the vasculature is intended. Although direct perfusion of the vasculature with a fixative agent may seem logical, a great potential exists for overdistention of the vessels with apparent loss of smooth muscle in the smaller vessels unless the pressures are controlled closely and consistent methodology is used [6]. The recommended technique is to infuse fixative into the lung through the bronchi or, in the case of a wedge biopsy, through needle injection directly into the lung. Even airway distention causes slight thinning of the tunica media of small vessels [7], probably as a result of traction on the vessels suspended within the parenchyma. Preparing lung tissue for optimal exposure of vascular architecture is best accomplished when the plane of section is perpendicular to the axial radiation of the vascular tree as it extends peripherally. This plane of section may not, however, be ideal for examination of other lung diseases such as interstitial pneumonitis. It is important to recognize that many vascular lesions, especially those of pulmonary hypertensive states, are often focal in their distribution; therefore, serial sections may be required for their identification.

In addition to hematoxylin and eosin, other histochemical stains are useful for demonstrating the subcomponents of the vascular wall. An elastic stain such as the Verhoff–van Gieson is indispensable when interpreting pulmonary vascular development and pathology. A more complex stain, such as the Movat pentachrome method, allows for visualization of the elastica as well as separate differentiation of smooth muscle, collagenous fibrous tissue, and acid mucopolysaccharide ground substances; many of the figures in this chapter use this stain. Other special stains for identifying amyloid, iron hemosiderin, fat, and microorganisms are periodically required.

Diseases of the pulmonary vasculature may be approached through etiology or morphology; congenital or acquired entities contribute in both instances. Many, but not all, discussions of pulmonary vascular disease focus on associations with the pulmonary hypertensive state, and the number of potentially culpable diseases is vast. In many cases, the pathologic expression of the developing or endpoint lesions overlaps multiple inciting causes, such as the presence of the arterial plexiform lesion in certain forms of primary pulmonary hypertension (PPH) and in hypertension secondary to congenital heart disease. When applied to the study of pulmonary vascular pathology, a morphologic approach results in a simple categorization of the ways in which the vessels are altered: 1) changes in the structure of the vessel wall, which may include pathological thickening, dilation, inflammation, necrosis, or accumulation of substances through altered metabolism or local excess production; 2) substances within the vascular lumen, most commonly thought of in the context of emboli, either endogenous (*eg*, thromboemboli, tumor, fat) or exogenous (*eg*, talc, iatrogenic substances); 3) abnormalities in structural connections, which embrace the scope of congenital cardiovascular lesions involving the lung and may also predicate certain lesions identified in items 1 and 2; 4) proliferative vascular disease, which is a limited form of change and essentially restricted to the entity known as pulmonary capillary hemangiomatosis (possibly overlapping with pulmonary venoocclusive disease) and the rare pulmonary angioma; and 5) traumatic disruption of a pulmonary vessel, either from iatrogenic cause or external injury.

This chapter concentrates on lesions of vascular wall structure and intraluminal substances, which together encompass the majority of diseases commonly involving the pulmonary vascular system. A short description of arteriovenous malformations is the only incursion into congenital lesions apart from the pulmonary hypertensive changes induced by them; the pathology of congenital heart disease is presented in chapter 2. Likewise, vasculitis is discussed elsewhere and is not repeated here. A complete clinical review of many of the diseases covered in this chapter may be found in volume III of the *Atlas of Heart Diseases* [8–12].

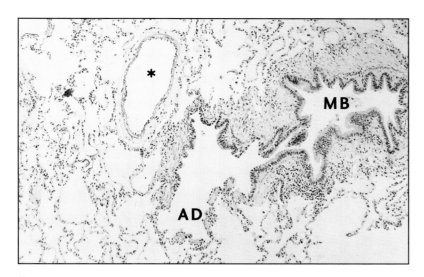

Figure 8-1.

Normal pulmonary artery and corresponding bronchiole. The walls of normal pulmonary arteries tend to be much thinner relative to the luminal diameter compared with their counterparts in the systemic circulation. This disparity becomes more confounding to the inexperienced observer when assessing the smaller vessels within the pulmonary acinus, where arteries may appear veinlike.

This photomicrograph depicts a normal pulmonary artery (*asterisk*) and its corresponding airway, which can be seen in transition between the terminal membranous bronchiole (MB) and alveolar duct (AD) levels. The media is composed of a thin layer of smooth muscle enclosed by both an internal and external elastic lamina; the thickness of the media is approximately 5% of the external diameter of the vessel.

In vessels with diameters larger than 66 μm, there is a complete muscular coat bound by internal and external elastic laminae. Below this diameter, however, the muscle layer becomes discontinuous, eventually disappearing and ultimately leaving a single remaining elastic lamina as the major wall structure. This transition occurs at the respiratory bronchiolar level, and vessels of this type are often referred to by some as pulmonary arterioles. The classification and nomenclature of these smaller pulmonary arterial vessels have been debated, and a wide range of criteria based on the presence of elastic laminae [13] or size [14] have been given. Physiologic alterations in pulmonary pressure may, however, affect vessel size and stimulate the acquisition of a smooth muscle coat where none previously existed, thus complicating the assessment of vessel classification. These factors, plus the requirement for multiple histologic sections and special stains, suggest to some that the term *pulmonary arteriole* should be abandoned [15].

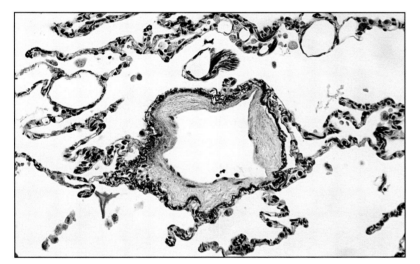

Figure 8-2.

Age-related venous intimal sclerosis. Acellular, hyaline thickening of the pulmonary venous intima is well recognized as an age-related phenomenon. Although this thickening may be brought about by pulmonary hypertension (PHT) and coexist with other lesions, by itself it should not be interpreted as a sign of PHT. Failure to recognize the structure as venous may lead to the erroneous diagnosis of arterial hypertensive change. The photomicrograph (from the same specimen as in Fig. 8-29) demonstrates the acellular fibrous intima and the elastic media with focal elastic reduplication.

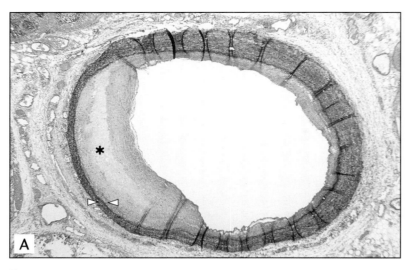

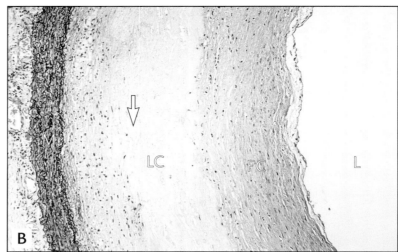

Figure 8-3.

Atherosclerosis. **A,** Low-power photomicrograph demonstrating the eccentric intimal thickening characteristic of atherosclerosis. The typical plaque architecture is also well represented with the lighter hypocellular central area denoting the necrotic lipid core (*asterisk*) and an overlying fibrous cap composed of dense fibrous tissue. Note the medial atrophy (between *arrowheads*) subjacent to the atherosclerotic plaque. The darker radially oriented bands represent an artefactual contraction of the arterial wall during histologic processing, most likely related to the elastic tissue content of the vessel. **B,** In a higher magnification of the same specimen, the components of the atherosclerotic plaque are identified. Directly underneath the endothelial layer, the fibrous cap (FC) is formed by compacted layers of collagen and cells of the smooth muscle myofibroblast type. External to this is a relatively hypocellular layer representing the necrotic lipid core (LC). The clear spaces within the core denote areas of cholesterol and lipid debris extracted through histologic processing. The lenticular or needle-shaped spaces are the so-called "cholesterol clefts" (*arrow*). Macrophages,

lymphocytes, and plasma cells form the mononuclear inflammatory cell population adjacent to the core. Atherosclerosis within the pulmonary system is not as common as in the systemic arterial system because of the lower pressures generated by the right-sided cardiac circulation and decreased susceptibility to abnormal turbulence and other physical forces potentially injurious to the endothelium. When present, however, the appearance is identical to the lesions found in the systemic circulation. Pulmonary atherosclerosis has been associated with advanced age, right ventricular hypertrophy and dilation, emphysema, and atherosclerosis of the aorta [16]. The presence of atherosclerosis in older patients probably reflects the effects of focal damage to the vascular wall secondary to turbulence from unfolding of the larger elastic arteries. The presence of atheromas within segmental or smaller vessels should lead to the investigation for other manifestations of pulmonary hypertension. Pulmonary artery atherosclerosis is almost universally present in cases of pulmonary hypertension from either congenital or acquired origin [17]. L—lumen; M—tunica media.

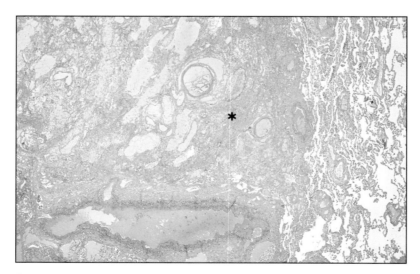

Figure 8-4.

Pulmonary infarct. The infarcted lung parenchyma is seen in the *center* and *left side* of the micrograph (*asterisk*). Although rem-

nants of parenchymal architectural detail may still be identified within the infarcted area, evidence of cell viability, such as nuclear staining, is lost. There is collapse of alveoli combined with hemorrhage and edema. Noninfarcted lung is present on the *right side* with a fairly sharp demarcation from the infarct. As documented histologically, the first stages of a pulmonary infarct are marked by capillary engorgement and intraparenchymal hemorrhage. By the second day, necrosis is visible and sections may show vascular damage with thrombosis involving all components of the peripheral pulmonary vascular system. At 1 week after infarction, organization begins and may progress for several weeks or months with progressive formation of granulation tissue from the periphery toward the center of the lesion, resolving as a fibroelastic scar. Reactive changes such as cuboidal cell and squamous cell metaplasia may accompany the healing process. In some cases, the physiologic events do not lead to the classical complete infarct but eventuate only in edema and hemorrhage that resolve without apparent distortion to the lung, termed an "incomplete" infarct [18].

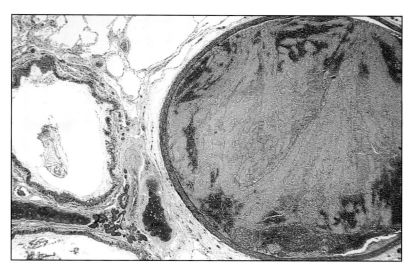

Figure 8-5.
Acute pulmonary thromboembolus. The musculoelastic pulmonary artery is distended by a recent thromboembolus that

occludes the lumen. Alternating layers of fibrin, platelets, leukocytes, and erythrocytes form the classic histologic pattern. Differences in the degree to which thromboemboli are composed of these elements depend on a variety of factors, such as blood flow, coagulation status, microvascular environment (both parent and receiving vessels), parenchymal disease, and chronology of formation. Thrombi that have formed for some time before embolization may be expected to display histologic evidence of organization at their periphery, derived from the in situ relationship with the parent vein. Those that have been present within the pulmonary artery for some time display changes of organization proportional to their duration at that site. In cases of death caused by acute pulmonary thromboembolism, little if any organization between the embolus and the pulmonary vessel will be present. Treated acute pulmonary thromboemboli rarely result in chronic thromboembolic pulmonary hypertension, and perfusion scans demonstrate return to normal perfusion within 1 year in 82% of patients [19].

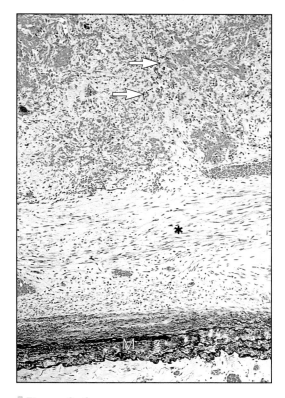

Figure 8-6.
The relationship of a thromboembolus to the vessel in which it has impacted. At the *bottom*, the native smooth muscle and elastic lamellae of the arterial media are identified. Superficial (luminal) to this there is a thickened intimal plaque composed of attenuated spindled myofibroblasts (*asterisk*) with an acid mucopolysaccharide matrix (*blue*). The overlying thrombus contains many small slitlike endothelial-lined channels (*arrows*) that represent neovascularization of the thrombus as part of the process of organization. An acid mucopolysaccharide ground substance matrix has replaced much of the mass of the thrombus. There are aggregates of erythrocytes throughout, which may be residual unresorbed cells from the initial mass or recent hemorrhage from the delicate infiltrating vessels.

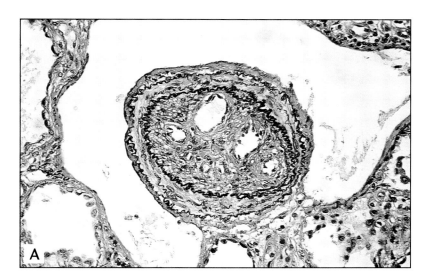

Figure 8-7.
Chronic arterial thrombus. **A,** A pulmonary artery in which the lumen is filled by a thrombus that has undergone advanced changes of organization so that small channels have formed ("recanalization"). Blood flow may resume to some extent through these channels. The substance of the thrombus at this point is composed of dense fibroelastic tissue with variable numbers of cells such as myofibroblasts. The rounded, punched-out appearance of the channels is responsible for the term "colander lesion." This feature is useful because it provides a distinction from the plexiform lesion of certain types of primary and secondary pulmonary hypertension (*see* Fig. 8-15). There is also muscular hypertrophy of the media. (*continued on next page*)

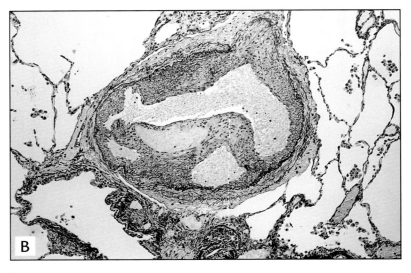

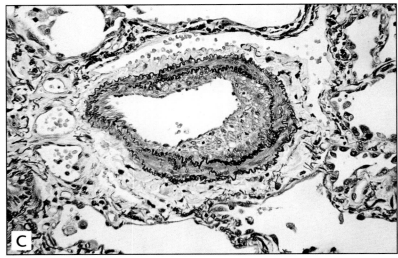

Figure 8-7. (*continued*)

B, In some cases, organization of a thrombus results in larger channels formed by definite septae that bridge the intima. In this example, the septae are composed of dense fibroelastic bands. The areas of acellular collagen indicate the chronicity of the process.

C, Micrograph demonstrating an eccentric intimal plaque. In small pulmonary arteries, such plaques are thought to represent the residual changes from subtotal thrombosis or small throm-

boemboli in which the thrombus and its subsequent organization have remained sessile rather than occlusive. Both of these lesions may be identified in certain forms of primary pulmonary hypertension (thrombotic type) as well as in secondary pulmonary hypertension from any of the thrombotic or embolic causes. (*Panel B* from English [76]; with permission.)

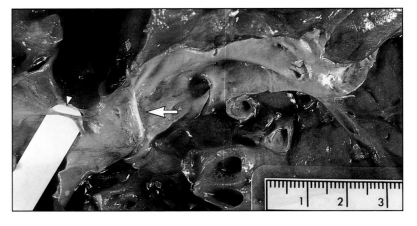

Figure 8-8.

Chronic recurrent pulmonary thromboemboli and webs. Larger elastic and musculoelastic pulmonary arteries rarely exhibit chronic occlusion by an organized thrombus or thromboembolus [20]. The residual tissue consists of fibrous band or webs (*arrow*) demonstrated by dissecting the proximal pulmonary arterial tree. In this example, the pulmonary artery has been dissected to display a transverse fibrous septum (*arrowhead*) and an intimal web crossing over the white marker.

Secondary Pulmonary Hypertension

HEATH-EDWARDS GRADING SYSTEM

Grade 1
  Medial hypertrophy of muscular arteries
  Muscularization of pulmonary arterioles
Grade 2
  Medial hypertrophy
  Cellular intimal proliferation
Grade 3
  Medial hypertrophy
  Intimal fibrosis
Grade 4
  Occlusive intimal fibrosis
  Dilation lesions
  Plexiform lesions
Grade 5
  Veinlike branches with rupture and hemorrhage
  Angiomatoid lesions
Grade 6
  Fibrinoid necrosis
  Arteritis

Figure 8-9.

Heath-Edwards grading system for secondary pulmonary hypertension (PHT). The spectrum of lesions of the pulmonary vasculature related to PHT is more diverse than in the equivalent systemic disease. Most pathologists are likely to confront these changes in the context of secondary PHT, commonly diseases associated with congestive heart failure, chronic lung disease, or areas of the lung involved by cancer. In these conditions, the pulmonary vascular changes are usually seen as combinations of medial hypertrophy, intimal proliferation or congestive vasculopathy involving veins and the capillary bed, possibly with acute or chronic alveolar hemorrhage. The large elastic arteries may demonstrate shallow atheromas that extend into the segmental arterial radicals. The lesions associated with secondary PHT caused by congenital heart disease are seen in practice settings that deal with a large pediatric patient population, and they exhibit a wide variety of appearances that may also denote disease progression.

In the 1950s, Heath and Edwards [21] published a description of the pulmonary arterial changes that were identified in the context of congenital heart defects and the association of these changes with PHT. These authors found six grades of lesions that reflected the progression of disease and, when present, could predict potential reversibility of the arterial lesions and reduction in PHT after correction of the cardiac defect [22]. Long-term follow-up studies have validated this concept [23]. In this concept of lesion formation, the earliest changes reflecting PHT begin with hypertrophy of the tunica media and muscularization of pulmonary arterioles. With progression of medial hypertrophy, intimal thickening occurs, first as

a cellular proliferation of myofibroblasts or smooth muscle cells, but subsequently with fibrosis that may be subtotal or severely narrow or occlude the vascular lumen, a change that heralds severe PHT. Appearance of the unique plexiform lesion with accompanying forms of arterial dilation indicates irreversibility. There is progressive arterial dilation to form veinlike branches that are fragile and give rise to hemorrhage. Fibrinoid necrosis or necrotizing vasculitis denotes the most severe grade. By convention, lung biopsies are assigned the highest grade observed. A range of lesions is usually present; for example, if a biopsy shows the presence of plexiform lesions (grade 4), then examples of medial hypertrophy, alone and in combination with intimal proliferation, should also be found elsewhere in the biopsy. The lesions of the Heath-Edwards scheme are identified in forms of PHT other than secondary to congenital heart defects with left-to-right shunts, but it must be stressed that the prognostic significance does not necessarily extend to those conditions and a grade designation may only serve as a descriptor. Clearly, however, the presence of plexiform lesions and fibrinoid necrosis indicates severe and irreversible PHT. As Wagenwoort [24] cautions, assessment of the pulmonary hypertensive state through morphology must include assessment of the capillary and venous portions of the circuit as well as the arteries.

In the years of use and scrutiny after publication of the Heath-Edwards grading scheme, several problems have arisen, as recounted by Kay [25]. First, fibrinoid arteriopathy has been documented in advance of the advent of plexiform lesions and presumably predicates their formation [26]. Rather than use this as evidence to negate the grading system, however, it is justified to distinguish areas of bland fibrinoid change within a segment of an arterial wall from the severe necrotic change associated with fulminant arteritis. A second defect in the original scheme was that it did not discriminate between degrees of laminar intimal fibrosis. This oversight is significant because mild intimal fibrosis is reversible [27], in contrast to the severe concentric form. Others [14,24] have emphasized that a qualitative description may not extract all the important information possible from a biopsy and suggest that a morphometric analysis provides a more complete assessment of the degree of pulmonary hypertensive changes. Other observations not considered in the Heath-Edwards scheme include noting the degree of fibrosis involving the media, which may predict response to vasodilator agents [28], and quantifying the number of peripheral arteries relative to alveolar density. This may be a useful index of disease in the first 2 years of life when the advanced lesions of the Heath-Edwards scheme are often not expressed even in the face of severe PHT [29]. Reduction of peripheral arteries has been shown to correlate with increased pulmonary vascular resistance [30].

Despite attempts at refining a more precise grading system than that offered by Heath and Edwards more than 40 years ago, the fact remains that the presence of any of the original grade 4 lesions or worse indicates severe and irreversible PHT. Furthermore, the presence of any one of the advanced lesions does not indicate a prognosis that is distinct from the other two [24]. (*Adapted from* Heath and Edwards [21].)

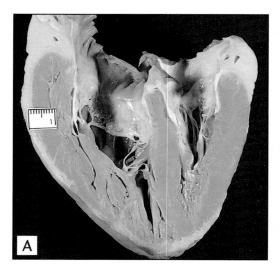
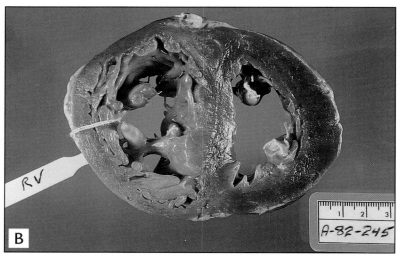

Figure 8-10.

Right ventricular hypertrophy. **A,** Explanted heart from a 29-year-old woman with primary pulmonary hypertension (PHT). This heart is sectioned in the four-chamber view (atria absent because of transplant procedure) and illustrates hypertrophy of the right ventricular wall, including prominent trabeculae and papillary muscles. The normal thickness of the right ventricular wall is 0.3 to 0.5 cm. In this case, the left ventricle is of normal size. **B,** Cross-section in the mid-ventricular plane of a heart removed at autopsy in a patient with multiple recurrent pulmonary emboli. The thickness of the hypertrophied right ventricle approximates that of the left ventricle. The section also demonstrates the characteristic straightening of the interventricular septum producing D-shaped ventricular cavities, replacing the normally crescent-shaped right ventricular cavity and the concentric left ventricular cavity.

Right ventricular hypertrophy and dilation caused by either primary pulmonary parenchymal or vascular hypertensive disease is termed *cor pulmonale* [31]. Although direct measurement of ventricular wall thickness is useful in noncritical documentation of obvious instances of right ventricular hypertrophy, a more precise methodology entails separation of the right ventricular free wall from the rest of the heart (including the fat and atria) and comparing the weight with the similarly dissected left ventricle and interventricular septum [32]. If the total ventricular weight is less than 250 g, acceptable right ventricular weights are less than 61 g for men and 50 g for women. In this context, ratios for right to left ventricular weights (LV + IVS/RV) are between 2.3:1 and 3.3:1. In older individuals, cases of coexistent valvular, systemic hypertensive, or ischemic disease, the left ventricular weight may be substantially altered, thus making it difficult to interpret the ratios. In this situation, an acceptable upper limit of normal right ventricular weight is about 71 g [33].

Primary Pulmonary Hypertension

PRIMARY PULMONARY HYPERTENSION

WHO	Burke *et al.* [53]	WHO Equivalent	Edwards *et al.* [37] and Pietra *et al.* [38]	WHO Equivalent
PPA	Arterial		PPA	
RPT	Plexiform type	PPA	Plexigenic type	PPA
PVOD	Primary medial or intimal type	PPA*	Thrombotic type	RPT
	Thrombotic type	RPT	Fibrotic type (concentric or occlusive)	RPT
	Orther rare forms		Fibrotic type (concentric laminar)	PPA
	Medial dysplasia	ND†	Isolated arteritis type	PPA
	Isolated arteritis	ND‡	Isolated medial hypertrophy type	PPA
	Venous		Rare forms	
	Veno-occlusive disease	PVOD	Medial defect type	ND
	Capillary hemangiomatosis	ND†	Misaligned vessel type	ND
			PVOD	PVOD
			Pulmonary capillary hemangiomatosis	ND†

*In many cases presumed to be antecedent of typical plexiform lesion development; may exist exclusive of other lesions.
†Not defined by WHO.
‡Not defined by WHO; designated as PPA equivalent by Edwards and coworkers [37] and Pietra and coworkers [38]

Figure 8-11.

Primary pulmonary hypertension (PPH). PPH is an uncommon disease of unknown etiology and variable vascular changes. It is a diagnosis of exclusion. The National Institutes of Health (NIH) registry diagnostic criteria include mean pulmonary artery pressure of greater than 25 mm Hg at rest or 30 mm Hg during exercise and no evidence of other known causes of pulmonary hypertension) (PHT), such as left-sided valvular disease, myocardial disease, congenital heart disease, chronic thromboembolic disease, or other chronic systemic or pulmonary disease [34]. For details regarding the clinical aspects of PPH, see Channick [8].

The pathogenesis of PPH is unknown; however, the commonly accepted view is that there is some element of vasoconstriction, either as a primary event or secondary to some injurious stimulus applied to the endothelium in a susceptible individual. Associated adverse events such as local thrombosis, cytokine and growth factor imbalance [35], and vasoconstrictor or vasodilator imbalance may then combine in various proportions to propagate the disease process, ultimately serving to reduce the pulmonary vasculature cross-sectional area and impair normal vascular response [36]. The assorted routes by which this state is achieved and the different potential susceptibilities of individuals to multiple forms of insult may explain the variable morphologic expressions witnessed in these patients. The pathology of PPH is, therefore, diverse, encompassing not only arterial lesions but also including distinct forms in which venous and capillary changes dominate. All arterial forms of PPH (and also secondary PHT) display medial thickening and intimal proliferation, but thrombosis, plexiform and dilation lesions, and arteritis are not present in all patients. This diversity is responsible for subdivision into morphologic classification systems. For comments on veno-occlusive disease and pulmonary capillary hemangiomatosis, *see* Figures 8-17 and 8-18, respectively. ND —not defined; PPA—plexogenic pulmonary arteriopathy; PVOD—pulmonary veno-occlusive disease; RPT—recurrent pulmonary thromboembolism; WHO—World Health Organization.

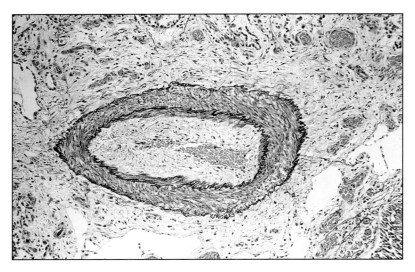

Figure 8-12.

Medial hypertrophy and cellular intimal hyperplasia. This artery demonstrates prominent medial hypertrophy, the thickness of the media being approximately 25% of the diameter of the vessel wall (external elastic lamina to external elastic lamina). Normally, the media is 5% or less of the total wall diameter. Medial hypertrophy is the most commonly identified vascular alteration in pulmonary hypertension (PHT) [39] and is not restricted to any particular etiology. Hypertrophy is caused by an increase in both size and

numbers of medial smooth muscle cells, and the degree of hypertrophy parallels physiologic values of hypertension [40] with 7% to 10% thickness of total vessel diameter representing mild, 10% to 15% moderate, and more than 15% severe hypertrophy [41]. The earliest demonstrable vascular alteration, which is considered to be the antecedent of subsequent lesions in PHT, is the formation of an obvious muscular media within the arterioles [29]. These structures, which are normally devoid of smooth muscle at the 66- to 100-μm diameter level, may exhibit a prominent muscle coat enclosed by internal and external elastic laminae and this coat may extend down to vessels of the 20- to 30-μm level [25]. Muscularization of the media of arterioles and arteries is assigned grade 1 in the Heath-Edwards classification [21].

The same vessel also depicts concentric cellular intimal hyperplasia, grade 2 in the Heath-Edwards scheme, and is thought to represent a potentially reversible change. This lesion consists of thickening of the tunica intima by a layer of media-derived smooth muscle cells [42] that progressively transform toward a myofibroblastic phenotype, insinuated between the internal elastic lamina and the endothelium. In the initial stages, the orientation of the axes of these cells is thought to be radial or irregular rather than circumferential (which suggests a more advanced lesion). The process begins in the smaller vessels, on the order of less than 300 μm [21] with progressively more severe alterations extending to larger muscular arteries.

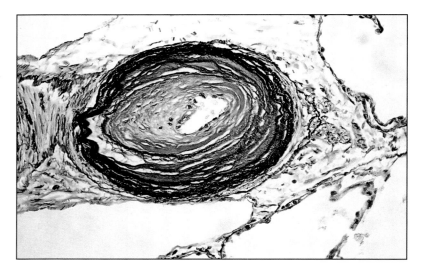

Figure 8-13.

Concentric laminar intimal fibrosis. The elastic stain used for this preparation demonstrates the features of concentric laminar intimal fibrosis (Heath-Edwards grade 3). The characteristic alteration consists of a circumferential lamellar deposition of fibrous and elastic tissue, often imparting an "onionskin" appearance to the vessel. Myofibroblasts also form part of the proliferating lesion. In severe examples, there may be atrophy of the tunica media. Because of the deposition of fibrous and elastic tissue, after it is established the occlusive change does not regress. Some believe that this lesion is the most reliable histologic indicator of the subset of primary pulmonary hypertension known as plexogenic pulmonary arteriopathy [43,44].

Figure 8-14.

Plexiform lesion. **A,** A cellular plexiform lesion close to a muscular pulmonary artery that displays medial hypertrophy and some intimal hyperplasia. The plexiform lesion consists of a conglomerate of cellular septae enclosing slitlike capillary channels imparting a "glomeruloid" appearance. The cellular constituents of the septae include myofibroblasts and smooth muscle and fibrillary cells [45]. A modified form of endothelial cell lines the channels. In older lesions, the septae may become less cellular and fibrotic and the lumens of the channels may widen, possibly causing confusion with the "colander" lesion of recanalized, luminal thrombosis (*see* Fig. 8-7A). Although not captured in the plane of this section, the plexiform lesion probably arises from the depicted muscular artery. (*continued on next page*)

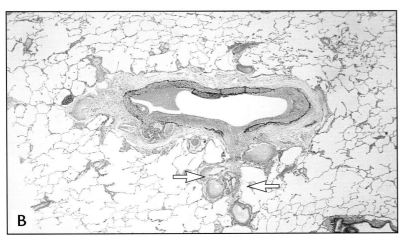

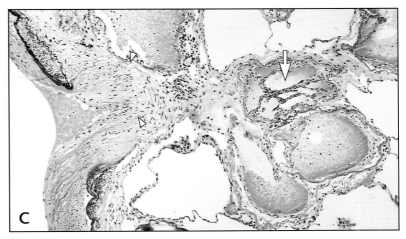

Figure 8-14. (*continued*)

B, Low-magnification photomicrograph of lung showing the origin of two plexiform lesions from a muscular pulmonary artery. At the origin of both lesions, note the discontinuity of the elastic lamina of the parent artery. There is intimal thickening around the neck of the origin of each plexiform lesion that immediately progresses to a dilated sac or cluster of angiomatoid vessels encompassing the smaller vascular channels (which are characteristic of the lesion). The large vessels extending from the plexiform lesions (*arrows*) represent one form of the entity known as the dilation lesion.

C, Higher magnification of *panel B.* This enlargement illustrates the prominent intimal hyperplasia of the parent muscular artery even as it extends down the side branch (*arrowheads*) giving rise to the plexiform lesion. Distal to the obstructed segment, there is a prominent dilated complex of vessels (*arrow*). The lumen of one of the dilated vessels is traversed by several thin septae. These are likely the residual septae of an older plexiform lesion in which the channels have widened. Adjacent to this structure are several aneurysmally dilated vessels, one of the manifestations of the so-called dilation lesion.

Plexiform lesions are designated, with their accompanying form of dilation lesions, as Heath-Edwards grade 4. They are present in pulmonary hypertensive states secondary to a number of etiologies such as congenital heart disease, portal hypertension, as well as in one of the types of unexplained or "primary" pulmonary hypertension. This lesion denotes the presence of severe pulmonary hypertension, although demonstration may require multiple histologic blocks and serial sections. Plexiform lesions are thought to arise from smaller branches of muscular pulmonary arteries close to their origin from a parent vessel [14] after focal fibrinoid degeneration of the vascular wall and aneurysmal dilation. Within this segment, the proliferating tuft of small vessels forms, causing arterial occlusion. The arterial segment just proximal to the plexiform nodule demonstrates fibroelastic narrowing [44].

The term "dilation lesion" encompasses a variety of alterations of the pulmonary arterial system, usually associated with plexiform and other high-grade hypertensive lesions. Heath and Edwards [21] identified four main forms: arterial dilation associated with plexiform lesions, 2) veinlike branches, 3) angiomatoid lesions, and 4) cavernous lesions.

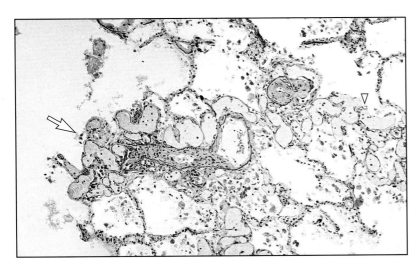

Figure 8-15.

Angiomatoid lesion with veinlike branches. The ectatic and dilated arterial branches that are associated with two plexiform lesions involving small pulmonary arteries are demonstrated here. Probably formed as either a poststenotic change or an attempt to bypass the stenosed region of plexiform lesion formation, these vessels are engorged with blood and because of the extreme thinning of the tunica media smooth muscle, take on the appearance of veins (hence the designation "veinlike branches"). This form of vascular ectasia extends directly to the alveolar capillaries (*arrowhead*). The discrete cluster of such vessels is called an *angiomatoid lesion* (*arrow*) [46] and is often witnessed as a tortuous array of vessels surrounding the obstructed pulmonary artery. Rupture of these fragile vessels gives rise to acute hemorrhage and hemosiderin deposits in lung tissue. Both the angiomatoid and veinlike lesions are labeled as grade 5 in the Heath-Edwards classification.

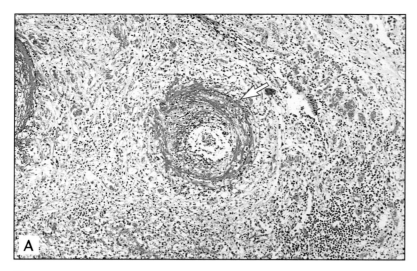

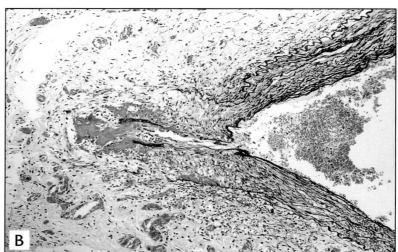

Figure 8-16.

Fibrinoid necrosis and necrotizing vasculitis. **A,** A pulmonary artery is totally involved by a necrotizing process that has resulted in the deposition of fibrinoid material (*arrow*) accompanied by severe arteritis. The inflammation, centered around the vessel cut in cross-section, has spread to the surrounding parenchyma. **B,** From the same patient, the process of fibrinoid necrosis involves a supernumerary preacinar artery close to its origin from a parent vessel. Fibrinoid material has become insinuated in all layers of the artery with destruction of the wall, including fragmentation of the elastic laminae. There is less inflammation than in *panel A*.

Fibrinoid necrosis and necrotizing vasculitis represent the most severe lesions in the classical Heath-Edwards grading system for

pulmonary hypertension associated with congenital heart defects causing left-to-right shunts [21] and indicate excessive arterial pressures. The spectrum of lesions within this category of pulmonary hypertensive changes ranges from focal fibrinoid degeneration involving only a segment of the arterial wall with degeneration of smooth muscle cells to frank necrosis with fulminant arteritis [6,60]. Necrotizing arteritis is not commonly encountered in sections. Fibrinoid degeneration of small pulmonary arteries at branch points is probably one of the precursor changes of plexiform and dilation lesions, causing aneurysmal weakening of the vessel wall and possibly stimulating the cellular proliferative response [46] eventuating in the characteristic plexiform morphology.

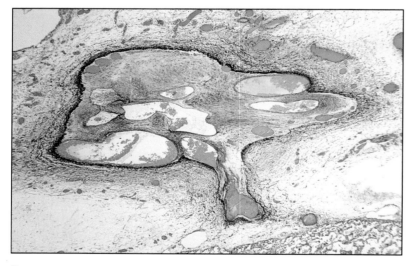

Figure 8-17.

Pulmonary veno-occlusive disease in a vein within the interlobular septum. The vein lumen is partitioned by multiple fibrous septae, which are the remnants of an organized thrombus. The dense fibrous nature of the lesion suggests it has been present for some time. There is also surrounding adventitial fibrosis and dilation of the periadventitial capillaries and other small vessels.

Pulmonary veno-occlusive disease is an uncommon cause of pulmonary hypertension and may present as primary pulmonary hypertension. The cause is unknown, but a number of cases have been recorded in association with antineoplastic chemotherapy, viral illnesses and other chest infections, oral contraceptives, bone marrow transplantation, and cardiomyopathy, among others [25]. Some have suggested that it represents a form of generalized pulmonary vaso-occlusion and is initiated by a number of factors [47]. Although the larger interlobular veins are most commonly involved, other smaller veins and venules may be affected. The identification of recently formed thrombi is uncommon; the recanalized intimal plaques may have a loose myxoid matrix or be predominately formed by mature collagen. Thickening and arterialization of the venous media are commonly seen [48]. There is generalized vascular dilation and associated hemorrhage and hemosiderosis. Capillary engorgement and proliferation may achieve proportions that suggest a diagnosis of pulmonary capillary hemangiomatosis (*see* Fig. 8-18), and many features of the two diseases appear to overlap [49]. Interstitial fibrosis and lymphatic dilation may be prominent. Plexiform and dilation lesions, components of other forms of primary and secondary pulmonary hypertension, are not present in this disease.

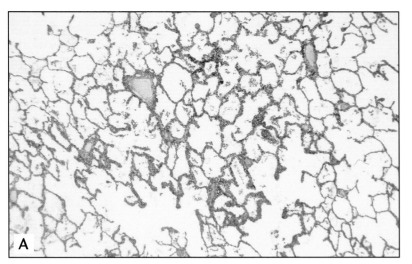

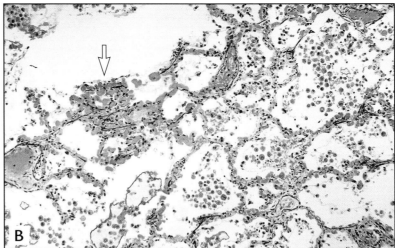

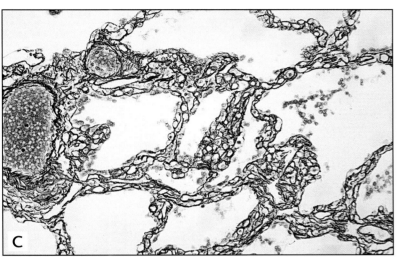

Figure 8-18.

Pulmonary capillary hemangiomatosis. **A,** One of the patchy lesions of pulmonary capillary hemangiomatosis. The low-magnification appearance is that of thickening of the alveolar septae with engorge-

ment of the capillary network. The gross appearance is often one of a spongelike area of congestion and hemorrhage [50], which may involve up to 20% of the lung [51]. **B,** At higher magnification, the capillaries clearly demonstrate dilation and engorgement but also show proliferative changes, evidenced by small clusters of vessels (*arrow*) and the presence of capillary loops on both sides of the alveolar septum. The alveolar spaces contain erythrocytes and hemosiderin-laden macrophages, evidence of acute and chronic hemorrhage. **C,** The reticulin stain highlights basement membrane proteins and outlines the capillaries to greater advantage.

This is a disease of unknown cause and is another rare cause of pulmonary hypertension. In addition to involving the acinar parenchyma, the vascular proliferation also affects the pleura and interlobular septae, bronchial, arterial, and venous walls. Infiltration of the walls of larger vessels may lead to thrombosis and luminal obstruction [52,53]. Hypertrophy of the arterial media and muscularization of the arterioles may be seen, but plexiform changes are not observed. There may be some degree of interstitial fibrosis. It is currently undecided whether this condition is a low-grade neoplasm or a reactive vascular proliferation.

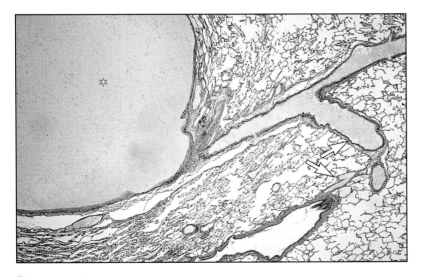

Figure 8-19.

Arteriovenous malformation. A dilated, ectatic vessel representing a portion of a pulmonary arteriovenous malformation (PAVM) (*asterisk*) is seen in this micrograph. Also present is a smaller vessel

that appears to connect with the ectatic structure, and continuity with a possible bronchial artery is seen (*arrows*). The walls of PAVMs contain variable amounts of collagen, elastin, and smooth muscle. Chronic dilation often causes sufficient compressive atrophy of these structures so that distinction between arterial and venous origin is impossible. Intimal fibrosis and luminal thrombosis may also be identified. The range of architectural appearances of these structures varies from single large ectatic vessels to a labyrinthine network of smaller telangiectatic lesions [54].

PAVMs are classified radiologically as large (> 8 mm in 20% of patients) or small (3 to 8 mm in 76% of patients) [55]. Most are single, and up to 42% are bilateral [25]. The larger lesions are usually found in the lower lobes subjacent to the visceral pleura. There is a strong association of PAVMs with hereditary hemorrhagic telangiectasia (HHT or Osler-Weber-Rendu disease) because 15% of affected individuals have PAVMs [54]; by comparison, 82% of patients with PAVMs have HHT [55]. These lesions may cause significant right-to-left shunts resulting in exercise intolerance and cerebral abscess. In 1% of cases, there is coexistent pulmonary hypertension.

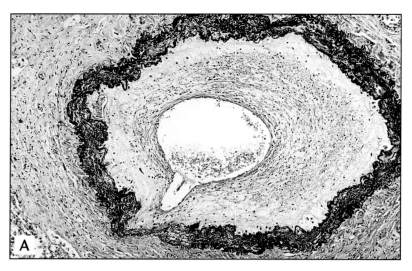

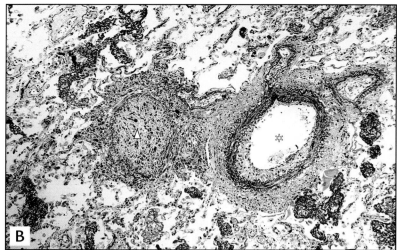

Figure 8-20.

Transplant vasculopathy. **A,** An elastic pulmonary artery showing concentric intimal hyperplasia with extreme stenosis of the lumen. The intimal plaque is composed of myofibroblasts within an acid mucopolysaccharide matrix. Older lesions may demonstrate more sclerosis. **B,** A smaller pulmonary artery (*asterisk*) and paired membranous bronchiole (*arrowhead*). The arterial intima demonstrates subtotal intimal stenosis with a mononuclear inflammatory cell component indicating ongoing transplant allograft vasculitis. The adjacent bronchiole is completely blocked by the granulation tissue of obliterative bronchiolitis.

The morphology of transplant pulmonary arterial vasculopathy is identical to that of allograft coronary disease and parallels the

progression of obliterative bronchiolitis to some degree, both changes being considered a form of chronic rejection. The appearance of the intimal thickening may range from active cellular proliferation with allograft vasculitis to relatively acellular fibrous lesions [56]. Also documented are atherosclerotic changes and associated attenuation of the muscular media. Veins may also be involved, but the pathology is usually one of concentric intimal sclerosis [57]. Despite evidence of pulmonary vasculopathy as early as 3 months after transplantation, the major concern in these patients still appears to be obliterative bronchiolitis, which is the primary factor in limiting long-term survival.

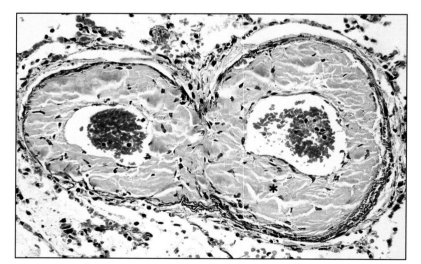

Figure 8-21.

Amyloidosis. Amyloid deposits typically involve and expand the media of small pulmonary arteries (*asterisk*), but all vessels, as well as the pulmonary interstitium, may be affected [58,59]. It is present as an amorphous, waxy substance containing very few cells within the deposit itself. On routine hematoxylin and eosin stains, the substance is eosinophilic. Classical identification is typically by demonstration of apple-green birefringence upon polarization of Congo red–stained material. Electron microscopy reveals the diagnostic feltwork arrangement of 7- to 10-nm fibrils. Whether identified primarily in vessel walls or within alveolar septae, amyloid imparts a rigid appearance, causes physical narrowing of the vessel lumen, and interrupts normal physiologic vascular constriction and dilation. The deposit may compress neighboring uninvolved structures. Pulmonary amyloid may be associated with pulmonary hypertension; however, these patients usually have coexistent cardiac involvement, which is usually the major cause of morbidity and mortality [60].

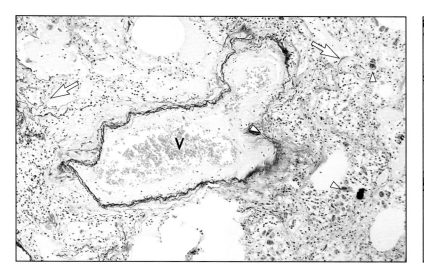

Figure 8-22.

Iron and calcium encrustation of vascular wall. Chronic pulmonary hemorrhage causes the elastic lamellae of vessel walls (and alveolar septae) to become impregnated with iron and calcium salts. This becomes pronounced in some cases, as shown here. The basophilic lamellae of the vein (V) in the hematoxylin and eosin–stained section represent composites of iron and calcium. Similar delicate deposits outline smaller vessels and alveolar walls (*arrows*). Hemosiderin-containing macrophages are visible within alveolar spaces (*arrowheads*).

Significant deposits of iron and calcium (termed "mineralizing pulmonary elastosis") are most frequently identified in idiopathic pulmonary hemosiderosis, pulmonary veno-occlusive disease, and other causes of recurrent pulmonary hemorrhage but rarely from chronic pulmonary venous congestion as a consequence of cardiac failure [61]. Medial hypertrophy and intimal hyperplasia may be associated findings. Specific differentiation of the iron moiety is accomplished through use of the Prussian blue staining method, and the calcium component stains positively with the von Kossa technique (*see* Fig. 8-23).

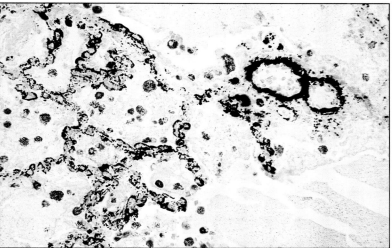

Figure 8-23.

Pulmonary calcification. The von Kossa stain (black reaction product) identifies calcium phosphate salts that have accumulated diffusely within the alveolar septae and the media of a small artery. The pattern is consistent with the observation that the elastic fibrils are the initial site of deposition [62].

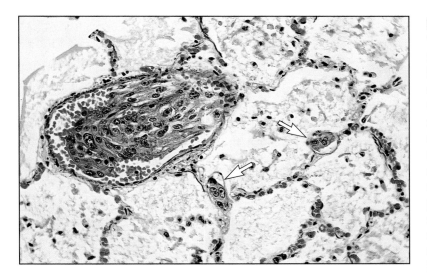

Figure 8-24.

Tumor emboli. Pulmonary tumor emboli are usually identified as small vessel lesions (shown here) rather than intralumenal masses involving the larger proximal vascular tree. The latter situation exists when there is extensive tumor growth into the vena cava or one of its larger tributaries. This example demonstrates a prominent cohesive cellular embolus within a small pulmonary arteriole as well as smaller cell clusters within two alveolar capillaries (*arrows*). In some cases, single neoplastic cells of metastatic carcinoma may be overlooked if the distribution is scarce and tumor cells are confined to capillaries. When discovered as an unknown primary diagnosis, a broad differential diagnosis including melanoma and lymphoma must be entertained. The most common tumors to give rise to intravascular emboli are adenocarcinomas of the breast (30%), lung (16%), prostate (13%), and stomach (9%) [63]. Lymphangitic carcinomatosis [63] and cor pulmonale [64] may be associated complications. Tumor emboli may take the form of pure cell aggregates, cells admixed with thrombus, or vessels containing thrombus only. Pulmonary tumor thrombotic microangiopathy encompasses microangiopathic hemolytic anemia and disseminated intravascular coagulation [65].

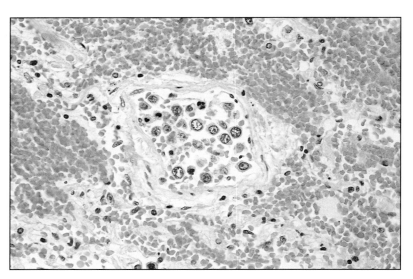

Figure 8-25.

Intravascular lymphomatosis ("malignant angioendotheliomatosis"). The *center* shows a pulmonary vessel within which a loose aggregate of atypical mononuclear cells with prominent nucleoli is present. In this case, the cells (*ie*, B lymphocytes) were confined to the vascular lumens of the organs, thus indicating the diagnosis. There is acute alveolar hemorrhage. Intravascular lymphomatosis is a rare form of lymphoma, usually of the B-cell type, in which the malignant cells are restricted to the lumen of the vessels [66]. Although significant pulmonary disease is less common than central nervous system or skin manifestations, patients occasionally present with features suggesting pulmonary hypertension or recurrent pulmonary thromboemboli [67]. The disease is often discovered only at autopsy [68], and the presence of malignant cells in the vessels should suggest the diagnosis along with the differential of metastatic carcinoma, melanoma, and leukemia.

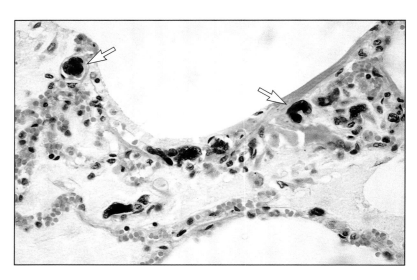

Figure 8-26.

Pulmonary megakaryocytes. The large, hyperchromatic nuclei of pulmonary megakaryocytes (*arrows*) may cause the inexperienced observer to consider them as neoplastic or virally altered cells. An intracapillary location can usually be appreciated, and the nuclei are characteristically hyperlobated. They are a normal component of lungs and are found in increased numbers in certain disease states such as adult respiratory distress syndrome, burn injuries, disseminated intravascular coagulation, and cancer metastatic to the lungs [69].

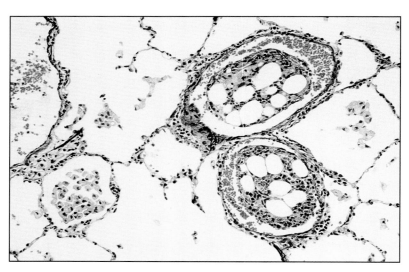

Figure 8-27.

Bone marrow embolus. Fragments of bone marrow are identified within two pulmonary arteries. The tissue is recognizable as a cohesive aggregate of cells within which clear spaces representing the lipid vacuoles of adipocytes are present. Higher magnification reveals myeloid and erythroid precursors and megakaryocytes comprising the closer-packed cellular elements. Occasional bone marrow emboli are ubiquitous findings in postmortem lungs or resections after major trauma, vigorous chest compressions during resuscitative efforts, or surgery involving the skeleton. Typical clinical symptoms and signs of the fat embolism syndrome notwithstanding, they are best considered incidental discoveries.

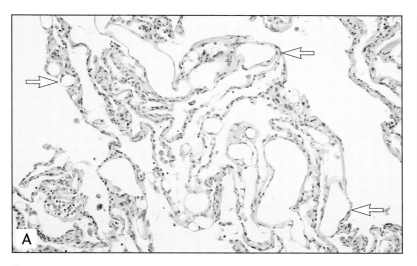

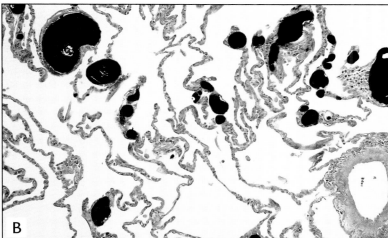

Figure 8-28.

Fat embolism. **A,** Acutely dispersed pulmonary fat emboli are often difficult to identify without a high index of suspicion. Routine tissue processing dissolves lipids, leaving only a clear vacuole or space. Sections typically show distended capillary lumens without any identifiable content (*arrows*). In frozen sections stained with the oil red–O method, the fat becomes visible; however, the preparations are often imperfect because the reaction product may become dislodged from the lumens. **B,** A more defin-

itive method is postfixation of formalin-fixed tissue blocks with osmium tetroxide, which immobilizes the fat droplets and produces a dense black reaction product [70].

Clinically, fat embolism syndrome manifests as respiratory insufficiency, petechial rash, and central nervous system abnormalities [71]. Diffuse alveolar damage and the adult respiratory distress syndrome are the result of the toxic action of free fatty acids liberated through the interaction of inflammatory cells, platelets, and lipases.

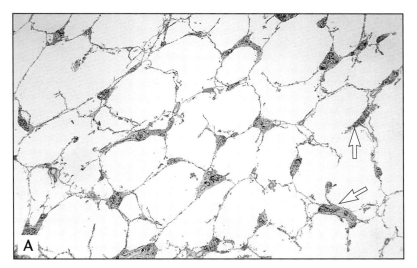

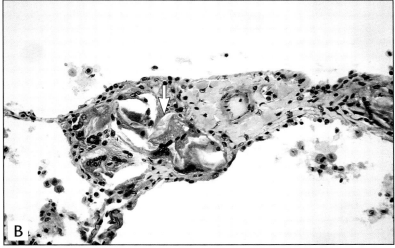

Figure 8-29.

Talcosis (intravenous drug abuse). **A,** Low-power photomicrograph of lung from an intravenous drug abuser. Foreign material (*ie,* talc) is diffusely distributed throughout the lung, residing in alveolar septae. The nodular thickenings (*arrows*) consist of numerous foreign body–type granulomatous reactions. In chronically involved lungs, as in this case, there is associated panacinar emphysema.

B, Higher-power micrograph demonstrating the features of the foreign body response. Multinucleated histiocytic giant cells engulf the characteristic plate-like fragments of talc (*arrow*). In this stain, the talc has a slight blue tint or is not stained; however, these substances demonstrate bright birefringence when exposed to polar-

ized light. In the *central portion,* a muscularized pulmonary arteriole is identified, and the surrounding alveolar wall has become fibrotic, a byproduct of the inflammatory process. Although talc and similar substances lodge initially within vascular lumens (possibly useful in determining chronology), they eventually become extruded into the interstitium [72]. Thrombosis, recanalized thrombi, intimal webs, and disruption of portions of the vessel wall and medial hypertrophy may be seen [73]. Pulmonary hypertension is a rare complication most likely as a result of progressive loss of the vascular bed and a decrease in diffusing capacity [74]. Plexiform lesions have not been linked with this condition.

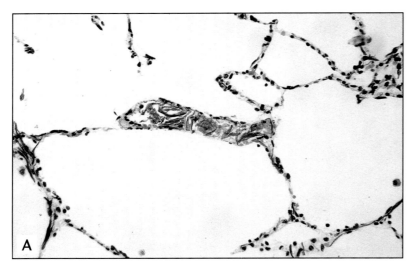

Figure 8-30.

Amniotic fluid embolus. **A,** Section demonstrating the classic finding of a plug of compacted fetal squames filling and distending an arteriole. The cells are often visualized on edge; therefore, the individual cell has a plate-like quality. When present in lesser numbers, they may be identified as separate linear structures, often incorporated within loose flocculent mucinous substance. **B,** A larger aggregate of mixed mucin and fetal squames.

In addition to epithelial squames and mucin, a variety of other substances of fetal origin may comprise the embolic tissue. Hairs (lanugo and scalp derived), sebaceous gland lipids, and bile may also be present [71]. Most amniotic fluid embolic events occur in

the peripartum period, although other predisposing conditions such as amniocentesis, hysterectomy, trauma, and abortions are known associations. Clinically, amniotic fluid embolus manifests as cardiovascular collapse, pulmonary edema, and anaphylactic shock. Amniotic fluid contains a number of thrombogenic and vasoactive substances, such as prostaglandins, which may combine with components of mechanical vascular obstruction or thrombosis, left ventricular dysfunction, and capillary leakage to produce the clinical-pathologic spectrum. The maternal mortality rate is high (> 80%), most deaths occurring within the first hour after childbirth [75].

REFERENCES

1. Reeves JT, Rubin LJ: The pulmonary circulation: snapshots of progress. *Am J Respir Crit Care Med* 1998, 157(suppl):101–108.

2. Dawes KE, Bishop JE, Peacock AJ, Laurent GJ: The role of the endothelium in vascular remodelling. In *Pulmonary Vascular Remodelling*. Edited by Bishop JE, Reeves JT, Laurent GJ. London: Portland Press; 1995:213–239.

3. Haworth SG, Hislop AA: Pulmonary vascular development: normal values of peripheral vascular structures. *Am J Cardiol* 1983, 52: 578–583.

4. Reid LM: The pulmonary circulation: remodelling in growth and disease. *Am Rev Respir Dis* 1979, 119:531–546.

5. Fritts HW, Harris P, Chidset CA, *et al.*: Estimation of flow rate through bronchial-pulmonary vascular anastomoses with use of T-1824 dye. *Circulation* 1961, 23:390–398.

6. Harris P, Heath D: *The Human Pulmonary Circulation: Its Form and Function in Health And Disease*, edn 3. New York: Churchill Livingstone; 1986.

7. Kuhn C: Normal anatomy and histology. In *Pathology of the Lung*, edn 2. Edited by Thurlbeck WM, Churg AC. New York: Thieme; 1995.

8. Channick RN: Primary pulmonary hypertension. In *Atlas of Heart Diseases, vol. III: Cardiopulmonary Diseases and Cardiac Tumors*. Edited by Braunwald E, Goldhaber SZ. Philadelphia: Current Medicine; 1995: 4.1–4.20.

9. Loh E: Cor pulmonale. In *Atlas of Heart Diseases, vol. III: Cardiopulmonary Diseases and Cardiac Tumors*. Edited by Braunwald E, Goldhaber SZ. Philadelphia: Current Medicine; 1995: 1.1–1.2.

10. Skibo L, Goldhaber SZ: Diagnosis of acute pulmonary embolism. In *Atlas of Heart Diseases, vol. III: Cardiopulmonary Diseases and Cardiac Tumors*. Edited by Braunwald E, Goldhaber SZ. Philadelphia: Current Medicine; 1995: 2.1–2.31.

11. Goldhaber SZ: Treatment of acute pulmonary embolism. In *Atlas of Heart Diseases, vol. III: Cardiopulmonary Diseases and Cardiac Tumors*. Edited by Braunwald E, Goldhaber SZ. Philadelphia: Current Medicine; 1995: 3.1–3.25.

12. Fedullo PF, Auger WR, Channick RN, *et al.*: A multidisciplinary approach to chronic thromboembolic pulmonary hypertension. In *Atlas of Heart Diseases, vol. III: Cardiopulmonary Diseases and Cardiac Tumors*. Edited by Braunwald E, Goldhaber SZ. Philadelphia: Current Medicine; 1995.

13. Brenner O: Pathology of the pulmonary circulation. *Arch of Intern Med* 1935, 56:211– 237.

14. Edwards WD: Pathology of pulmonary hypertension. *Cardiovasc Clin* 1988, 18:321–359.

15. Miller RR, Müller NL, Thurlbeck WM: Diffuse diseases of the lungs. In *Principles and Practice of Surgical Pathology and Cytopathology*. Edited by Silverberg SG. New York: Churchill Livingstone; 1997:1099–1187.

16. Moore GW, Smith RRL, Hutchins GM: Pulmonary artery atherosclerosis. Correlation with systemic atherosclerosis and hypertensive pulmonary vascular disease. *Arch Pathol Lab Med* 1982, 106:378–380.

17. Heath D, Wood EH, Dushane JW, Edwards JE: The relation of age and blood pressure to atheroma in the pulmonary arteries and thoracic aorta in congenital heart disease. *Lab Invest* 1960, 9:259–272.

18. Hampton AO, Castleman B: Correlation of postmortem chest tele-roentgenograms with autopsy findings with special reference to pulmonary embolism and infarction. *AJR Am J Roentgenol* 1940, 43:305–325.

19. Rich S, Levitsky S, Brundage BH: Pulmonary hypertension from chronic pulmonary thrombo-embolism. *Ann Intern Med* 1988, 108:425–434.

20. Moser KM, Auger WR, Fedullo PF, Jamieson SW: Chronic thromboembolic pulmonary hypertension: clinical picture and surgical treatment. *Eur Respir J* 1992, 5:334–342.

21. Heath D, Edwards JE: The pathology of hypertensive pulmonary vascular disease: a description of six grades of structural changes in the pulmonary arteries with special reference to congenital cardiac septal defects. *Circulation* 1958, 18: 533–547

22. Heath D, Helmholz HF, Burchell HB, *et al.*: Graded pulmonary vascular changes and hemodynamic findings in cases of atrial and ventricular septal defect and patent ductus arteriosus. *Circulation* 1958, 18:1155–1166.

23. Braunlin EA, Moller JH, Patton C, *et al.*: Predictive value of lung biopsy in ventricular septal defect: long-term follow-up. *J Am Coll Cardiol* 1986, 8:113–118.

24. Wagenwoort CA: Grading of pulmonary vascular lesions: a reappraisal. *Histopathology* 1981, 5: 595–598.

25. Kay JM: Vascular disease. In *Pathology of the Lung*, edn 2. Edited by Thurlbeck WM, Churg AC. New York: Thieme; 1995:931–1066.

26. Saldana ME, Harley RA, Liebow AA, Carrington CB: Experimental extreme pulmonary hypertension and vascular disease in relation to polycythemia. *Am J Pathol* 1968, 52:935–981.

27. Wagenwoort CA, Wagenwoort N, Draulans-Noe Y: Reversibility of plexogenic pulmonary arteriopathy following banding of the pulmonary artery. *J Thorac Cardiovasc Surg* 1984, 87:876–886.

28. Palevsky HI, Schloo BL, Pietra GG, *et al.*: Primary pulmonary hypertension: vascular structure, morphometry, and responsiveness to vasodilator agents. *Circulation* 1989, 80:1207–1221.

29. Rabinovitch M, Haworth SG, Castaneda AR, *et al.*: Lung biopsy in congenital heart disease: a morphometric approach to pulmonary vascular disease. *Circulation* 1978, 58:1107–1122.

30. Rabinovitch M: New concepts in pulmonary vascular disease. In *Atlas of Heart Diseases, vol. XII: Congenital Heart Disease*. Edited by Freedom RM, Braunwald E. Philadelphia: Mosby; 1997: 22.2–22.10.

31. Chronic cor pulmonale: report of an expert committee. *Wld Hlth Org Tech Rep Ser* 1961, 213:1.

32. Fulton RM, Hutchinson EC, Jones AM: Ventricular weight in cardiac hypertrophy. *Br Heart J* 1952, 14:413–420.

33. Lamb D: Chronic bronchitis, emphysema and the pathological basis of chronic obstructive pulmonary disease. In *Spencer's Pathology of the Lung*, edn 5. Edited by Hasleton PS. New York: McGraw-Hill; 1996:597–629.

34. Rich S, Dantzker DR, Ayers SM *et al.*: Primary pulmonary hypertension: a national prospective study. *Ann Intern Med* 1987, 107:216–223.

35. Tuder RM, Voelkel NF. Pulmonary hypertension and inflammation. *J Lab Clin Med* 1998, 132:16–24.

36. Rubin LJ, *et al.*: Primary pulmonary hypertension: ACCP consensus statement. *Chest* 1993, 104:236–250.

37. Edwards BS, Weir EK, Edwards WD, *et al.*: Coexistent pulmonary and portal hypertension: morphologic and clinical features. *J Am Coll Cardiol* 1987, 10:1233–1238.

38. Pietra GG, Edwards WD, Kay JM, *et al.*: Histopathology of primary pulmonary hypertension: a qualitative and quantitative study of pulmonary blood vessels from 68 patients in the National Heart, Lung and Blood Institute, primary pulmonary hypertension registry. *Circulation* 1989, 80:1198–1206.

39. Wagenvoort CA, Wagenvoort N: *Pathology of Pulmonary Hypertension*. New York: Wiley & Sons; 1977.

40. Yamaki S, Wagenwoort CA: Plexogenic pulmonary arteriopathy: significance of medial thickness with respect to advanced pulmonary vascular lesions. *Am J Pathol* 1981, 105: 70–75.

41. Wagenwoort CA, Mooi WJ: *Biopsy Pathology of the Pulmonary Vasculature*. London: Chapman and Hall; 1989.

42. Wagenwoort CA, Wagenwoort N: Primary pulmonary hypertension: a pathologic study of the lung vessels in 156 clinical diagnosed cases. *Circulation* 1970, 42:1163–1184.

43. Pietra, GG: Histopathology of primary pulmonary hypertension. *Chest* 1994; 105(suppl.):2–6.

44. Smith P, Heath D: Electron microscopy of the plexiform lesion. *Thorax* 1979, 34: 177–186.

45. Heath D: Pulmonary vascular disease In *Spencer's Pathology of the Lung*, edn 5. Edited by Hasleton PS. New York: McGraw-Hill; 1996:649–693.

46. Wagenvoort CA: Pulmonary veno-occlusive disease: entity or syndrome? *Chest* 1976, 69:82–86.

47. Wagenvoort CA, Wagenvoort N, Takahashi T: Pulmonary veno-occlusive disease: involvement of the pulmonary arteries and review of the literature. *Hum Pathol* 1985, 16:1033–1041.

48. Petitpretz P, Brenot F, Azarian R, *et al.*: Pulmonary hypertension in patients with human immunodeficiency virus infection: comparison with primary pulmonary hypertension. *Circulation* 1994, 89:2722–2727.

49. Eltorky MA, Headley AS, Winer-Muram H, *et al.*: Pulmonary capillary hemangiomatosis: a clinicopathologic review. *Ann Thorac Surg* 1994, 57:772–776.

50. Ishii H, Iwabuchi K, Kameya T, Koshino H: Pulmonary capillary hemangiomatosis. *Histopathology* 1996, 29:275–278.

51. Magee F, Wright JL, Kay JM, *et al.*: Pulmonary capillary hemangiomatosis. *Am Rev Respir Dis* 1985, 132: 922–925.

52. Tron V, Magee F, Wright JL, *et al.*: Pulmonary capillary hemangiomatosis. *Hum Pathol* 1986, 17:1144–1150.

53. Burke CM, Safai C, Nelson DP, Raffin TA: Pulmonary arteriovenous malformations: a critical update. *Am Rev Respir Dis* 1986, 134:334–339.

54. Lee DW, White RI, Egglin TK, *et al.*: Embolotherapy of large pulmonary arteriovenous malformations: long term results. *Ann Thorac Surg* 1997, 64:930–940.

55. Yousem SA, Burke CM, Billingham ME: Pathologic pulmonary alterations in long-term human heart-lung transplantation. *Hum Pathol* 1985, 16:911–923.

56. Yousem SA, Paradis IL, Dauber JH, *et al.*: Pulmonary arteriosclerosis in long-term human heart-lung transplant recipients. *Transplantation* 1989, 47:564–569.

57. Hui An, Koss MN, Hochholzer L, Wehunt WD: Amyloidosis presenting in the lower respiratory tract. *Arch Pathol Lab Med* 1986, 110:212–218.

58. Smith RRL, Hutchins GM, Moore GW, Humphrey RL: Type and distribution of pulmonary parenchymal and vascular amyloid: correlation with cardiac amyloidosis. *Am J Med* 1979, 66:96–104.

59. Shiue S-T, McNally DP: Pulmonary hypertension from prominent vascular involvement in diffuse amyloidosis. *Arch Intern Med* 1988, 148:687–689.

60. Pai U, McMahon J, Tomashefski JF: Mineralizing pulmonary elastosis in chronic cardiac failure: endogenous pneumoconiosis revisited. *Am J Clin Pathol* 1994, 101:22–28.

61. Bestetti-Bosisio M, Cotelli F, Schiaffino E, *et al.*: Lung calcification in long-term dialysed patients: a light and electron microscopic study. *Histopathology* 1984, 8:69–79.

62. Bassiri AG, Haghighi B, Doyle RL, *et al.*: Pulmonary tumor embolism. *Am J Respir Crit Care Med* 1997, 155:2089–2095.

63. Soares FA, Pinto AP, Landell GA, de Oliveira JAM: Pulmonary tumor embolism to arterial vessels and carcinomatous lymphangitis: a comparative clinicopathological study. *Arch Pathol Lab Med* 1993, 117:827–831.

64. Soares FA, Landell GA, de Oliveira JAM: Pulmonary tumor embolism to alveolar septal capillaries: a prospective study of 12 cases. *Arch Pathol Lab Med* 1991, 115:127–130.

65. Case records of the Massachusetts General Hospital (Case 19-1995). *N Engl J Med* 1995, 332:1700–1707.

66. Wick MR, Mills SE: Intravascular lymphomatosis: clinicopathological features and differential diagnosis. *Semin Diagn Pathol* 1991, 8:91–101.

67. Snyder LS, Harmon KR, Estensen RD: Intravascular lymphomatosis (malignant angioendotheliomatosis) presenting as pulmonary hypertension. *Chest* 1989, 96:1199–1200.

68. Demirer T, Dail DH, Aboulafia DM: Four cases of intravascular lymphomatosis and a literature review. *Cancer* 1994, 73:1738–1745.

69. Soares FA: Increased numbers of pulmonary megakaryocytes in patients with arterial pulmonary tumor embolism and with lung metastases seen at autopsy. *J Clin Pathol* 1992, 45:140–142.

70. Abramowsky CR, Pickett JP, Goodfellow BC, Bradford WD: Comparative demonstration of pulmonary fat emboli by "en bloc" osmium tetroxide and oil red O methods. *Hum Pathol* 1981, 12:753–755.

71. Dudney TM, Elliot CG: Pulmonary embolism from amniotic fluid, fat, and air. *Prog Cardiovasc Dis* 1994, 36:447–474.

72. Waller BF, Brownlee WJ, Roberts WC: Self-induced pulmonary granulomatosis: a consequence of intravenous injection of drugs intended for oral use. *Chest* 1980, 78:90–94.

73. Tomashefski JF, Hirsch CS: The pulmonary vascular lesions of drug abuse. *Hum Pathol* 1980, 11:133–145.

74. Overland ES, Nolan AJ, Hopwell PC: Alteration of pulmonary function in intravenous drug misusers. *Am J Med* 1980, 68:231–237.

75. Kobayashi H, Ooi H, Hayakawa H, *et al.*: Histological diagnosis of amniotic fluid embolism by monoclonal antibody TKH-2 that recognizes NeuAc 2-6GalNac epitope. *Hum Pathol* 1997, 28:428–433.

76. English JC: Pulmonary Vascular Lesions. In *Diagnostic Pulmonary Pathology*. Edited by Cagle PT. New York: Marcel Dekker, Inc.; 359–411.

Genetic, Idiopathic, and Toxic Cardiomyopathies

H. Thomas Aretz

Although epicardial coronary artery disease, valvular heart disease, and systemic diseases involving the heart cause the majority of cardiomyopathic syndromes, "true" cardiomyopathies are defined as primary disorders of cardiac muscle. They have been traditionally divided into dilated (DCM), hypertrophic (HCM), and restrictive (RCM) forms, a useful classification despite the fact that it is a somewhat curious mixture based in part on morphologic (DCM, HCM) and in part on functional (RCM) characteristics. For instance, an entity such as arrhythmogenic right ventricular dysplasia has no place in this classification scheme. The figures in this chapter follow the traditional classification scheme, but the brief introduction proposes a more pathophysiologic approach. The heart is a pump, itself reliant on adequate vascular supply and orderly electrical stimulation; thus, idiopathic, genetic, and toxic cardiomyopathies may be classified as those primarily 1) affecting cardiac contraction (systolic dysfunction), 2) impairing myocardial relaxation (diastolic dysfunction), 3) leading to disturbances of the microcirculation (microinfarction), and 4) causing electrical instability (arrhythmias, sudden death).

The morphological paradigm of primary systolic dysfunction is idiopathic dilated cardiomyopathy characterized by four-chamber dilatation and secondary eccentric hypertrophy, endocardial thrombosis, and variable fibrosis. Because membrane depolarization, cellular metabolism, and the myofibrillar apparatus all play crucial roles in myocyte contraction, genetic abnormalities and toxins affecting any of these elements can result in contractile dysfunction. Inherited dilated cardiomyopathies, which may account for 20% to 25% of cases, can be broadly divided into disorders involving energy metabolism (*ie*, defects in fatty acid oxidation or mitochondrial oxidative phosphorylation) and those affecting the contractile apparatus (*ie*, X-linked muscular dystrophies, neuromuscular disorders, familial cardiomyopathies). Toxins and deficiency states that suppress myocyte function (*eg*, alcohol), cause myocyte degeneration (*eg*, adriamycin, potassium deficiency), or lead to toxic myocarditis (*eg*, diphtheria toxin) can all cause depressed systolic function. In addition, there is evidence for a genetic predisposition to the development of autoantibodies in patients with DCM. Antibodies directed against sarcolemmal pump constituents, adrenergic receptors, mitochondrial components, and contractile proteins have all been identified and may be the possible consequence of prior myocarditis or cardiac damage.

One of the pathologic hallmarks of a "stiff," physiologically restrictive ventricle is atrial dilatation in the face of a normally sized ventricular cavity and normal or exaggerated ventricular function. Causes include myocardial hypertrophy (*eg*, HCM, idiopathic RCM); abnormal myocardial structure (*eg*, HCM, idiopathic RCM); increased cardiac fibrosis, either myocardial (*eg*, HCM, radiation changes) or endocardial (*eg*, EFE, EMF); and infiltrative diseases involving interstitial substances (*eg*, amyloidosis), interstitial cellular infiltrates (*eg*, Gaucher's disease), or intracellular accumulation of various substances (*eg*, hemochromatosis, storage diseases). The fact that HCM (despite exhibiting an obstructive pattern in 25% of cases) presents predominantly with diastolic dysfunction emphasizes the crucial role normal myocardial morphology and function play in adequate ventricular filling. Recent molecular studies have shown the genetic lesions to be related to contractile proteins: β-myosin heavy chain, cardiac troponins T and I, α-tropomyosin, cardiac myosin binding protein-C, and myosin light chains. Amyloidosis, which includes hereditary forms, is the most common infiltrative cardiomyopathy and is more frequently found at autopsy as the population ages. Chloroquine cardiotoxicity is an example of a toxic cardiomyopathy mimicking a storage disease (*ie*, Fabry's disease). It should be noted that with time many restrictive cardiomyopathies develop an element of dilatation, thus leading to a mixture of systolic and diastolic dysfunction.

Multiple foci of contraction band necrosis, with or without sparse inflammation, myocyte dropout, and multiple microscopic scars are the acute to chronic spectra of pathologic findings related to microinfarction. Causes include microvascular spasm (*eg*, from catecholamines, cocaine), microvascular thrombosis (*eg*, from venoms), or microvascular endothelial injury (*eg*, from radiation, cyclophospamide, venoms). This form of cardiomyopathy is mostly a result of toxic injury, although systemic diseases such as diabetes mellitus, thrombotic thrombocytopenic purpura, or the antiphospholipin antibody syndrome may cause this type of myocardial damage. Abnormal intramyocardial vessels are also present in patients with HCM.

Arrhythmogenic right ventricular dysplasia (ARVD), a familial cardiomyopathy, exemplifies many of the pathologic features associated with arrhythmogenic myocardial tissue: intermingling of myocardium with fat or fibrous tissue, often with entrapped myocytes; myocyte degeneration; and inflammatory infiltrates. These features are often seen in the much more common conditions leading to arrhythmias, such as ischemia, myocarditis, and myocardial fibrosis. The variable incidence of sudden cardiac death in patients with HCM, which may possibly be related to the amount of myocyte disarray, is another indication that morphologically disordered myocardium provides an arrhythmogenic substrate. It is also interesting to note that the risk of sudden death in patients with HCM varies greatly as a function of the specific genetic defect.

Finally, it is important to reiterate that in the chronic phase, many of the cardiomyopathies may be quite indistinguishable on morphologic grounds because primary dilated cardiomyopathies develop secondary hypertrophy, and hypertrophic and restrictive forms may develop dilatation and systolic failure. In addition, myocyte degeneration, ischemia, and fibrosis are common findings in end-stage heart disease; in other words, it is difficult to determine the cause of death. Because morphologic findings may be inconclusive, the taking of a careful clinical, family, and social history often plays an important role in determining the cause of cardiomyopathy.

DILATED CARDIOMYOPATHY

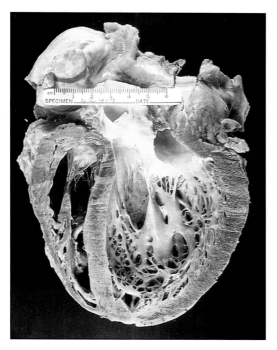

Figure 9-1.
Bivalved cardiac specimen from a patient with dilated cardiomyopathy (DCM) corresponding roughly to an echocardiographic four-chamber view showing the typical globoid shape of the left ventricle. The interventricular septum is deviated to the right and the prominent trabeculations in the left ventricle serve as evidence of the marked secondary hypertrophy despite the normal thickness of the ventricular walls. In addition, mural thrombi are a common finding. (The specimen was injected with blue and red radio-opaque dye solutions into the left and right coronary arteries, respectively.)

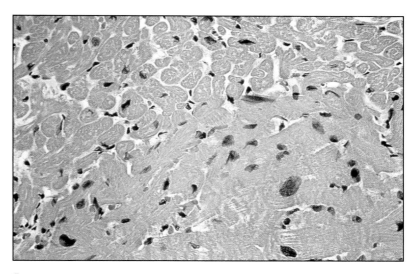

Figure 9-2.
An example of endomyocardial biopsy from a patient with dilated cardiomyopathy illustrating patterns of myocyte hypertrophy. In cross-section, the myocytes are of varying sizes but are on the average enlarged with often angular and bizarre nuclei.

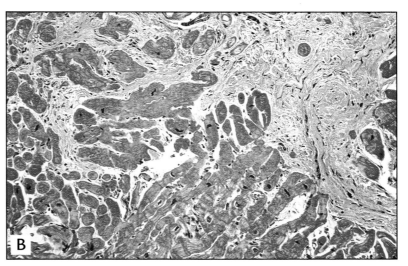

Figure 9-3.
Fibrosis in dilated cardiomyopathy (DCM). This fibrosis may be quite variable; its patterns can vary widely. **A,** Perivascular, interstitial (a severe case). **B,** Replacement (Masson's trichrome stain) and subendocardial fibrosis. These patterns are all seen in DCM, particularly in the later stages of the disease. The amount of fibrosis on endomyocardial biopsy seems to correlate with the amount of fibrosis in the right ventricular free wall but not the left ventricle [1].

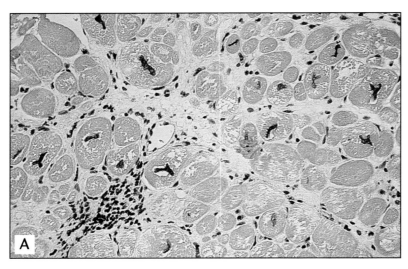

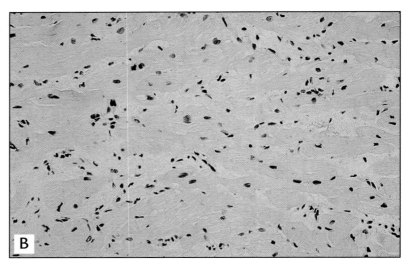

Figure 9-4.

Small foci of inflammatory cells (*panel A*), mostly lymphocytes, may be present in the interstitium or within scars. Increased interstitial cellularity (*panel B*), usually a mixture of inflammatory and mesenchymal cells, is also not uncommon in specimens from patients with dilated cardiomyopathy. These findings should not be confused with those seen in patients with myocarditis [2].

GENETIC CARDIOMYOPATHIC DISORDERS

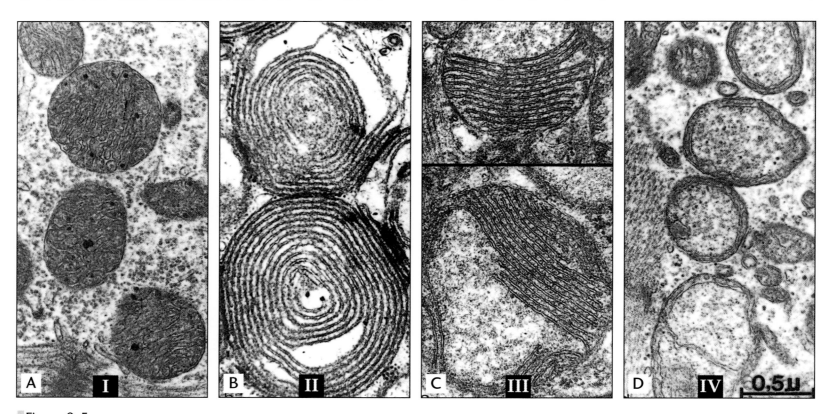

Figure 9-5.

Ultrastructural features of normal and abnormal cardiac mitochondria from patients with Kearns-Sayre syndrome. The genetics of mitochondrial cardiomyopathies have recently been elucidated; both mutations and deletions in the mitochondrial DNA have been associated with dilated cardiomyopathy (DCM) [3,4]. Kearns-Sayre syndrome is a rare mitochondrial myopathy characterized by ptosis, chronic progressive external ophthalmoplegia, abnormal retinal pigmentation, and conduction system abnormalities. Fewer than 20% of patients have cardiac involvement manifesting either as conduction system disease or cardiomyopathy. **A,** The appearance of normal mitochondria with closely packed cristae and granules. **B,** Mitochondrial abnormalities, with huge mitochondria with concentric cristae. **C,** Enlarged mitochondria with transverse cristae. **D,** Small vacuolated mitochondria. These abnormalities were found in seven of nine patients with the syndrome, demonstrating that mitochondrial cardiomyopathy is part of this condition. (*Adapted from* Schwarzkopff and coworkers [5]; with permission.)

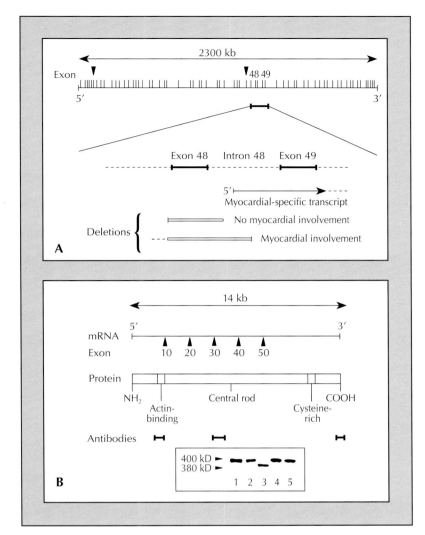

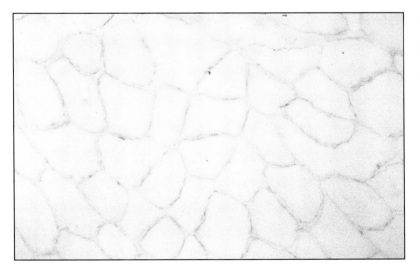

Figure 9-6.
Neuromuscular disorders associated with cardiomyopathy and mutations in the dystrophin gene. The dystrophin gene codes for a cytoskeletal protein found both in striated and cardiac myocytes. Mutations of this gene cause both Duchenne and Becker muscular dystrophy. Duchenne muscular dystrophy is associated with complete absence of dystrophin, and Becker muscular dystrophy shows decreased levels of the protein (*see* Fig. 9-7). Cardiac involvement has been noted in more than 80% of patients with Duchenne and about 50% of patients with Becker muscular dystrophy. Recently, X-linked cardiomyopathies without neuromyopathic symptoms have been described and linked to dystrophin gene mutations [6,7].

A, The dystrophin gene. Exons are indicated by *vertical bars*, and *arrowheads* mark the sites where deletion breakpoints occur most often in Duchenne and Becker dystrophy. Melacini *et al.* [8] described an association between cardiac involvement and intragenic deletions that include exons 48 and 49 in patients with Becker dystrophy. The finding that patients with deletions only in exon 48 have no cardiac involvement has led to the hypothesis that a myocardium-specific transcript exists whose 5' end is located within intron 48. Deletions of this sequence could be crucial in the development of cardiomyopathy in patients with muscular dystrophy.

B, The 14-kb dystrophin mRNA with exon numbers indicated and its corresponding protein product. Several domains of the protein are indicated: NH_2(amino-terminal) domain, actin-binding domain, central-rod domain, cysteine-rich domain, and COOH (carboxy-terminal) domain. Using antibodies to various locations of the protein (*inset*), Western blotting can be used to demonstrate the abnormal lower molecular weight protein (lane 3, 380 kD) in a patient with Becker muscular dystrophy compared with the normal 400-kD dystrophin in lanes 1,2,4, and 5. (**A** and **B** *adapted from* Melacini and coworkers [8]; with permission.)

Figure 9-7.
A skeletal muscle biopsy specimen from a patient with Becker muscular dystrophy stained for dystrophin by the immunoperoxidase method. There is noticeable reduction in the intensity of dystrophin staining in the patient's specimen. Immunohistochemical staining using an antibody directed against dystrophin can help make the diagnosis of dystrophin-related myopathies. Decreased staining for dystrophin has been demonstrated in endomyocardial biopsy specimens in patients with X-linked cardiomyopathy [9] and Becker muscular dystrophy [10]. (*From* Jones and de la Monte [11]; with permission.)

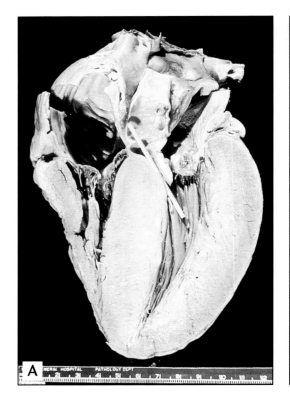

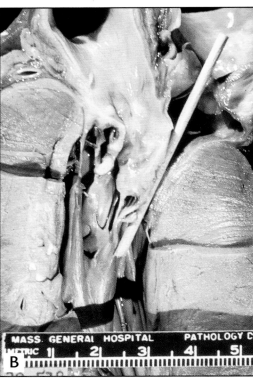

Figure 9-8.

Gross pathology of hyptertrophic cardiomyopathy (HCM). The asymmetric form of HCM, previously called idiopathic hypertrophic subaortic stenosis, was described originally. It is characterized by disproportionate septal hypertrophy. The symmetrical form (*panel A*) may be more difficult to recognize pathologically. The "comma-shaped" left ventricle and thick apex are helpful gross features. One of the most useful findings relates to the presence of a fibrous plaque on the upper left ventricular septal endocardial surface, which is caused by the systolic anterior motion (SAM) of the anterior leaflet of the mitral valve. In addition to the septal plaque, the anterior leaflet of the mitral valve is thickened (*panel B*). A probe was placed in the left ventricular outflow tract for illustration purposes.

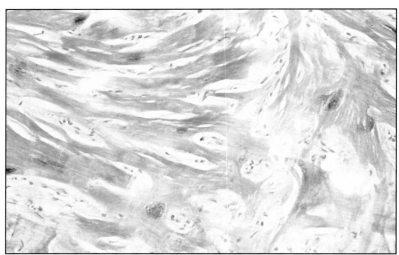

Figure 9-9.

Histologic findings in hypertrophic cardiomyopathy (HCM). These findings include markedly hypertrophied and bizarre myocytes with intra- and intercellular disarray, often in association with prominent interstitial fibrosis. Additional histologic features include inflammatory interstitial infiltrates and thickened small intramyocardial arteries. Myocyte disarray per se is not diagnostic of HCM, but it is seen to a greater extent in patients with HCM when compared with hypertrophy caused by other factors [12]. The majority of endomyocardial biopsy specimens and about 50% of septal myomectomy specimens show only myocyte hypertrophy without disarray [13]. (*Courtesy of* Frederick J. Schoen, Boston, MA.)

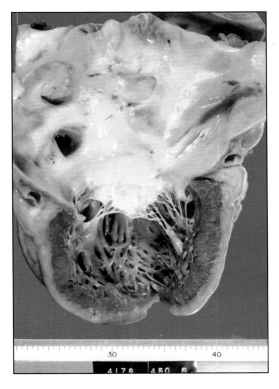

Figure 9-10.

Gross anatomy of restrictive cardiomyopathy (RCM). The left atrium is markedly dilated in this case of idiopathic RCM, and the thickness of the left ventricle is within normal limits. Both of these morphologic features are generally found in cases of RCM. The left ventricular endocardium is normal and cavity obliteration is not present [14]. In other cases, the endocardium may by mildly thickened.

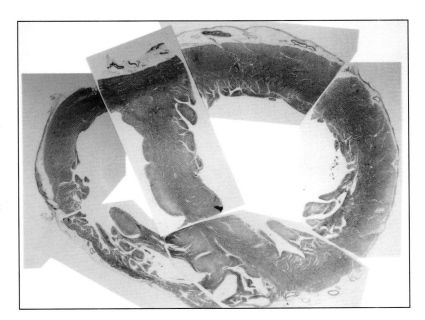

Figure 9-11.

A cross-sectional view of the right and left ventricles with low-power magnification showing diffuse and fine interstitial fibrosis in the left ventricle without replacement fibrosis or hypertrophy of the wall. The left ventricular cavity is of normal size (Mallory-azan stain).

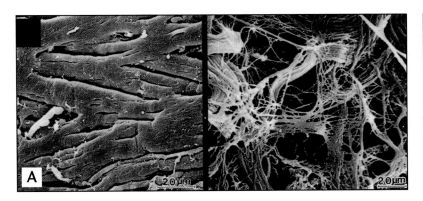

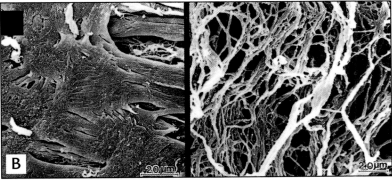

Figure 9-12.

Scanning electron micrographs of the myocytes (*left*) and interstitial collagen fibers (*right*) of two hearts of patients with restrictive cardiomyopathy (RCM) (*panels A and B*). Hypertrophy of the myocytes is prominent in both restrictive and cardiomyopathic hearts compared with the normal heart [14–16]. Bizarrely shaped myocytes, fre-

quently seen in hypertrophic cardiomyopathy (HCM), are present in *B* [16–18]. The thick collagen fibers are abundant and often form three-dimensional reticular networks in RCM [14–16, 4]. Many of these features are similar to those seen in HCM [18], which raises the question of whether these two disorders are related.

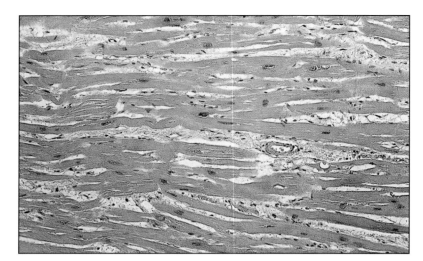

Figure 9-13.
High-power view of the free wall of the left ventricle demonstrating prominent fibrosis and moderate to marked myocardial disarray.

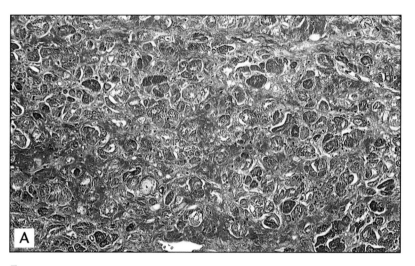

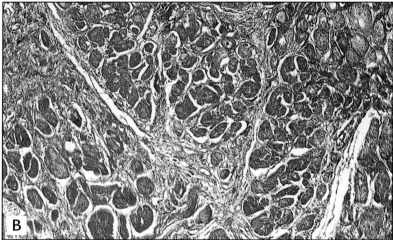

Figure 9-14.
Cross-sectional view of myocytes surrounded by fibrous tissue (Mallory-azan stain). Whereas severe interstitial fibrosis is seen in both *panel A* and *panel B*, fibrous tissue surrounds each myocyte in *panel A*, and fibrous tissue surrounds bundles or fascicles of the myocytes in *panel B*.

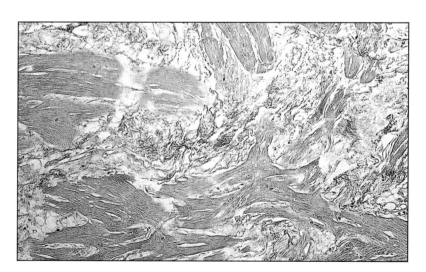

Figure 9-15.
Myocyte disarray with elastic fiber proliferation (elastic van Gieson's stain). Surrounding the bizarrely shaped myocytes, proliferation of fine elastic fibers can be seen in the area of fibrosis.

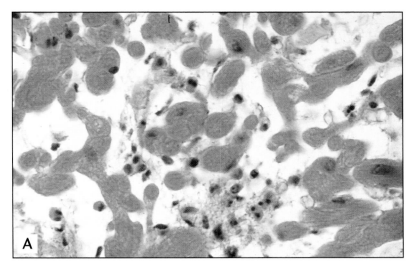

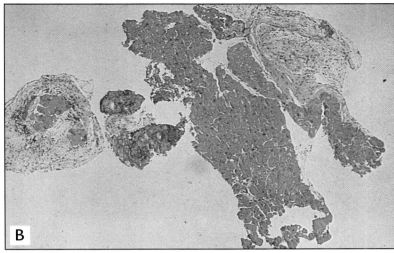

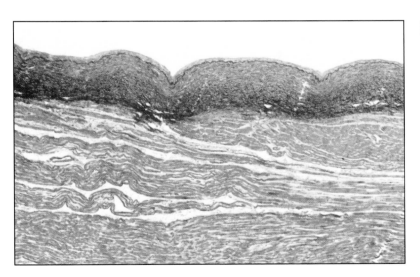

Figure 9-16.

Löffler's disease. This disease is caused by myocardial damage secondary to hypereosinophilia of any etiology. It can be divided into three stages [20]: **A,** The *inflammatory stage* is characterized by myocarditis or endomyocarditis often with a prominent eosinophilic infiltrate. The endocardial and myocardial damage is related to the eosinophile granule product [21]. The *thrombotic (second) stage* is characterized by endocardial thrombosis, predominantly in the inflow portions of both ventricles. **B,** An endomyocardial biopsy from a patient with eosinophilic leukemia. It demonstrates the endocardial proliferation and organizing ventricular thrombus. The patient died 11 months later. **C,** The transition to the *fibrotic phase* in its fully developed form is characterized by endocardial thickening and marked fibrosis of the subendocardial myocardium (Gomori's trichrome stain).

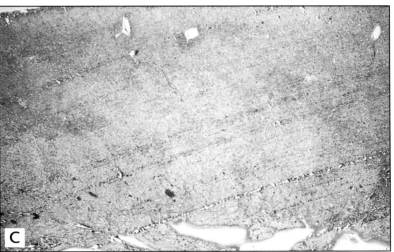

Figure 9-17.

Endocardial fibroelastosis. Photomicrograph of tissue stained for elastin demonstrating marked endocardial thickening rich in highly layered elastic tissue (elastic van Gieson's stain) [22]. The subendocardium also shows some fibrosis, but it is not as deep and pronounced as that seen in endomyocardial fibrosis. The muscle fibers are mildly hypertrophied, and inflammatory infiltrates are usually absent. This rare disorder is seen in infants and children and is believed to be the result of fetal viral myocarditis or a manifestation of idiopathic dilated cardiomyopathy.

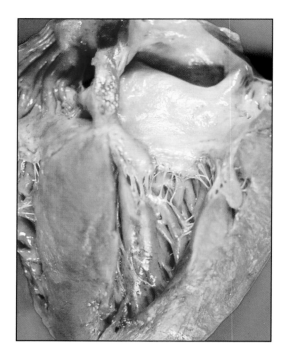

Figure 9-18.

Gross pathology of cardiac amyloidosis. This disorder may look quite inconspicuous. The ventricular cavity is often normal in size, and the myocardium may appear normal or hypertrophied. This heart came from a woman who had undergone liver transplantation for familial amyloidosis. The heart was hypertrophied and "stiff," and the atrial endocardium was granular secondary to multiple endocardial amyloid deposits.

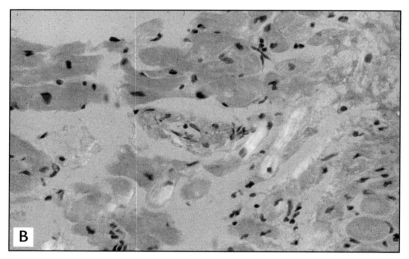

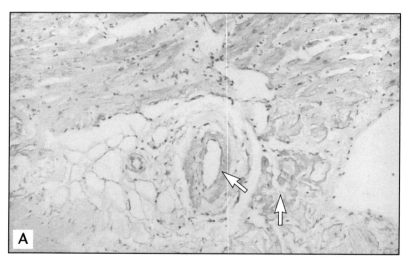

Figure 9-19.

Specimens from the myocardium of patients with amyloidosis. Amyloid stains red with the Congo red stain (*panel A*). The staining here is prominent in the vascular walls and the interstitium. Viewed under polarized light, amyloid stained with Congo red exhibits the characteristic "apple-green" birefringence, in contrast to the white birefringence exhibited by collagen and myocytes (*panel B*). Ultrastructurally, amyloid is characterized by nonbranching fibrils that are 7 to 10 nm wide (*panel C*).

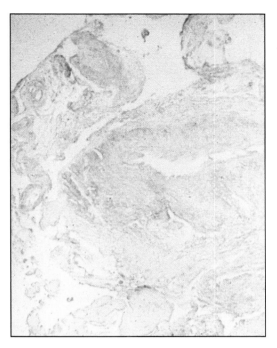

Figure 9-20.

Amyloidosis of the heart. Frozen section of an endomyocardial biopsy specimen from a patient with AL-type amyloidosis, stained with an antibody against λ-light chains. The positive staining results identify the amyloid deposits as being derived from λ-light chain molecules, usually their variable portions. A similar staining pattern may also be found in light chain disease, but light chain deposits are ultrastructurally amorphous and not fibrillary like amyloid deposits are.

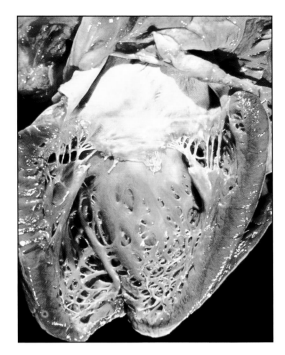

Figure 9-21.

Hemochromatosis. Although hemochromatosis initially presents with a restrictive physiology, a conjuction of restriction and dilatation is seen in the later stages of the disease. This is is well demonstrated in the heart from a thalassemic patient who died of congestive failure. The cut surface of the myocardium reveals its prominent bronze color. Staining of the myocardium with Prussian blue would demonstrate the extensive iron deposits in the myocytes. Any amount of intracellular iron in myocytes is considered to be pathologic. One cannot distinguish between primary and secondary forms on morphologic grounds alone. Additional work-up is therefore required to establish the cause in patients who do not have obvious predisposing conditions.

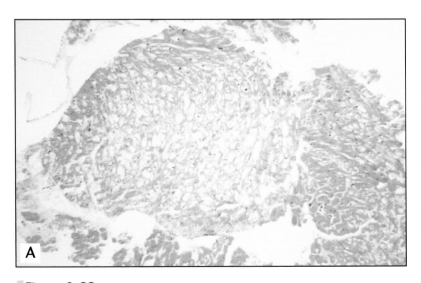

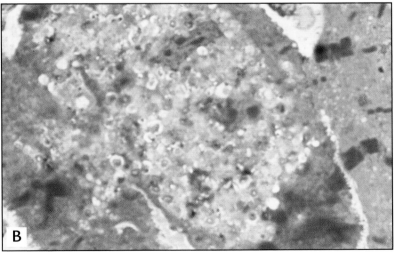

Figure 9-22.

Fabry's disease. This X-linked lysosomal storage disease is caused by the absence of α-galactosidase A, which results in the accumulation of ceramide trihexoside in certain cells. It may mimic hypertrophic cardiomyopathy (HCM) in heterozygous female patients [23]. **A,** An endomyocardial biopsy from such a patient demonstrates vacuolated myocytes in some areas; other myocytes, because of lyonization, may appear quite normal. Because routine tissue fixation and processing dissolve water-soluble substances and certain lipids, attention needs to be paid to preserving the tissues in the appropriate fixatives. Water-soluble substances (eg, glycogen) can be preserved in absolute alcohol solutions, and plastic embedding and ultrastructural examination should always be performed if storage diseases are strongly suspected. **B,** These principles are very well demonstrated by the 1-μ-thick plastic-embedded section (Toluidine blue stain) of the biopsy shown in *panel A*. The apparently "empty" spaces are filled with metachromatic rounded structures, which showed the classical lamellar bodies seen in Fabry's disease on electron microscopy.

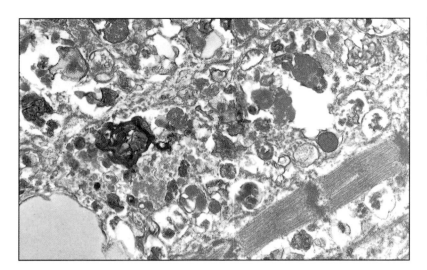

Figure 9-23.
Chloroquine cardiotoxicity. Tissue from myocardium shows findings similar to Fabry's disease. The cells are vacuolated and lamellar structures bound to phospholipid membranes are seen by ultrastructural examination [24].

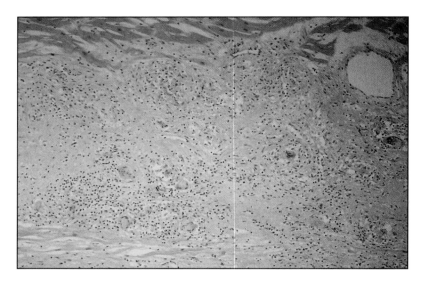

Figure 9-24.
Sarcoidosis involving the myocardium. This finding has been seen at autopsy in about 25% of patients with the disease [25]. It often presents with conduction disturbances, and preferential involvement of the upper septum is common. An endomyocardial biopsy specimen from a patient with sarcoidosis showing the typical granulomatous inflammation with giant cells—which needs to be distinguished from giant cell myocarditis. Immunohistochemical tissue typing of the inflammatory infiltrate has shown that sarcoid lesions consist mostly of CD4+ T-cells in contrast to giant cell myocarditis, which exhibits a predominantly CD8+ T-cell population [26]. Cardiac sarcoidosis leads to a mixture of dilated and restrictive cardiomyopathy, and the granulomas are replaced by fibrous tissue in the final stages, making the diagnosis difficult. In this section taken from the explanted heart of a patient, the marked increase in fibrosis and decrease in the inflammatory infiltrate are readily apparent.

TOXIC AND DRUG-RELATED CARDIOMYOPATHIES

MORPHOLOGIC PATTERNS OF TOXIN- AND DRUG-RELATED MYOCARDIAL INJURY WITH EXAMPLES

Myocarditis

Hypersensitivity

Aminoglycosides	Chloramphenicol	Horse serum	Phenindione	Smallpox vaccine	Tetracycline
Ampicillin	Digitalis/digoxin	Hydrochlorothiazide	Phenylbutazone	Streptomycin	Carbamazine
Amphotericin B	Dobutamine	Isoniazid	Phenytoin	Sulfonamides	Para-amino-salicylic acid
Cocaine	(IV preservative)	Methyldopa	Procainamide	Sulfonylureas	
Clozapine	Furosemide	Penicillin	Quinidine	Tetanus toxoid	Oxyphenbutazone

Toxic

Amphetamines	Antimony	Catecholamines	Emetine hydrochloride	Lithium carbonate	Quinidine
Anthracyclines	Arsenicals	Cocaine	Immunosuppressives	Paraquat	Rapeseed oil
Antihypertensives	Barbiturates	Cyclophosphamide	Interleukin-2	Phenothiazines	Theophylline
	Caffeine	Diptheria toxin		Plasmocid	

Vasculitis

Nonnecrotizing

Allopurinol	Chlorothiazide	Cromolyn sodium	Griseofulvin	Oxyphenbutazone	Quinidine
Ampicillin	Chloropropamide	Dextran	Indomethacin	Penicillin	Spironolactone
Bromide	Chlortetracycline	Diphenhydramine	Isoniazid	Phenylbutazone	Sulfonamides
Carbamazepine	Chlorthalidone	Diphenylhydantoin (phenytoin sodium)	Levamisole	Potassium iodide	Tetracyclines
Chloramphenicol	Colchicine		Methylthiouracil	Procainamide	Trimethadione

Necrotizing

Arsenic	Bismuth	Cyclophosphamide	Gold	Methamephetamine	Sulfonamides

Vascular Spasm/Thrombosis and Microinfarction

Catecholamines	Cocaine	Epinephrine	Scorpion sting	Snake bites	Radiation

Lupus-like Syndrome

Carbamazepine	Diphenylhydantoin	Isoniazid	Phenylbutazone
Chloropromazine	D-Penicillamine	Methyldopa	Procainamide

Cardiomyopathy and Myocyte Degeneration

Adriamycin	? Interferon-γ	Potassium deficiency	Sodium azide	5-Fluorouracil
Ethanol	Selenium deficiency	Magnesium deficiency	Paracetamol	

Intracellular Inclusions

Chloroquine	Amiodarone

Endocardial Fibrosis

Ergotamine	Fen-phen	Methysergide (serotonin)

Figure 9-25.

Morphologic patterns of toxin- and drug-related myocardial injury with examples. The list is not all-inclusive, and many more drugs and synthetic or natural substances may exhibit cardiac toxic effects. Many of these may depress myocardial function or lead to electrical disturbances, but they may not show any morphologically recognizable changes, making the diagnosis of acute toxic cardiac injury difficult in many instances [27–33]. IV—intravenous.

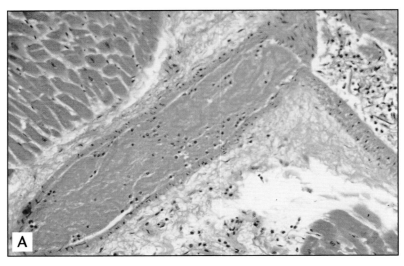

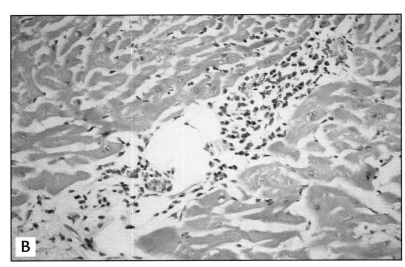

Figure 9-26.

Two lesions associated with cocaine use. **A,** Coronary vascular thrombosis. **B,** Hypersensitivity myocarditis. In addition, multiple foci of contraction band necrosis (see Fig. 9-28) may be seen acutely, which develop into multiple microscopic myocardial scars. (*Courtesy of* Renu Virmani, AFIP, Washington, DC.)

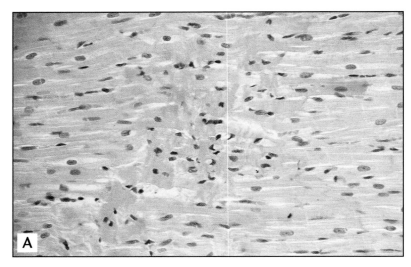

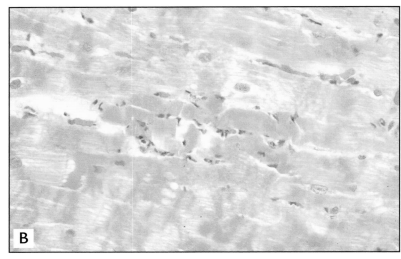

Figure 9-27.

Myocardial catecholamine (or pressor) lesions. **A,** A group of myocytes exhibiting contraction band necrosis. This section was obtained from the heart of a dog 2 hours after a subarachnoid hemorrhage was created experimentally. The lesions are thought to be related to vascular spasm and increased myocardial catecholamine levels [34]. **B,** An endomyocardial biopsy specimen from a patient with severe heart failure who was treated with high-dose pressor agents demonstrating a later stage of the lesion. There is a focus of myocardial coagulation necrosis surrounded by a scant mixed inflammatory infiltrate. The contraction bands seen in the surrounding "normal" myocardium are an artifact of the biopsy procedure, and they are only seen as an artifact in viable myocytes.

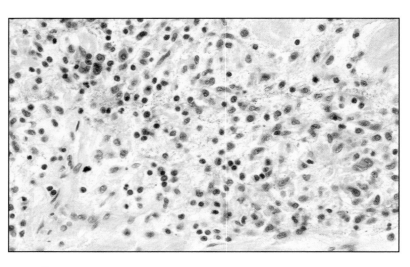

Figure 9-28.

Hypersensitivity myocarditis. This specimen was obtained from a patient who underwent placement of a left ventricular assist device while awaiting cardiac transplantation. He had been treated with intravenous (IV) dobutamine for several weeks before the procedure. The apical myocardium removed at the time of the device insertion showed a marked interstitial mixed inflammatory infiltrate, which contained a prominent eosinophilic component typical of hypersensitivity myocarditis. The sodium bisulfate preservative in some IV dobutamine preparations is thought to be the inciting agent [35]. When the patient received a cardiac allograft a few weeks later, the explanted heart showed almost total resolution of the infiltrate.

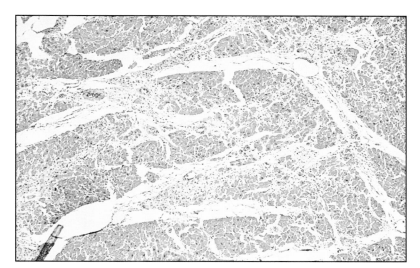

Figure 9-29.

Toxic myocarditis caused by diphtheria toxin. Myocyte degeneration and an interstitial inflammatory infiltrate are typical morphologic features of this toxic myocarditis. Diphtheria toxin causes
marked myocyte degeneration with fatty change and myocytolysis,
associated with a secondary inflammatory infiltrate. The mechanism is related to the inhibition of protein synthesis. In more
chronic exposures to cardiotoxic substances, lesions of varying
ages (*ie*, chronic, healing, and acute) may be seen, a feature that is
not found in hypersensitivity myocarditis.

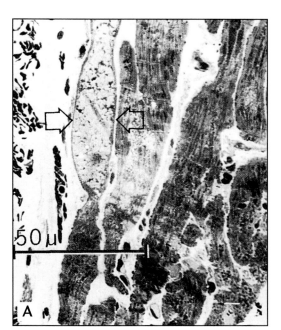
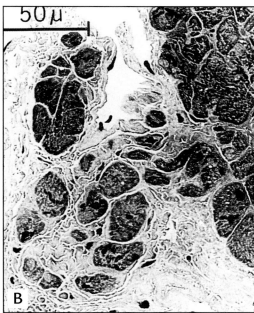
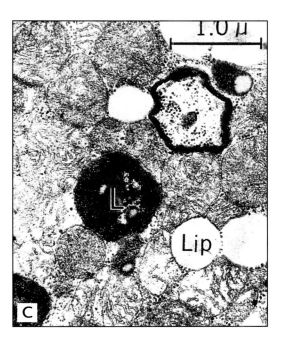

Figure 9-30.

Microscopic and ultrastructural findings in alcoholic cardiomyopathy. The findings are generally not specific and parallel those found
in dilated cardiomyopathy. **A,** Myocyte degeneration. **B,** Interstitial
fibrosis. Fat stains (*eg*, oil red O) and electron microscopy (*panel
C*) can demonstrate intracellular lipids. Myocardial damage may be
related in part to disturbances in cellular lipid metabolism [36].

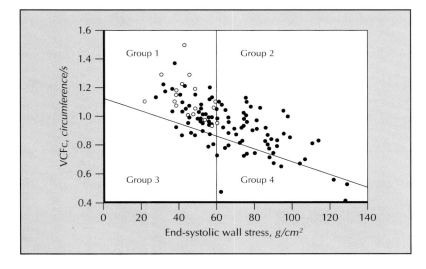

Figure 9-31.

Relationship of anthracycline dose and myocardial dysfunction.
Lipshultz *et al.* [37] studied 115 patients 1 to 15 years after treatment for acute lymphoblastic leukemia with a chemotherapeutic
regimen that included doxorubicin. Of 18 patients who received a
single dose (45 mg/m^2; *open circles*) of doxorubicin, none had
decreased contractility (group 1). However, among patients
receiving multiple doses (median, 360 mg/m^2; *closed circles*),
many had increased afterload (group 2), decreased contractility
(group 3), or both (group 4). Cumulative doxorubicin dose predicted cardiac function. The *diagonal line* indicates the lower 95%
CI for left ventricular contractility, and the *vertical line* indicates
the upper limit of normal end-systolic wall stress for adults.
VCFc—velocity of circumferential fiber shortening. (*Adapted from*
Lipshultz and coworkers [37]; with permission.)

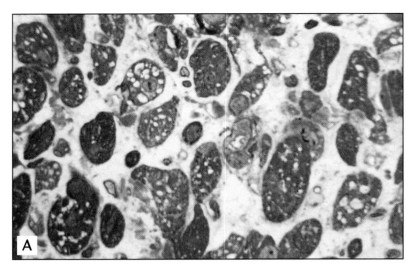

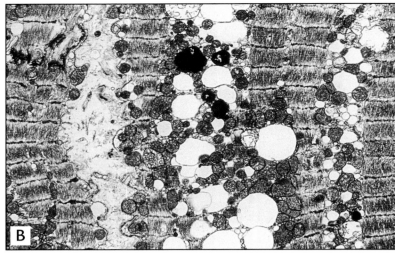

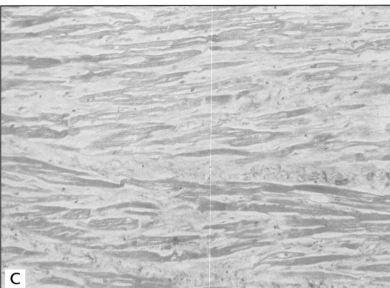

Figure 9-32.

Morphologic changes associated with anthracycline cardiotoxicity. **A,** Myocyte vacuolization is evident and easily appreciated in a 1-u-thick plastic-embedded section (Toluidine blue stain). A grading scheme has been developed that allows for prognostic information. (A grade 3 lesion is demonstrated here). **B,** Dilatation of the sarcoplasmic reticulum is a structural change, as is the loss of myofibrils. **C,** In the chronic stage, the histopathologic changes are indistinguishable from the ones seen in idiopathic dilated cardiomyopathy. (*Panels A and B courtesy of* Margaret Billingham, Stanford University, CA.)

GRADING SYSTEM FOR ANTHRACYCLINE CARDIOTOXICITY

Grade	Morphology
0	Normal myocardial morphology
1.0	Isolated myocytes affected by distended sarcotubular system (vacuolization) or early myofibrillar loss; damage to <5% of all myocytes
1.5	Changes similar to those in grade 1 but with damage to 6%–15% of myocytes
2.0	Clusters of myocytes affected by myofibrillar loss or vacuolization, with damage to 16%–25% of myocytes overall
2.5	26%–35% of myocytes affected by vacuolization or myofibrillar loss
3.0	Severe and diffuse involvement with >35% of myocytes having vacuolization or myofibrillar loss

Figure 9-33.

Grading system for adriamycin cardiotoxicity based on the examination of 10 or more 1-μ-thick plastic-embedded tissue blocks from an endomyocardial biopsy specimen. Grading is based on the extent of myocyte alterations, as outlined here. The light microscopic observations need to be confirmed by electron microscopy, and both elements are essential for accurate grading. Thus, for the evaluation of anthracycline cardiotoxicity, all biopsy specimens need to be submitted in a fixative suited for electron microcopy. At grade 2.5, more doses of adriamycin should not be given without further evaluation; at grade 3.0, no more treatment should be administered. (*Adapted from* Billingham [38]; with permission.)

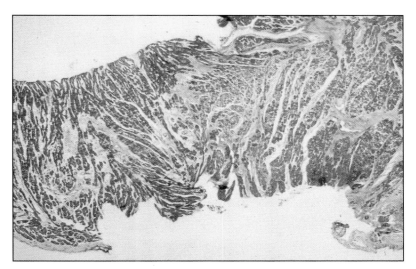

Figure 9-34.

Right ventricular endomyocardial biopsy (Masson's trichrome stain) from a patient who received mediastinal radiation for Hodgkin's disease more then 10 years before this biopsy was obtained. The patient presented with restrictive physiology disproportionate to the pericardial disease evident by imaging studies. Perivascular, endocardial, and interstitial fibrosis along with prominent small vessels are present. These findings are typical for radiation-induced myocardial damage, but similar findings may also be present in dilated cardiomyopathy. Prominent small vessels with adventitial fibrosis or duplication of the basement membranes seen on electron microscopy are more specific features indicative of radiation-related damage [39].

ARRHYTHMOGENIC RIGHT VENTRICULAR CARDIOMYOPATHY

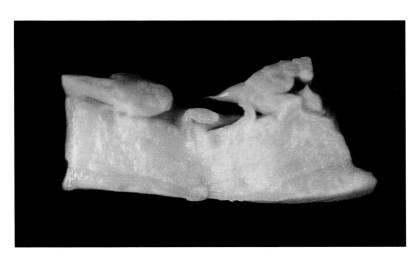

Figure 9-35.

Arrhythmogenic right ventricular dysplasia. This disorder occurs most often in young men and presents with arrhythmias and sudden death. It is familial in about one third of the cases, with an autosomal dominant pattern of inheritance, the gene mapping to chromosome 14q23-q24 [40]. It is characterized pathologically by marked fatty and fibrofatty replacement of the right ventricular free wall, often with dilatation.

REFERENCES

1. Angelini A, Vescovo G, Calliari I, *et al.*: Correlation between endomyocardial biopsies and full-thickness samples in dilated cardiomyopathy: a study of myocytes and fibrosis. *Cardiovasc Pathol* 1994, 3:167–171.

2. Aretz HT, Billingham ME, Edwards WD, *et al.*: Myocarditis: a histopathologic definition and classification. *Am J Cardiovasc Pathol* 1987, 1:3–14.

3. Zeviani M, Gellara C, Antozzi C, *et al.*: Maternally inherited myopathy and cardiomyopathy: associated with mutation in mitochondrial DNA tRNA$^{Leu(UUR)}$. *Lancet* 1991, 338:143–147.

4. Suomalainen A, Paetau A, Leinonen H, *et al.*: Inherited idiopathic dilated cardiomyopathy with multiple deletions of mitochondrial DNA. *Lancet* 1992, 340:1319–1320.

5. Schwartzkopff B, Frenzel H, Breithardt G, *et al.*: Ultrastructural findings in endomyocardial biopsy of patients with Kearns-Sayre syndrome. *J Am Coll Cardiol* 1988, 12:1522–1528.

6. Towbin JA, Hejtmancik JF, Brink P, *et al.*: X-linked dilated cardiomyopathy: molecular evidence of linkage to the Duchenne muscular dystrophy (dystrophin) gene at the Xp21 locus. *Circulation* 1993, 87:1854–1865.

7. Muntoni F, Cau M, Ganua A, *et al.*: Deletion of the dystrophin muscle-promoter region associated with X-linked dilated cardiomyopathy. *N Engl J Med* 1993, 329:921–925.

8. Melacini P, Fanin M, Danieli GA, *et al.*: Cardiac involvement in Becker muscular dystrophy. *J Am Coll Cardiol* 1993, 22:1927–1934.

9. Franz WM, Cremer M, Herrmann R, *et al.*: X-linked cardiomyopathy: novel mutation of the dystrophin gene. *Ann N Y Acad Sci* 1995, 732:470–491.

10. Maeda M, Nakao S, Miyazato H, *et al.*: Cardiac dystrophin abnormalities in Becker muscular dystrophy assessed by endomyocardial biopsy. *Am Heart J* 1995, 129:702–707.

11. Jones H, Royden de la Monte SM: Weekly Clinicopathologic Exercises: case 22-1998. *N Engl J Med* 1998, 339:182–190.

12. Van der Bel-Kahn J: Muscle fiber disarray in common heart disease. *Am J Cardiol* 1977, 40:355–364.

13. Tazelaar HD, Billingham ME: The surgical pathology of hypertrophic cardiomyopathy. *Arch Pathol Lab Med* 1987, 111:257–260.

14. Keren A, Billingham ME, Weintraub D, *et al.*: Mildly dilated congestive cardiomyopathy. *Circulation* 1985, 72:302–309.

15. Katritsis D, Wilmshurst PT, Wendon JA, *et al.*: Primary restrictive cardiomyopathy: clinical and pathologic characteristics. *J Am Coll Cardiol* 1991, 18:1230–1235.

16. Hirota Y, Shimizu G, Kita Y, *et al.*: Spectrum of restrictive cardiomyopathy: report of the national survey in Japan. *Am Heart J* 1990, 120:188–194.

17. Yutani C, Imakita M, Ishibashi-Ueda H, *et al.*: Quantitative analysis of myofiber disorganization and fibrosis in patients with idiopathic cardiomyopathy characterized by restrictive physiology. In *Cardiomyopathy Update 3. Restrictive Cardiomyopathy and Arrhythmias.* Edited by Olsen EGJ, Sekiguchi M. Tokyo: University of Tokyo Press; 1990:291–302.

18. Angelini A, Cazolari V, Thiene G, *et al.*: Morphologic spectrum of primary restrictive cardiomyopathy. *Am J Cardiol* 1997, 80:1046–1050.

19. Maisch B, Brilla C: Restrictive cardiomyopathy. *Curr Opin Cardiol* 1993, 8:447–453.

20. Spry CJF, Tai PC: Clinical studies on endomyocardial fibrosis in patients with hypereosinophilia: a historical review. In *Cardiomyopathy Update 3. Restrictive Cardiomyopathy and Arrhythmias.* Edited by Olsen EGJ, Sekiguchi M. Tokyo: University of Tokyo Press; 1990:81–98.

21. Sasano H, Virmani R, Patterson RH, *et al.*: Eosinophilic products lead to myocardial damage. *Hum Pathol* 1989, 20:850–857.

22. Neustein HB, Lurie PR, Fujit AM: Endocardial fibroelastosis found on transvascular endomyocardial biopsy in children. *Arch Pathol Lab Med* 1979, 103:214–219.

23. Colucci WS, Lorrell BH, Schoen FJ, *et al.*: Hypertrophic obstructive cardiomyopathy due to Fabry's disease. *N Engl J Med* 1982, 307:926–928.

24. Ratliff NB, Estes ML, Myles JL, *et al.*: Diagnosis of chloroquine cardiomyopathy by endomyocardial biopsy. *N Engl J Med* 1987, 316:191–193.

25. Ratner S, Fenoglio JJ Jr, Ursell PC: Utility of endomyocardial biopsy in the diagnosis of cardiac sarcoidosis. *Chest* 1986, 90:528–533.

26. Litovsky SH, Burke AP, Virmani R: Giant cell myocarditis: an entity distinct from sarcoidosis characterized by multiphasic myocyte destruction by cytotoxic T-cells and histiocytic giant cells. *Mod Pathol* 1996, 9:1126–1134.

27. Burke AP, Saenger J, Mullick F, Virmani R: Hypersensitivity myocarditis. *Arch Pathol Lab Med* 1991, 115:764–769.

28. Fenoglio JJ Jr, McAllister HA, Mullick F: Drug related myocarditis: I. Hypersensitivity myocarditis. *Hum Pathol* 1981, 12:900–907.

29. Mullick FG, McAllister HA Jr, Wagner BM, Fenoglio JJ Jr: Drug related vasculitis: clinicopathologic correlations in 30 patients. *Hum Pathol* 1979, 10:313–325.

30. Fenoglio JJ Jr: The effects of drugs on the cardiovascular system. In *Cardiovascular Pathology*, vol 2. Edited by Silver MD. New York: Churchill Livingstone; 1983: 1085–1107.

31. Aretz HT: Diagnosis of myocarditis by endomyocardial biopsy. *Med Clin North Am* 1986, 70:1215–1225.

32. Aretz HT: Myocarditis, drug-induced. In *Diagnostic Criteria for Cardiovascular Pathology: Acquired Diseases.* Edited by Bloom S. Philadelphia: Lippincott-Raven; 1997:69–70.

33. Wayne J, Braunwald E: The cardiomyopathies and myocarditides. In *Heart Disease: A Textbook of Cardiovascular Medicine*, edn 5. Edited by Braunwald E. Philadelphia: WB Saunders; 1997:1445–1449.

34. Elrifai AM, Bailes JE, Shih S-R, *et al.*: Characterization of the cardiac effects of acute subarachnoid hemorrhage in dogs. *Stroke* 1996, 27:737–742.

35. Spears GS: Eosinophilic explant carditis with eosinophilic hypersensitivity to dobutamine infusion. *J Heart Lung Transplant* 1995, 14:755–760.

36. Diamond I: Alcoholic myopathy and cardiomyopathy. *N Engl J Med* 1989, 320:458–460.

37. Lipshultz SE, Colan SD, Gelber RD, *et al.*: Late cardiac effects of doxorubicin therapy for acute lymphoblastic leukemia in childhood. *N Engl J Med* 1991, 324:808–815.

38. Billingham ME: Role of endomyocardial biopsy in diagnosis and treatment of heart disease. In *Cardiovascular Pathology*, edn 2. Edited by Silver MD. New York: Churchill Livingstone; 1991:1465–1486.

39. Virmani R, Atkinson JB: Endomyocardial biopsy in the diagnosis of heart disease. In *Cardiovascular Pathology*. Edited by Virmani R, Atkinson JB, Fenoglio JJ. Philadelphia: WB Saunders; 1991:220–245.

40. McKenna WJ, Thiene G, Nava A, *et al.*: Diagnosis of arrhythmogenic right ventricular dysplasia/cardiomyopathy. Task Force of the Working Group Myocardial and Pericardial Disease of the European Society of Cardiology and of the Scientific Council on Cardiomyopathies of the International Society and Federation of Cardiology. *Br Heart J* 1994, 71:215–218.

41. Mallat Z, Tedqui A, Fontaliran F, *et al.*: Evidence of apoptosis in arrrhythmogenic right ventricular dysplasia. *N Engl J Med* 1996, 335:1190–1196.

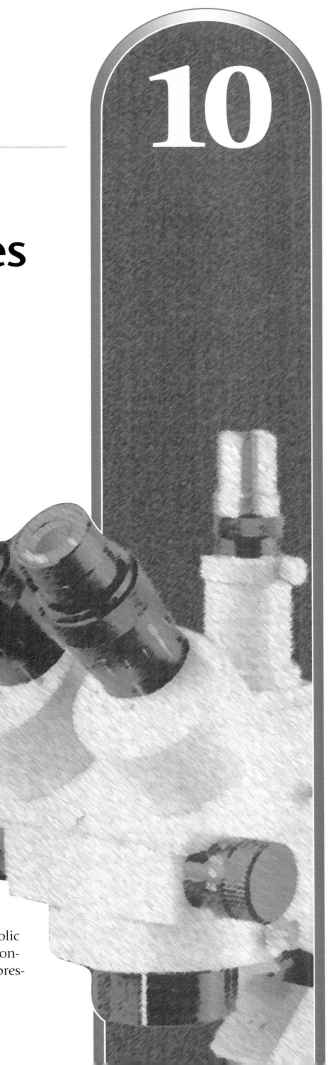

Metabolic and Hereditary Myopathies of Childhood

Glenn P. Taylor
E. Rene Rodriguez

Cardiomyopathy accounts for only a small fraction of cardiovascular disease in infants and children. At the Hospital for Sick Children in Toronto, Ontario, for instance, less than 2% of patients admitted to the cardiac services ward present with cardiomyopathy. However, this group requires consideration of a wide spectrum of metabolic conditions, inherited and acquired, not usually included in the evaluation of adult patients with cardiomyopathy. This spectrum comprises storage disorders, mitochondriopathies, disorders of cardiac substrate utilization, some neuromuscular diseases, and conditions resulting from abnormal intrauterine maternal influences or neonatal iatrogenic factors. These disorders often also have clinical importance beyond the affected individual, with implications for close relatives and family planning. Appropriate management and counseling for these diseases requires specific diagnosis. To determine the definitive diagnosis, pathologic examination is often necessary, either absolutely or as significant adjunct to other laboratory and clinical studies. This chapter presents morphologic features of inherited and acquired metabolic heart muscle disease affecting children.

Many inherited disorders of metabolism primarily cause neurologic or hepatic disease with heart involvement minor or rare. Cardiac manifestations often are vascular or endocardial rather than myocardial. Even when a disorder significantly affects skeletal muscle, myocardial injury may be minimal. However, a myopathic inherited or metabolic disorder can have clinical presentation dominated by heart disease, and a few conditions manifest only in the heart. Depending on the diversity of somatic expression of the disorder, tissue required for the clinical investigation of a presumed inherited metabolic cardiomyopathy varies from peripheral blood (*ie*, for lymphocyte inclusions) at one end of invasiveness to endomyocardial biopsy (or possibly even an explanted heart) at the other end. The tissue is precious, and its dispensation must consider the importance of morphologic assessment weighed by the pathologist and clinician against the potential usefulness of biochemical and molecular investigations. Unfortunately, presentation with sudden unexpected death occurs in pediatric cardiomyopathy, often without any antemortem clinical investigation. In such circumstances, autopsy examination of the heart and other organs, despite all caveats related to autolytic change, becomes essential for diagnosis.

The gross phenotype of cardiomyopathy caused by metabolic disease can be hypertrophic, dilated, or restrictive, with or without superimposed endocardial fibroelastosis [1,2]. Although many disorders in this group have nonspecific histologic findings, light and electron microscopy are useful for diagnosing numerous conditions. Ancillary morphologic studies such as histochemistry and immunostaining can confirm or define a diagnosis. The morphologic workup of these cases requires systematic full use of the contemporary pathology laboratory. Interpretation of morphologic findings must also incorporate the normal age-related variations of gross, light microscopic, and ultrastructural features of the heart in the fetus, infant, and child.

STORAGE DISORDERS

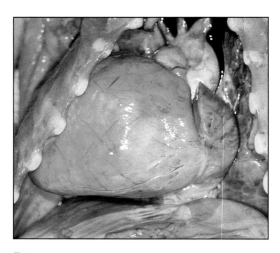

Figure 10-1.
Marked cardiomegaly in a 3-month-old boy with Pompe disease, an autosomal recessive disorder. All chambers are hypertrophied, and the heart has a pale tan color because of an accumulation of glycogen in the cardiac myocytes. Myocardial involvement is prominent in the infantile form of glycogen storage disease (GSD) type II (Pompe disease, GSD IIa); rare in the juvenile form (GSD IIb), in which presentation occurs after 2 years of age; and not a feature of the adult form (GSD IIc). Classic Pompe disease presents within the first few weeks or months of life with hypotonia, feeding difficulties, and respiratory distress. Cardiomegaly, hepatomegaly, and macroglossia develop early. Death usually occurs before the patient reaches 2 years of age.

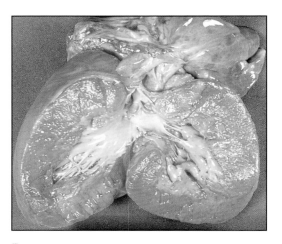

Figure 10-2.
Opened heart from an infant with Pompe disease demonstrating greatly thickened left ventricle including distorted papillary muscles and septal endocardial fibroelastosis. The cardiomegaly is progressive, with thickening also of the right ventricle and interventricular septum. Left ventricular outflow tract obstruction may develop. At death, patients with Pompe disease can have hearts up to seven times their expected weight. About 20% of cases show endocardial fibroelastosis [3].

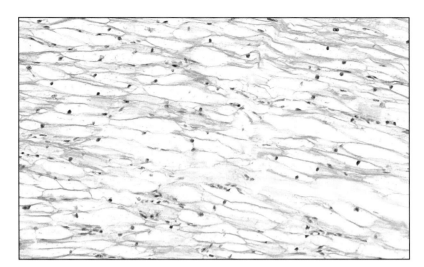

Figure 10-3.

Cardiac myocytes in Pompe disease. Hematoxylin and eosin–stained cardiac myocytes in Pompe disease have a swollen and vacuolated appearance because of the accumulation of glycogen that peripherally displaces contractile elements. The change is not confined to one zone such as the subendocardium but rather occurs throughout the myocardium. This histologic appearance also is seen with glycogen storage disease III (Cori disease) and cardiac phosphorylase B kinase deficiency.

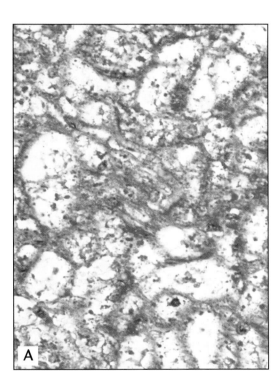

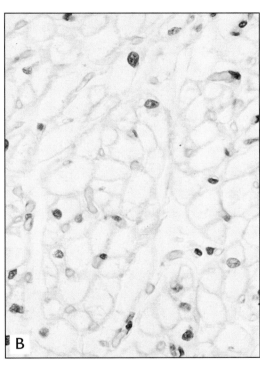

Figure 10-4.

Glycogen accumulated in Pompe disease. This accumulation stains positively with periodic acid–Schiff (PAS) stain (*panel A*) and digests with diastase (*panel B*), as does that occurring with glycogen storage disease III. Glycogen is lost during paraffin section processing, and the amount of cytoplasmic glycogen may be underrepresented in routinely processed histology sections. Myocardial glycogen content in suspected Pompe disease must be compared with that of the normally well-glycogenated fetal and infantile myocardium.

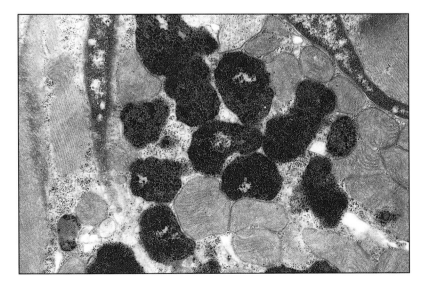

Figure 10-5.

Intralysosomal glycogen storage in Pompe disease. Ultrastructurally, the glycogen storage in Pompe disease is intralysosomal. This is because of a deficiency of acid α-glucosidase (acid maltase), which normally hydrolyzes glycogen. The glycogen is retained as β-particles. Free cytosolic and intranuclear β-particle glycogen also occurs, presumably from disruption of storage lysosomes. Storage lysosomes are widely distributed in Pompe disease, including in peripheral blood lymphocytes (where buffy coat ultrastructural examination can be used for diagnosis) and in endothelial, smooth muscle, skeletal muscle, and liver cells. The condition "lysosomal glycogen storage disease without acid maltase deficiency" is a rare disorder presenting in older children and adolescents with myotonia, concentric hypertrophic cardiomegaly, and intellectual impairment. It has similar ultrastructural features to Pompe disease, with lysosomal and free β-particle glycogen accumulation in cardiac and skeletal myocytes. However, acid maltase activity is normal [4].

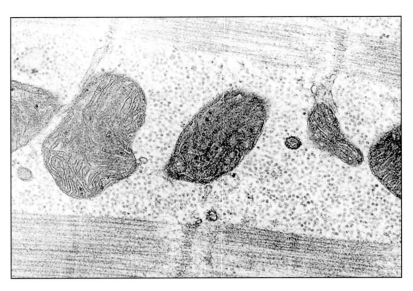

Figure 10-6.
Electron micrograph of a cardiac myocyte in glycogen storage disease (GSD) III (Cori disease) showing excessive free cytosolic beta particles and some intramitochondrial glycogen. Intranuclear glycogen also occurs. The hematoxylin and eosin–stained light microscopy appearance of swollen and vacuolated cardiac myocytes in GSD III is similar to that of Pompe disease. The abnormal storage results from deficiency of glycogen debrancher enzyme (amylo-1,6-glucosidase), inherited as an autosomal recessive condition. Glycogen storage is widespread in GSD III but is found primarily in skeletal muscle and hepatic tissues. Cardiac involvement is frequent but most often clinically silent, with only a minority of patients having cardiomegaly or heart failure [5]. Hypertrophic cardiomyopathy can develop, but heart enlargement is not as marked as with Pompe disease.

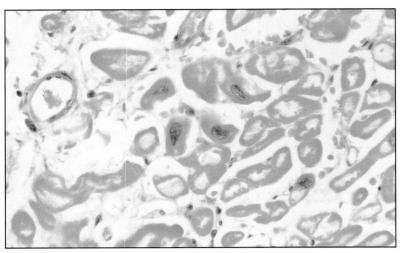

Figure 10-7.
Hematoxylin and eosin–stained myocardium in a 13-year-old boy with glycogen storage disease (GSD) IV (Andersen disease). Glassy pale basophilic inclusions swell cardiac myocytes and displace the contractile elements and nuclei. The appearance resembles that of basophilic myofiber degeneration seen in hearts from adults. Although the primary impact of GSD IV, an autosomal recessive condition caused by a deficiency of branching enzyme (α-1,4-glucan: α-1,4 glucan 6-glycosyltransferase) is on the liver, tissue deposits are generalized. Rarely, cardiac involvement predominates [6]. In children receiving liver transplants for GSD IV, cardiomyopathy can become clinically significant in time.

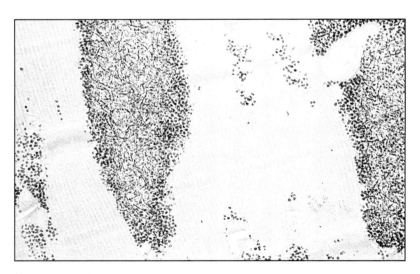

Figure 10-8.
Abnormal glycogen accumulated in glycogen storage disease IV. This glycogen accumulation has a fibrillar ultrastructural appearance and is not membrane bound. β- and α-particulate glycogen accompany the fibrillar aggregates. The fibrils are 5 to 6 nm thick. Similar fibrillar aggregates occur with Lafora disease and in the inclusions of basophilic myofiber degeneration.

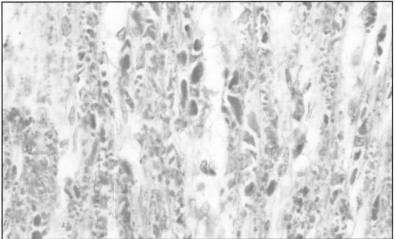

Figure 10-9.
Diastase predigested periodic acid–Schiff–stained myocardium from a stillborn fetus with glycogen storage disease IV demonstrating the relative resistance of the abnormal glycogen to diastase. The glycogen molecule has long outer branches, conferring the enzymatic resistance. The storage product is preserved sufficient for histologic identification despite maceration of the myocardium.

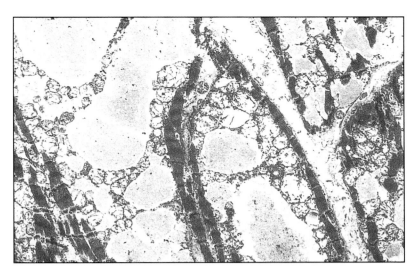

Figure 10-10.
Ultrastructural examination of the myocardium from a macerated
fetus with glycogen storage disease IV. This examination satisfac-
torily identifies the fibrillar glycogen aggregates even though cells
show advanced autolysis with loss of organelle ultrastructural
details. Maceration or long postmortem intervals do not preclude
special morphologic studies in metabolic cardiomyopathies.
However, the diagnostic value of the autopsy of a child who died
from a clinically suspected metabolic disorder is maximized when
relevant tissues are obtained with the shortest postmortem interval
possible. This is the basic principle of the "metabolic autopsy,"
and it requires coordination with clinicians, communication and
empathy with the child's family, and a willingness of the pathologist to be readily available.

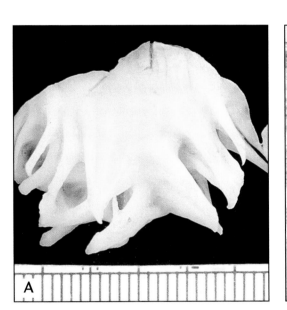
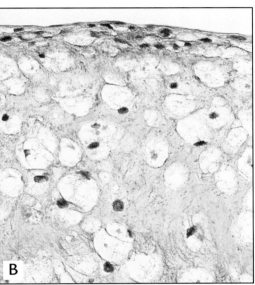

Figure 10-11.
Vascular and endocardial involvement illustrated by a thickened dysplastic mitral valve
leaflet and chordae from a patient with Scheie syndrome (a subtype of mucopolysaccharidosis I) (*panel A*). Vascular and endocardial involvement overshadow myocardial disease

in most mucopolysaccharidose, mucolipi-
dose, and gangliosidose diseases affecting
the cardiovascular system. These conditions result from deficiency of various
degradative enzymes causing lysosomal
storage. They are histologically characterized by cytoplasmically cleared or vacuolated cells, such as those seen in this
Movat-stained section of the mitral valve
in Scheie syndrome (*panel B*), infiltrating
endocardium, vessel walls, or the fibrous
interstitium of the heart. Vessels are narrowed, leading to myocardial ischemic
injury. In addition, valves are thickened,
resulting in dysfunction and secondary
myocardial hypertrophy. The vacuolated
cells generally do not have specific morphology or histochemical staining characteristics to distinguish the various conditions by light microscopy, although the
spectrum of affected cell types may narrow
the differential diagnosis.

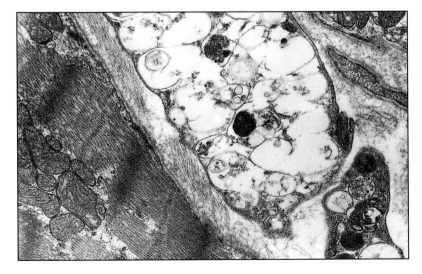

Figure 10-12.
Electron micrograph of heart in a patient with Hurler syndrome
(another subtype of mucopolysaccharidosis [MPS] I) shows an
interstitial cell filled with distended lysosomes that appear nearly
empty or contain relatively sparse granular, fibrillar, or membranous structures. This type of inclusion is also seen in Scheie syndrome, MPS VI, MPS VII, mucolipidosis II (I cell disease), and
GM1 gangliosidosis as well as in other types of lysosomal storage
disorders that do not significantly affect the heart. The involvement of myocardial interstitial cells can lead to hypertrophic or
dilated cardiomyopathy.

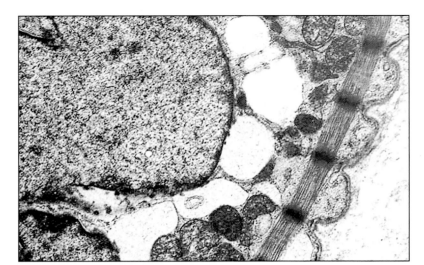

Figure 10-13.

Lysosomal storage within cardiac myocytes in GM1 gangliosidosis. This occurs in only a few conditions, which also include Hurler syndrome, mucolipidosis II, GM2 gangliosidosis (Sandhoff disease), and Fabry disease.

MITOCHONDRIOPATHIES

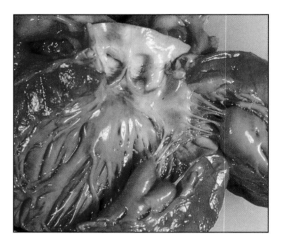

Figure 10-14.

Gross morphologic features of lethal infantile mitochondrial cardiomyopathy. Left ventricle from a 3-month-old baby who died with congestive failure and lactic acidosis demonstrating myocardial hypertrophy (highlighted by the thick papillary muscles) and an abnormal tan-red color. This is one entity in the spectrum of mitochondrial myopathy, defined as "muscle disease characterized by structurally or numerically abnormal mitochondria and/or abnormally functioning mitochondria" [7]. The abnormalities relate to mutations in the genes coding for mitochondrial function and structure, mainly of mitochondrial DNA rather than nuclear DNA. Abnormalities of mitochondrial DNA are associated with highly variable phenotypic expressions. Initial symptoms, organ involvement, and rate of disease progression vary from patient to patient. Diagnosis can be made on the basis of morphologic, respiratory enzyme, and molecular genetic analyses. Histologic study revealing ragged red fibers in type 1 skeletal muscle cells is helpful in the differential diagnosis of inborn errors of metabolism but may not always be present. Electron microscopic examination is more sensitive and shows abnormalities in the number and ultrastructure of mitochondria. Biochemical analyses of respiratory chain enzymes are often abnormal but are not specific. More recently, molecular mitochondrial DNA analysis has shown that specific point mutations and deletions are associated with particular clinical entities within this clinically heterogeneous group of diseases.

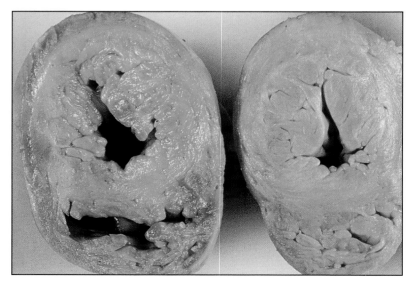

Figure 10-15.

Transverse sections of heart from a 1-month-old baby who died from mitochondriopathy showing concentric biventricular hypertrophy. The myocardium is pale tan rather than the usual red-brown, which is a fairly common gross observation. Mitochondrial cardiomyopathies of early life range in presentation from sudden death, a clinical picture dominated by arrhythmias, or heart failure with cardiomyopathy. The hearts in early infantile presentations usually have hypertrophic morphology. These types of "hypertrophic" hearts should not be confused with the familial type of hypertrophic cardiomyopathy characterized by myofiber disarray and mutations in genes that code for sarcomeric proteins. Superimposed endocardial fibroelastosis of the ventricles may be present. Older patients often have dilated cardiomyopathy.

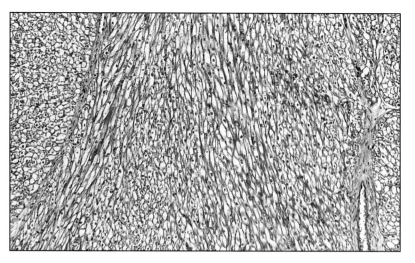

Figure 10-16.

Myocyte hypertrophy and perinuclear vacuolar swelling in mitochondrial cardiomyopathy. This is the histologic hallmark of mitochondrial cardiomyopathy, best appreciated with trichrome stain. It is the myocardial equivalent of "ragged red fibers" seen in skeletal muscle mitochondriopathies and is one cause of cytoplasmically cleared cardiac myocytes encountered in infantile myocardium.

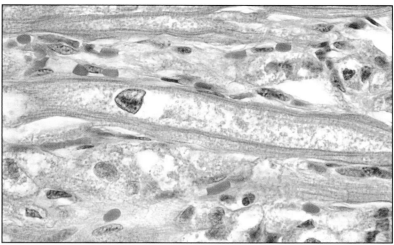

Figure 10-17.

Higher magnification light microscopy of myocardium in mitochondrial cardiomyopathy. Even with hematoxylin and eosin–stained sections, eosinophilic granules occupying the perinuclear space are demonstrated. The granules are deep magenta with Masson's trichrome stain and represent abnormal mitochondria. The mitochondrial accumulations displace contractile elements peripherally. Subsequently, depending on the amount of cell edema and glycogen, the perinuclear cytoplasm appears either "empty" or granulated. Transversely sectioned myocytes may have a glassy cytoplasm imparted by densely packed central mitochondria.

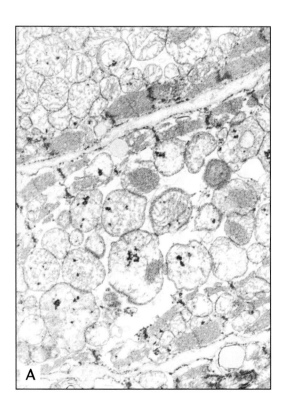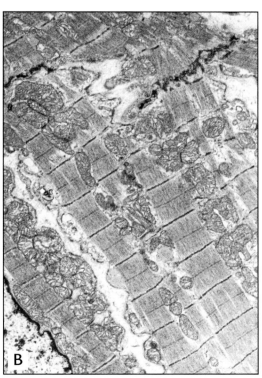

Figure 10-18.

Marked hyperplasia and variation in size and shape of mitochondria in mitochondriopathy. There is an increase in number and variability in morphology of the mitochondria in mitochondriopathy. These electron micrographs, one of myocardium obtained about 60 minutes after the infant died with mitochondrial cardiomyopathy (*panel A*) and the other of myocardium from a control patient matched by age, postmortem interval, and magnification power (*panel B*) illustrate the marked hyperplasia and variation in size and shape of mitochondria. Also apparent are displacement and atrophy of sarcomeres. The mitochondria can have ring, ameboid, or pleomorphic form and may be giant, up to 3 μm in diameter. Perimitochondrial lipid vacuoles may be prominent.

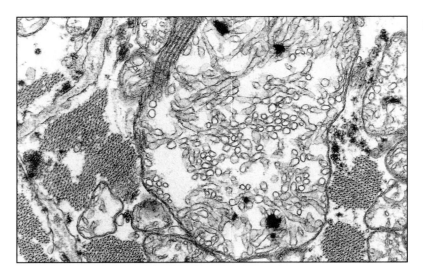

Figure 10-19.
Mitochondrial internal structural abnormalities. These abnormalities, such as tubular rather than plate-like cristae and parallel "stacks" of cristae seen in this higher power electron micrograph, can be identified despite presence of autolysis. However, excessive autolysis masks mitochondrial morphologic abnormalities. When the diagnosis of mitochondrial cardiomyopathy must be established on the basis of explanted or autopsy myocardium, efforts should be made to obtain the tissue with the shortest interval possible after explantation or death; this facilitates biochemical and molecular genetic studies as well as the ultrastructural examination.

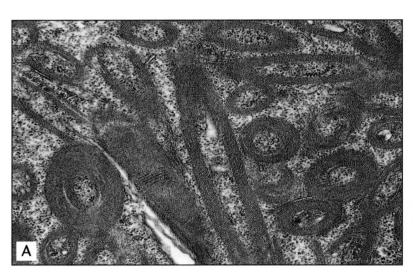

Figure 10-20.
Mitochondrial alteration. Mitochondrial alterations like "fingerprint" or "onion skinning" mitochondria (*panel A*), but less commonly paracrystalline inclusions (*panel B*), demonstrated in these electron micrographs from skeletal muscle biopsies, can also be found in myocardial mitochondria of patients with mitochondriopathy. Although morphologic abnormalities such as these and tubular cristae strongly suggest a mitochondrial DNA defect involving the oxidative phosphorylation system, they are not completely specific [8] nor is there clear correlation with specific mitochondrial biochemical defects. In addition, myopathies with biochemically proven mitochondrial defects may have morphologically normal mitochondria, although these usually result from nuclear mutations rather than mitochondrial DNA mutations. Cardiac myocyte hypertrophy from any cause results in increased numbers of mitochondria, a change that must be considered when evaluating a diagnostic endomyocardial biopsy. However, the morphology in such secondary mitochondrial hyperplasia remains normal.

The variability in morphologic manifestations of mitochondriopathy reflects the variability in clinical severity and syndromes seen with mitochondriopathies. The heterogenous nature of mitochondrial disorders can be explained on the basis of some unique features of mtDNA genetics. MtDNA is a closed circular molecule of 16,569 base pairs with three to 10 copies located in the mitochondrial matrix. Because of their extranuclear location, an individual's mtDNA is practically derived only from the oocyte cytoplasm and thus is strictly maternally inherited. There are thousands of copies of mtDNA in each cell, which can either be pure wild or mutant type, a condition termed *homoplasmy*. Occurrence of mutation, however, yields a mixed population of wild and mutant molecules, or *heteroplasmy*. During mitosis or meiosis, segregation of mutant and wild type mtDNA between daughter cells is a random event.

Consequently, proportions of wild versus mutant mtDNA vary from tissue to tissue and from individual to individual within a pedigree, accounting for intrafamilial and interfamilial phenotypic variation of mitochondrial diseases. In addition to the relative amount of mutant versus wild type mtDNA in cells and tissues, the clinical phenotype of the affected individual is also determined in part by the threshold energy requirement of different organ systems. Deficiency in energy production caused by alterations in the mtDNA constitution of the cell, eventually resulting in specific organ dysfunction when expression threshold is reached, are expected to manifest early in tissues with high metabolic energy requirement. Mitochondrial diseases, therefore, preferentially affect the brain, skeletal muscle, eyes, ears, heart, liver, kidney, and pancreas.

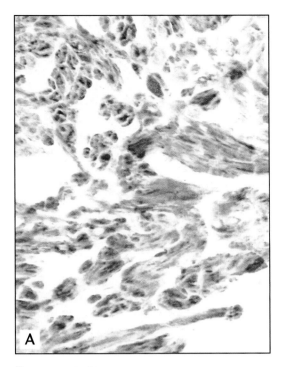

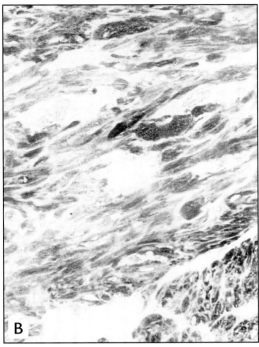

I. Complexes IV and III are the most frequently reported complexes identified abnormal in mitochondrial cardiomyopathy [8]. Normal succinic dehydrogenase (SDH) staining of an endomyocardial biopsy frozen section (*panel B*) demonstrates adequate function of complex II. Defects in complex II components reduce SDH activity. However, endomyocardial biopsies may show increased SDH staining because of mitochondrial hyperplasia if the mitochondriopathy affects another complex. Complex I defects are evaluated by NADH-reductase histochemical staining. This also tests the overall ability of the oxidative phosphorylation system to oxidize NADH and can point to defects in complexes III, IV, and V. Analytical biochemical testing can also be applied to snap-frozen endomyocardial biopsy, explant myocardium, or autopsy myocardium to further define a mitochondriopathy, although this technique has been substantially superseded by mitochondrial DNA molecular genetic studies to identify the various point mutations, deletions, or duplications associated with the mitochondriopathy syndromes [10].

▍Figure 10-21.

Histochemical staining of endomyocardial frozen sections can be applied to the investigation of mitochondrial cardiomyopathy [9]. Normal intensity cytochrome C oxidase staining demonstrated in endomyocardial biopsy frozen section (*panel A*) indicates satisfactory function of complex IV of the mitochondrial respiratory chain. Significantly diminished or absent cytochrome C oxidase histochemical staining implicates that complex, although cytochrome C oxidase deficiency can accompany a defect of complex

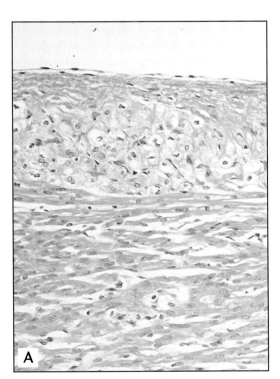

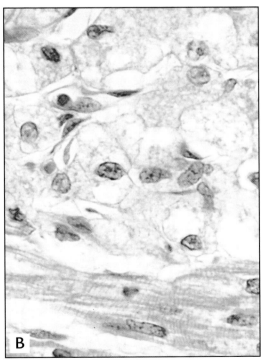

▍Figure 10-22.

Focal oncocytic transformation of cardiac myocytes characterizes the histology of histiocytoid cardiomyopathy, a rare pediatric disorder primarily affecting girls under 2 years of age [11]. About 70 cases have been reported. **A,** The histiocytoid cells, which have been demonstrated to be altered myocytes, form distinct nodules chiefly in the subendocardium. **B,** The cells are polygonal and have foamy or granular eosinophilic cytoplasm. The disease presents in infancy or early childhood with intractable tachyarrhythmias or, in about 20% of cases, with sudden death. Females account for 75% of reported cases. Grossly, the heart is hypertrophied and studded with tan-yellow endocardial nodules up to 5 mm in diameter. Nodular infiltrates also occur in deeper myocardium, the subepicardium, conducting system regions, and in the cardiac valves.

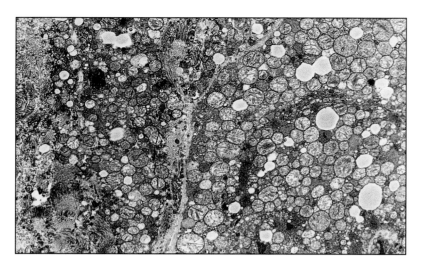

Figure 10-23.
Ultrastructural examination showing the abnormal cells of histiocytoid cardiomyopathy filled with mitochondria. The cells contain lipid microvacuoles, few or no sarcomeres, and no T-tubular system. The mitochondria vary somewhat in size but are generally round. Tubular cristae or stacked whorled arrays of cristae are uncommon and paracrystalline inclusions, as seen with mitochondriopathy, are not found. Some mitochondria contain round electron-dense inclusions [12]. Association with mitochondriopathy has been made on the basis of reports indicating a defect in oxidation phosphorylation complex III [13]. Previously suggested causes include localized cardiac glycogen or lipid storage disorder, Purkinje cell hamartoma, and viral-induced cytopathic effect. Histiocytoid cardiomyopathy has been associated with the syndrome microphthalmia with linear skin defects, and X-linked chromosomal disorder.

DISORDERS OF CARDIAC SUBSTRATE UTILIZATION

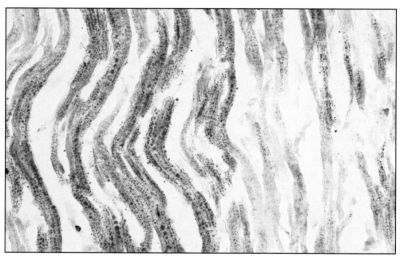

Figure 10-24.
Cardiac myocyte lipid accumulation demonstrated in an oil-red-O–stained frozen section from the heart of an infant who died suddenly. This type of accumulation is a feature of cardiomyopathies caused by abnormalities in fatty acid β-oxidation. Mitochondrial β-oxidation is the primary myocardial energy system after birth.

Metabolic abnormalities in this system can result from deficiencies of either enzymes or transport factors involved in the β-oxidation of fatty acids. Carnitine is required for transport of long-chain fatty acids into the matrix space of mitochondria, where β-oxidation occurs. Deficiencies of carnitine, either primary or secondary, cause early childhood onset of skeletal muscle weakness, liver dysfunction, and cardiomyopathy [14,15]. Physiologic stresses such as fasting or infections exacerbate the clinical severity and may precipitate acute heart failure. Administration of carnitine may reverse the acute illness. Hypertrophic cardiomyopathy with superimposed endocardial fibroelastosis can develop. Primary carnitine deficiency results from impaired liver synthesis. Cardiomyopathy also results from defects in the transport of carnitine into cells and with mitochondrial enzyme carnitine palmitoyltransferase II deficiency. Lipid accumulation occurs in a wide spectrum of cell types. Ultrastructurally, the lipid is microvacuolar and often closely associated with mitochondria. Defects in long-chain fatty acid oxidative enzymes also cause hypertrophic or dilated cardiomyopathy with myocyte lipid accumulation. Medium- and short-chain fatty acid oxidation defects are not associated with cardiomyopathy but can, like long-chain fatty acid defects, cause sudden unexpected death.

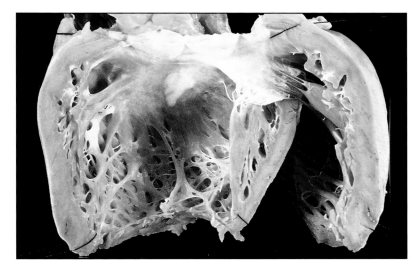

Figure 10-25.

Cardiomyopathy in an explanted dilated heart from a 12-year-old boy with congenital fiber type disproportion. Cardiomyopathy accompanies skeletal muscle disease in various congenital myopathies, muscular dystrophies, myotonic disorders, and neuromuscular conditions. Heart disease usually presents in adolescents and adults rather than in infants and young children. With most patients, the cardiac involvement is clinically overshadowed by the skeletal muscle pathology, but in some patients, such as those with Becker muscular dystrophy, cardiomyopathy occasionally predominates. The majority of conditions in this group are associated with dilated cardiomyopathy, but some are hypertrophic. Gross morphologic features generally are not distinguishing, except that Duchenne muscular dystrophy shows characteristic posterobasal left ventricular free wall subepicardial fibrosis and Friedreich's ataxia has hypertrophic cardiomyopathy with asymmetric ventricular septal hypertrophy that is often obstructive. Microscopy also is usually nonspecific, with hypertrophic changes, interstitial fibrosis, and fatty infiltration.

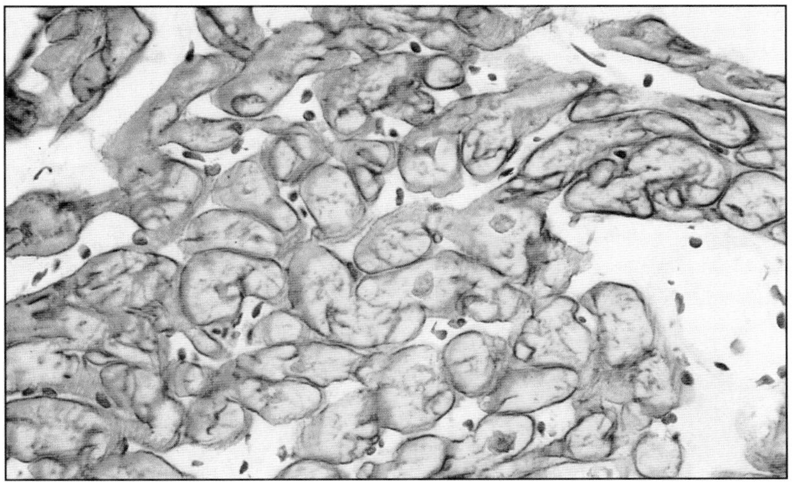

Figure 10-26.

The normal continuous cell membrane dystrophin immunohistochemical staining pattern in a frozen section of an endomyocardial biopsy from a boy with dilated cardiomyopathy. Dystrophin staining is valuable in the assessment of childhood idiopathic dilated cardiomyopathy because dystrinopathy can clinically present with cardiomyopathy alone, molecular genetic study results are negative in about one third of muscular dystrophy cases, and cardiomyopathy can occur in female carriers [16]. As with the evaluation of skeletal muscle biopsies, N-terminus, C-terminus, and midrod dystrophin antisera should be applied. Affected myocardium shows either complete absence of membrane staining or a mosaic or discontinuous pattern [17].

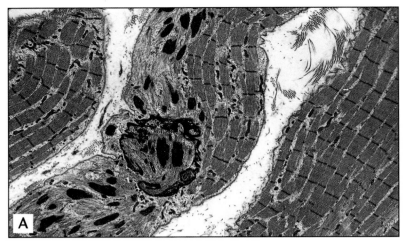

Figure 10-27.

Nemaline myopathy. This disorder is characterized by presence of short rod–shaped cytoplasmic inclusions within striated muscle cells. These are not well appreciated in hematoxylin and eosin–stained sections but are easily seen with modified Gomori trichrome stain and in toluidine blue–stained thick epon–embedded sections. They are seen easily on electron microscopy as electron-dense structures occurring in foci of sarcomeric disruption

(*panel A*). Heart involvement is rare, but childhood presentation with dilated cardiomyopathy occurs [18]. The rods are rectangular or oval, up to 7 μm long, and lie in continuity with Z bands. An internal lattice-like structure can be seen, and thin filaments stream from the rods (*panel B*). Immunohistochemical staining reveals α-actinin content. Similar structures can rarely be found in other myopathic conditions.

PEDIATRIC METABOLIC CARDIOMYOPATHY RELATED TO MATERNAL AND IATROGENIC FACTORS

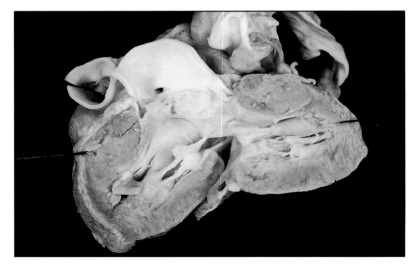

Figure 10-28.

Heart from an infant of a diabetic mother showing marked left ventricular hypertrophy with subaortic prominence caused by asymmetric septal thickening. The hypertrophic cardiomyopathy is acquired by the fetus from the abnormal metabolic state resulting from maternal hyperglycemia. Fetal hyperinsulinemia occurs in response to the mother's diabetes. The growth-promoting effects of insulin lead to fetal macrosomia, including cardiomegaly [19]. The asymmetric septal hypertrophy can be recognized antenatally, with the septal-free wall ratio, measured by fetal echocardiography, generally larger than 1.5 (the ratio may be up to 3.9). Newborns present with congestive heart failure, but the condition is usually transient, with failure resolving within a few weeks of birth and septal hypertrophy regressing within a few months. Rarely, the cardiomyopathy leads to death in infancy [20]. The heart at autopsy in such cases is up to four times the expected weight and shows right and left ventricular hypertrophy accompanying the septal hypertrophy. Similar hypertrophic changes can occur in babies given dexamethasone for treatment of bronchopulmonary dysplasia [21].

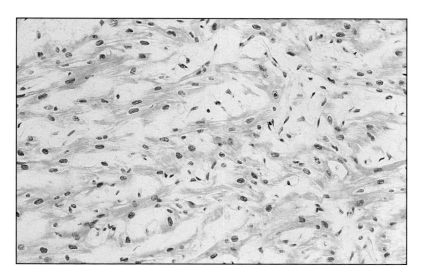

Figure 10-29.

Myocardium from an infant of a mother with insulin-dependent diabetes mellitus (IDDM) demonstrating disarray resembling that seen in autosomal dominant familial hypertrophic cardiomyopathy (HCM). However, the extent of disarray in IDDM is significantly less than in HCM. This is best evaluated in a full-thickness section of the mid-interventricular septum taken through the horizontal plane. In HCM, even in infants, myocardial disarray occupies more than 5%, and as much as 30%, of the surface area of such a section. The disarray found in IDDM covers less than 5% of the surface area and is generally confined to the ends of the septum at the confluence of septum and free right and left ventricular walls [20,22]. It should be noted that normal hearts also have focal myocardial disarray at the ventricular confluences.

MORPHOLOGIC CONSIDERATIONS IN PEDIATRIC CARDIOMYOPATHY

Endocardial Fibroelastosis

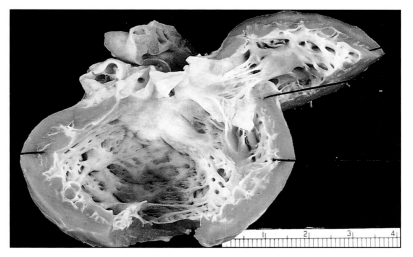

Figure 10-30.

Explanted heart from a neonate receiving a transplant for congenital dilated cardiomyopathy showing diffuse endocardial fibroelastosis (EFE) of the left ventricle. The lesion, which develops in the immature heart, consists of a white rubbery layer up to 3 mm thick that coats the luminal surface of the affected cardiac chamber. It smooths the surface features of trabeculae and papillary muscles and may thicken and shorten chordae tendineae. Within a chamber, thickness varies but usually is greatest at the outflow tract. Mural thrombus occurs in up to 6% of cases in which EFE is superimposed on a dilated cardiomyopathy. The left ventricle is most commonly involved, but the right ventricle, with or without the left, and the atria can also be affected. Atrial involvement can lead to antenatal closure or stenosis of the foramen ovale, which is associated with hydrops fetalis.

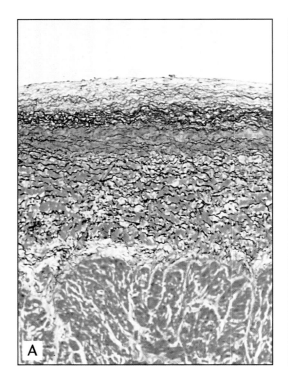

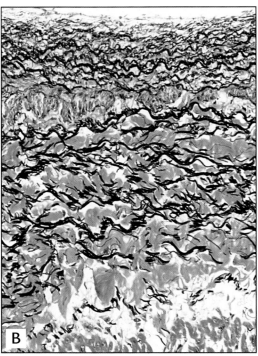

Figure 10-31.
Microscopic appearance of endocardial fibroelastosis (EFE). This appearance consists of relatively hypocellular fibrous tissue with multiple lamellae of elastic fibers arranged parallel to the luminal surface, as demonstrated in these trichrome-stained sections. The lower-power photomicrograph (*panel A*) illustrates the relatively sharp border between EFE and myocardium and the lack of inflammation. The underlying myocardium may show hypertrophic change or degrees of vacuolar degeneration. Occasionally, a few mononuclear inflammatory cells are scattered in the adjacent myocardium. The higher-power view (*panel B*) shows the constituent collagen, elastic lamellae, and spindle interstitial cells. Also demonstrated is a zone of smooth muscle cells just beneath the endocardial surface—a frequent finding.

Vacuolated Cardiac Myocytes

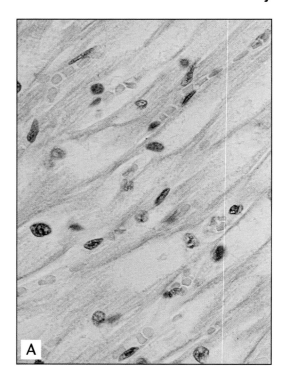

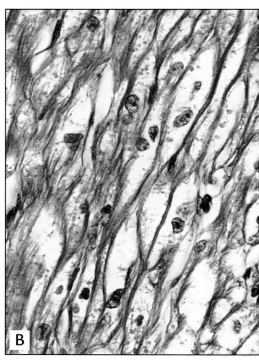

Figure 10-32.
Histologic appearance of vacuoloated cardiac myocytes. The histologic hallmark of metabolic cardiomyopathy is the vacuolated myocyte, as seen in Pompe disease (*panel A*) and mitochondrial cardiomyopathy (*panel B*). However, swollen and "cleared" myocytes are seen in other forms of cell injury and are not pathognomonic of a metabolic disorder. (*continued on next page*)

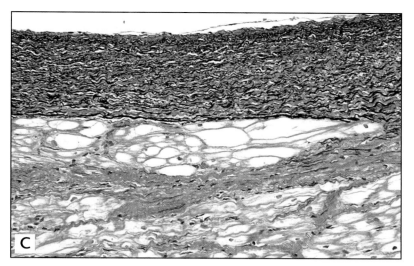

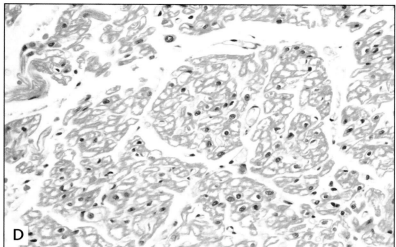

Figure 10-32. (*continued*)

For example, hypoxic cell injury to myocytes immediately beneath the relative diffusion barrier of endocardial fibroelastosis (*panel C*) causes vacuolar degeneration with cytoplasmic clearing. This can be seen in the myocardium of a fetus stillborn after being stressed by an idiopathic congenital cardiomyopathy and confound interpretation of the heart at autopsy. In contrast to glycogen storage diseases, the periodic acid–Schiff stain in this circumstance shows diminished myocyte positivity. Immature cardiac myocytes have a relative paucity of organelles, including contractile elements in addition to increased glycogen stores. During fetal development, the organelle complement and density of sarcomeres increase. However, fetal or neonatal myocardium normally has a vacuolated character, as demonstrated in this hematoxylin and eosin–stained myocardium from a stillborn premature fetus (*panel D*). This needs consideration in the histologic evaluation of a possible fetal or neonatal cardiomyopathy.

REFERENCES

1. Schwartz ML, Cox GF, Lin AI, *et al.*: Clinical approach to genetic cardiomyopathy in children. *Circulation* 1996, 94:2021–2038.

2. Servidei S, Bertini E, DiMauro S: Hereditary metabolic cardiomyopathies. *Adv Pediatr* 1994, 41:1–32.

3. Dincsoy MY, Dincsoy HP, Kessler AD, *et al.*: Generalized glycogenosis and associated endocardial fibroelastosis: report of 3 cases with biochemical studies. *J Pediatr* 1965, 67:728–740.

4. Riggs JE, Schochet SS, Jr, Gutmann L, *et al.*: Lysosomal glycogen storage disease without acid maltase deficiency. *Neurology* 1983, 33:873–877.

5. Moses SW, Wanderman KL, Myroz A, Frydman M: Cardiac involvement in glycogen storage disease type III. *Eur J Pediatr* 1989, 148:764–766.

6. Servidei S, Riepe RE, Langston C, *et al.*: Severe cardiopathy in branching enzyme deficiency. *J Pediatr* 1987, 111:51–56.

7. Sengers RCA, Stadhouders AM, Trijbels JMF: Mitochondrial myopathies: clinical, morphological and biochemical aspects. *Eur J Pediatr* 1984, 141:192–207.

8. Marin-Garcia J, Goldenthal MJ: Mitochondrial cardiomyopathy: molecular and biochemical analysis. *Pediatr Cardiol* 1997, 18:251–260.

9. Trijbels JMF, Sengers RCA, Ruitenbeek W, *et al.*: Disorders of the mitochondrial respiratory chain: clinical manifestations and diagnostic approach. *Eur J Pediatr* 1988, 148:92–97.

10. Kiechle FL, Kaul KL, Farkas DH: Mitochondrial disorders: methods and specimen selection for diagnostic molecular pathology. *Arch Pathol Lab Med* 1996, 120:597–603.

11. Shehata BM, Patterson K, Thomas JE, *et al.*: Histiocytoid cardiomyopathy: three new cases and a review of the literature. *Pediatr Dev Pathol* 1998, 1:56–69.

12. Kearney DL, Titus JL, Hawkins EP, *et al.*: Pathologic features of myocadial hamartomas causing childhood tachyarrhythmias. *Circulation* 1987, 4:705–710.

13. Papadimitriou A, Neustein HB, DiMauro S, *et al.*: Histiocytoid cardiomyopathy of infancy: deficiency of reducible cytochrome b in heart mitochondria. *Pediatr Res* 1984, 18:1023–1028.

14. Pons R, De Vivo DC: Primary and secondary carnitine deficiency syndromes. *J Child Neurol* 1995, 10(suppl 2):8–24.

15. Winter S, Jue K, Prochazka J, *et al.*: The role of L-carnitine in pediatric cardiomyopathy. *J Child Neurol* 1995, 10(suppl 2):45–51.

16. Oldfors A, Eriksson BO, Kyllerman M, *et al.*: Dilated cardiomyopathy and the dystrophin gene: an illustrated review. *Br Heart J* 1994, 72:344–348.

17. Maeda M, Nakao S, Miyazato H, *et al.*: Cardiac dystrophin abnormalities in Becker muscular dystrophy assessed by endomyocardial biopsy. *Am Heart J* 1995, 129:702–707.

18. Ishibashi-Ueda H, Imakita M, Yutani C, *et al.*: Congenital nemaline myopathy with dilated cardiomyopathy: an autopsy study. *Hum Pathol* 1990, 21:77–82.

19. Fowden AL: The role of insulin in fetal growth. *Early Human Development* 1992, 29:171–181.

20. McMahon JN, Berry PJ, Joffe HS: Fatal hypertrophic cardiomyopathy in an infant of a diabetic mother. *Pediatr Cardiol* 1990, 11:211–212.

21. Israel BA, Sherman FS, Guthrie RD: Hypertrophic cardiomyopathy associated with dexamethasone therapy for chronic lung disease in preterm infants. *Am J Perinatol* 1993, 10:307–310.

22. Maron BJ, Sato N, Roberts WC, *et al.*: Quantitative analysis of cardiac muscle cell disorganization in the ventricular septum: comparison of fetuses and infants with and without congenital heart disease and patients with hypertrophic cardiomyopathy. *Circulation* 1979, 60:685–96.

23. Lurie PR: Endocardial fibroelastosis is not a disease. *Am J Cardiol* 1988, 62:468–470.

11

Myocarditis

Bruce M. McManus
Reinhard Kandolf

Myocarditis is defined, pathologically, as cell necrosis or cell injury with associated inflammation of the heart muscle, in the absence of ischemic phenomena [1]. The cause may or may not be known. Myocarditis frequently underlies acute dilated cardiomyopathy in humans, and may be a precursor to chronic dilated cardiomyopathy [2,3]. Clinically, myocarditis is difficult to diagnose because of the range of presentations—from subclinical, virtually innocuous, to fulminant, with profound pump failure or lethal arrhythmias. Endomyocardial biopsy may allow a more or less definitive diagnosis in life; however, bioptome sampling of myocarditis has limited sensitivity [4,5].

Myocarditis can result from infection, or from toxic or allergic or hypersensitivity responses [6]. Viruses are the most common infectious causes of myocarditis acquired in the community, although many additional agents (including bacteria, protozoa, and fungi) can produce myocarditis. The latter forms of myocarditis are more often seen in immunodeficient or immune-compromised patients. Viruses most commonly associated with human myocarditis include picornaviruses, influenza viruses, HIV-1, herpesviruses, and adenoviruses. Of patients with clinical myocarditis, nearly half have had or currently have an enteroviral infection. Most current work on the pathogenesis and consequences of viral myocarditis has focused on the Coxsackie B group of viruses, which have the highest likelihood of causing clinical cardiovascular disease (30 to 40 cardiovascular diagnoses per 1000 serologically documented virus infections [7]).

Molecular techniques have been applied successfully in the detection of enteroviral RNA and other viral RNA in patients with myocarditis or idiopathic dilated cardiomyopathy (IDC). Thus, RNA blotting, reverse transcriptase polymerase chain reaction (RT-PCR), and in situ hybridization together have shown that up to 70% of adult myocarditis patients and up to 45% of IDC patients in certain populations may be positive for viral genome [8]. The average overall frequency of myocardial positivity for enteroviral genome in adult patients with myocarditis and IDC is 25%. The frequency is much higher in fatal myocarditis of infancy. Other viruses have been solidly implicated in viral heart disease when investigations have used sensitive molecular detection strategies [9,10].

Perhaps the most long-standing hypothesis regarding the pathogenesis of enteroviral heart disease is that coxsackievirus (CVB3) induces autoimmune responses including cellular constituents of the immune system that are lytic for uninfected cells (as bystanders), as well as for infected heart cells. A second hypothesis proposes that the humoral limb of the immune response causes chronic tissue pathology through autoreactive antibodies and molecular mimicry. A third and current hypothesis implicates extensive, direct, virus-mediated injury of infected tissues, particularly evident prior to cellular immune infiltrates. Persistent low-level replication of the virus may elicit long-term antiviral immune responses, as well as virus-induced loss of cardiocyte function and cell death accompanied by an inflammatory response [11,12]. Certainly, the early predominance of the virus in the myocarditic process, and the inherent differences in virulent properties of different viral strains, profoundly influence the nature and severity of myocardial damage and the subsequent immune and inflammatory sequelae.

Using in situ hybridization to determine the presence, locale, and persistence of viral RNA in murine tissues following infection has yielded entirely new insights into the systemic nature of enteroviral disease. The results of TUNEL (TdT-mediated dUTP nick end labeling of fragmented cellular DNA) and other complementary electrophoretic and biochemical techniques, when interpreted cautiously, can be used to evaluate cell death mechanisms underlying pathologic processes in CVB3 infection of heart muscle. TUNEL-positive cells are typically positive for viral RNA, as determined by in situ hybridization on adjacent sections [13]. The diffuse cellular nature of TUNEL labeling in such cells suggests a necrotizing mechanism of death in cardiocytes, whereas other biochemical indices indicate that apoptotic injury is also involved.

The myocardial consequences of viral interactions with immune cells in the spleen or other lymphoid organs are not completely understood; however, the phenomenon of virus being retained in the spleen and lymph nodes has been documented in many different types of viral infections. Factors that determine target organ virulence beyond interactions of the virus with immune cells must be accounted for, including viral receptor distribution, host cell proteins, and viral genetics [13].

Definitive therapies for viral myocarditis are not available. Treatment of patients with histopathologic myocarditis requires multiple potential approaches depending on the stage of disease at detection, the nature of the cellular infiltrate, and the age of the patient. Immunosuppression and immunodeficiency are neutral-to-adverse to outcome, whereas antiviral and immunologically augmentive therapy and cardiologic support of ventricular dysfunction may be particularly beneficial in certain patients. Neither pathologic, serologic, nor hemodynamic descriptors of myocarditis are now sufficient for characterization of the disease process. Molecular, immunologic, genetic, metabolic, and microvascular considerations must also be made.

In this chapter we present information regarding causes of myocarditis, key events in the evolution of clinical and scientific understanding of myocarditis, diagnostic approaches, the pathologic spectrum of disease, and in situ hybridized human myocardium illustrating the distributive features of infection. We then provide a synopsis of human data regarding enteroviral positivity in the heart, and pathologic, molecular, and biochemical aspects of the disease process as determined or hypothesized on the basis of model systems in vivo and in vitro.

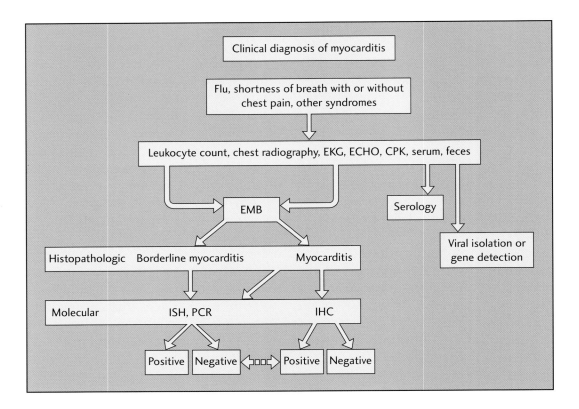

Figure 11-1.

Clinical diagnosis of myocarditis. It is widely appreciated that the clinical manifestations of myocarditis are protean and variable, even when induced by the same agent or cause. In general, a flulike illness may be accompanied by shortness of breath, with or without chest pain. Other presentations, however, are also observed; one of these, rather unsettlingly, is sudden cardiac death. Thus, sudden collapse with an unexpected dysrhythmia is a frequent cause of near death or mortal events. The clinical diagnostic approach, beyond physical examination and historical observations, includes peripheral blood leukocyte count, chest radiography, electrocardiogram (EKG), echocardiogram (ECHO), serum creatinine phosphokinase (CPK), viral serology, and fecal isolation of virus or genome. The leukocyte count will be elevated in certain patients and depressed in others. This latter group probably constitutes 20% of all patients who are studied clinically for suspected myocarditis. The cardiac shadow may be enlarged on chest radiography or when examined by other image modalities, and an ECHO may reveal diminished global or regional myocardial function. The ECG is often associated with sinus tachycardia, but may reveal a variety of rhythm disturbances or conduction blocks. CPK of cardiac origin may be elevated in the blood of 10% of such patients. Viral serology may be useful in demonstrating acute-to-convalescent changes in neutralizing antibody titers against certain viral antigens. A major caveat exists, however, in that the immunologic response to an infection by a given virus may include polyclonal elevations in antibodies to viruses that are antigenically similar to the one in question. As such, serologic information has been helpful, but not without its significant limitations or misleading nature. The isolation of virus or detection of genome in fecal material is very helpful when positive, but because of a number of logistical and timing issues, such an approach may not reveal the myocarditic pathogen.

The endomyocardial biopsy (EMB) specimen brings the diagnosis of myocarditis to the anatomic pathology laboratory [14]. The sensitivity of endocardial biopsy in the detection of myocarditis has been questioned [4,15]. Thus, the sensitivity of detection of active myocarditis in human hearts is perhaps 45% to 50% when four to five pieces of right ventricular endomyocardium are obtained and submitted to histopathologic evaluation by a knowledgeable cardiovascular pathologist. This diagnostic sensitivity is based on the application of the Dallas criteria developed in support of the National Institutes of Health–sponsored myocarditis treatment trial [1]. These criteria distinguish absence of myocarditis from borderline myocarditis (localized inflammatory infiltrate without myocyte death), which is, in turn, distinguished from myocarditis (infiltrate plus myocyte damage). Certainly, the histopathologic detection of myocarditis by an EMB is limited by the amount of tissue available for examination and by the variable nature of infiltrates and of cell damage (see Fig. 11-2). With more intensive evaluation of EMB tissue by in situ hybridization (ISH), gene amplification, or immunohistochemistry (IHC) of viral antigens, the possibility exists that a biopsy may be histopathologically negative but molecularly positive. The possibility also exists for the biopsy to be rather strikingly abnormal from a histopathologic point of view, but negative for potentially cardiotropic human viruses. Thus, the package that encompasses a diagnosis of myocarditis is now much more complex and challenging than ever before. We have numerous indices, but the precise definition may be clinical, pathologic, virologic, or immunologic. Reconciliation of divergent results within a given patient requires further study; in the meantime, EMB remains a useful tool, particularly at referral centers where patients with new and sometimes profound heart muscle failure are strongly considered for EMB in the process of diagnostic evaluation [16]. PCR—polymerase chain reaction.

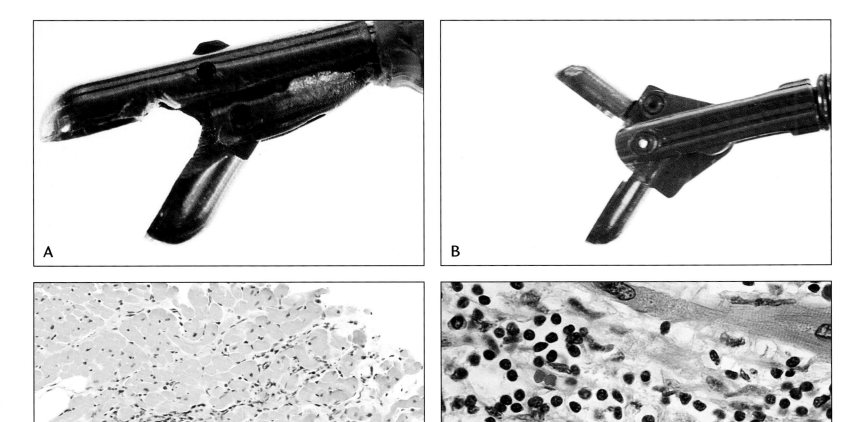

Figure 11-2.

The endomyocardial biopsy procedure. **A,** A close-up of the biting jaws of a Scholten bioptome, which is frequently used for the endomyocardial biopsy procedure. One jaw is fixed whereas the other is mobile and hinged. The biopsy specimen is captured in a small "chamber" after being resected by the cutting jaws. **B,** In contrast, the Cordis bioptome has two mobile hinged jaws with a smaller cutting surface. Tissues acquired by either of these bioptomes may yield tissue sufficient for a histopathologic diagnosis of myocarditis [1]. Other effective bioptomes are also on the market. **C,** An endomyocardial biopsy fragment with focal adipocytes also has an area of scant interstitial cellular infiltrate associated with limited myocyte damage. When such an infiltrate is viewed at higher magnification, its cellular constituents and the minor degree of localized injury may be documented (mild myocarditis, barely exceeding borderline myocarditis). **D,** In serious myocarditis, the associated edema and myocyte disruption cause loss of myocytes and consequent loss of ventricular function. The histologic picture of early-healing myocarditis 5 weeks after a diagnosis and isolation of coxsackievirus B4, beyond continued lymphocyte infiltrates, is associated with early fibrosis, and macrophages with brown pigment. The latter include those with lipofuscin from engulfed dying myocytes and hemosiderin from localized hemorrhages.

PRINCIPLES AND PRACTICE OF ENDOMYOCARDIAL BIOPSY IN FAILING NATIVE OR ALLOGRAFT HEARTS

Essentials for Optimal Diagnoses	Mimickers and Artifacts	Caveats
Adequate tissue: generally 3–5 pieces of tissue for paraffin sections (rarely fixed for ultrastructural analyses)	Contraction bands	Amount of fibrous and adipose tissue will vary considerably from biopsy to biopsy
Rapid and consistent tissue triage, tissue or damp sterile saline-soaked gauze, immediately fixed	Compression (squeeze)	Sensitivity of detection is disease-specific (detection of myocarditis is much less sensitive then acute rejection[45% vs 98% using ≥4 pieces of tissue])
Representative section:adequate levels and number of slides	Hemorrhage	In tertiary referral centers, expect approximately 20% specific diagnoses (nonreferral centers may have even fewer specific diagnoses)
Appropriate use of stains, molecular probes, primers	Edema	
Freeze biopsy tissue	Telescoped blood vessels	
Obtain serum and leukocytes	Healed biopsy sites	
History of drug use, other clinical factors	Catheter lesions	
	Vasopressor lesions	
	Ischemia	
	Endocardial fibrous tissue	
	Adipocytes	
	Myocardial calcification	
	Tangenital sections	
	Nonendomyocardial tissue	
	Opportunistic infections	
	Endocardial infiltrates: "Quilty effects"	
	MICE	

Figure 11-3.

Principles and practice of endomyocardial biopsy in failing native or allograft hearts. With currently available bioptomes, a minimum of three to five pieces of endomyocardial tissue measuring approximately 2 × 2 × 3 mm in greatest dimension are required for routine processing, paraffin sections, and histopathologic examination. The preparation of at least three glass slides with at least three levels of tissue per slide would be considered conventional practice. A number of centers prepare additional levels, whereas others "cut through the block" in preparing glass slides. Arguably, the use of a trichrome stain or another connective tissue stain to delineate elements of the interstitium and endocardium, in addition to defining small blood vessels and cardiac myocytes, may be helpful in extending interpretation beyond what is possible by hematoxylin and eosin staining alone.

Certainly, immunohistochemical stains that demarcate cardiac myocytes (eg, muscle myosin, muscle actin) and define immune cell type or origin (eg, CD68 for giant cells; B-cell markers to distinguish deep Quilty lesions from rejection in allograft biopsies) will improve the value of a biopsy review. On occasion, the use of molecular probes and primers may be helpful diagnostically, although apart from the search for viruses, more frequently such tools are reserved for clinical investigation. Given the need to preserve the integrity of proteins and nucleic acids in biopsy tissue, the obligation for rapid, standardized processing of specimens cannot be overemphasized. Flash-freezing should also be carried out in a standardized fashion with ample embedding compound to assure preservation of tissue architecture. Rapid freezing of unembedded tissues is crucial for the protection of nucleic acids that can later be extracted for genetic analysis. Liquid nitrogen is the best means for achieving rapid and reliable freezing. The archive of serum and cells from peripheral blood may render valuable material for diagnostic investigation. Clinical history, including therapeutic and illicit drug use, exposures to pathogens or other toxins, as well as age, sex, and cardiac history (eg, heart failure, chest pain) will enhance the use of this clinicopathologic tool.

The use of endomyocardial biopsy is not without limitations. Numerous confounding architectural features may prevent accurate diagnoses. With experience, these features are accounted for and discounted from the diagnostic result. The presence of opportunistic infections or endocardial infiltrates is particularly a feature of biopsy specimens from heart allografts [17]. Finally, considering the somewhat heterogeneous nature of the endomyocardium, it is crucially important that inherent variabilities in tissue constituency, diagnostic sensitivity for given diseases, and expected specific results in certain patient groups are acknowledged. Satisfaction with the "yield" of diagnostically discriminating information will be enhanced by appreciation of these limitations. A search continues for new analytical approaches to the biopsy of heart tissues and to the use of tissue once obtained. MICE—mesothelial/monocytic incidental cardiac excrescence.

CLINICAL CLASSIFICATION OF MYOCARDITIS

	Fulminant	Acute	Chronic	Resolved
Initial presentation	Cardiogenic shock; severe LV dysfunction; heart block; arrhythmias	CHF; LV dysfunction	CHF; LV dysfunction	No CHF; usually normal LV function
Initial EMB	Multiple foci of active myocarditis	Active or borderline myocarditis	Active, borderline, or healing myocarditis	Borderline or inactive, healed myocarditis
Clinical natural history	Complete recovery or death	Incomplete recovery or DCM	DCM	Normal LV function

Figure 11-4.

Clinical classification of myocarditis. A classification scheme for myocarditis based on both clinical and pathologic information has been published and revised [18,19]. In this figure we present yet another rendering in which myocarditis categories are defined as fulminant, acute, chronic, and resolved. This classification scheme recalls that of Lustock et al. [20]. The system also provides a framework for addressing the needs of patients with myocarditis. Correlation of endomyocardial biopsy (EMB) findings with initial presentation or natural history must be considered essential, because the composite of findings will be unique for a given patient. Even within inbred strains of mice infected with human and murine cardiotropic coxsackievirus strains, there is consider-

able variation in presentation, histopathology, and outcome of the disease [21]. Part of this variability relates to the fact that myocarditis is a systemic illness [13]. Other organs may be more or less predominantly involved by active infection with pathologic consequences (eg, liver, pancreas), and the host outcome may be determined more by involvement of such targets than the myocardium itself. Supportive cardiovascular therapy remains the mainstay of myocarditis management, reflecting in part the lack of definitive evidence from controlled clinical trials for an effective therapy and in part the high likelihood of spontaneous clinical remission in such patients. CHF—congestive heart failure; DCM—dilated cardiomyopathy; LV—left ventricular.

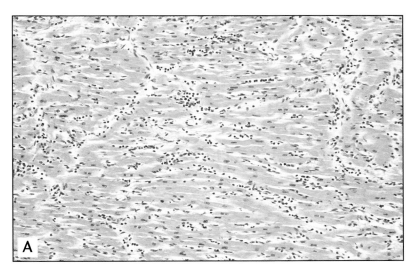

Figure 11-5.

Patterns of human myocarditic cellular infiltrates. These can vary widely among cases of fatal myocarditis and even within a given heart. This series of photomicrographs highlights the extent of variability. **A,** This widely dispersed interstitial infiltrate tracks along tissue planes and is associated with apparent extracellular

edema. **B,** The image in *panel A* compares with more localized aggregates of mononuclear cells in this panel and with even more prominent focal infiltrates and associated edema. (*continued on next page*)

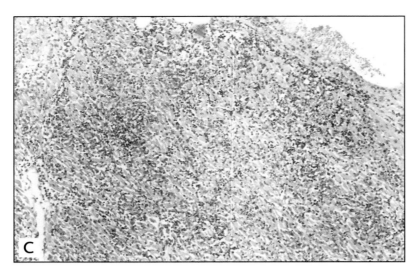

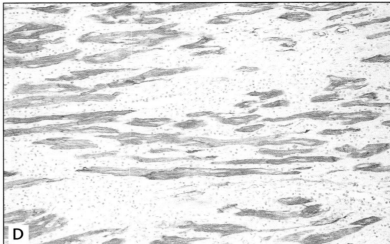

Figure 11-5. (*continued*)

C, Ultimately, the infiltrate may be diffuse and confluent, virtually effacing myocardial architecture (*panel D*). Chronicity of the process may be reflected by continued cellular infiltrates with associated edematous connective tissue. (In *panels A through C*, hematoxylin and eosin stain, × 125; *panel D*, HHF-35 stain, × 125.)

Several inflammatory lesions of ventricular myocardium may masquerade as myocarditis. Cocaine abuse may produce a focal polymorphic infiltrate in a perivascular distribution with direct involvement of microvessels. The infiltrate in this instance is associated with localized myocyte coagulation and contraction band changes suggestive of ischemic damage. In end-stage cardiomyo-

pathic hearts explanted at the time of transplantation, there is often extensive scarring with inflammatory infiltrates responsive to tissue injury and repair. As well, the infiltration of myocardium by lymphomatous cells may be associated with tissue disruption, edema, and widespread cellularity. Such infiltrates are not uncommon accompaniments of systemic lymphoma or leukemia and may be seen as myocardial involvement of posttransplant lymphoproliferative disease (PTLD) [22]. Such cardiac infiltration by PTLD may in the latter case be associated with Epstein-Barr virus infection and a B-cell lymphomatous process.

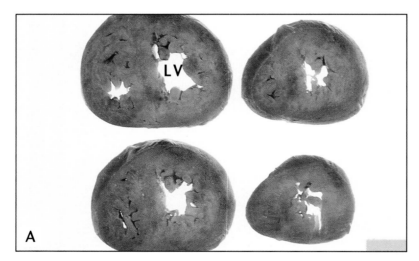

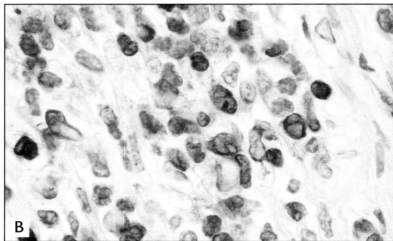

Figure 11-6.

Pathological findings in severe myocarditis. An infant girl presented with profound ventricular dysfunction, arrhythmias, and cyanosis. She had echocardiographic evidence of wall motion abnormalities that were nonuniform throughout the left ventricular free wall. Dysfunction progressed and she died within days of presentation in severe heart failure. **A,** Subserial ventricular myocardial sections of the autopsy heart revealed marked diffuse thickening of both the right and left ventricular free walls and the ventricular septum. The

myocardium was generally mottled, soft, and focally hemorrhagic. Both ventricular cavities were dilated, particularly the left. The histologic picture included a diffuse cellular infiltrate with marked destruction of cardiac myocytes and pronounced edema. **B,** Immunohistochemical labeling of the inflammatory infiltrate revealed numerous T cells and many macrophages (CD68-positive). (*continued on next page*)

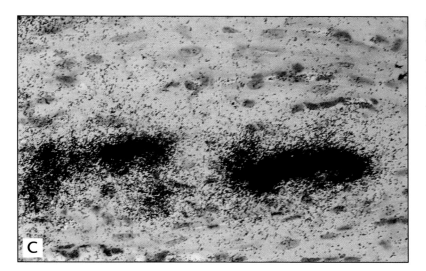

Figure 11-6. (*continued*)

C, In addition, there was readily detectable enteroviral RNA on in situ hybridization with a full-length ³⁵S-labeled cDNA probe (hematoxylin and eosin stain on hybridized slide). This in situ hybridization positivity corresponded to high titers of cardiac virus detected on plaque assay. An echovirus was isolated and characterized. LV—left ventricle.

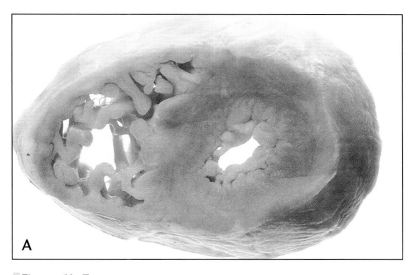

Figure 11-7.

Morphology of fatal myocarditis in childhood. For very young infants acquiring myocarditis in the peripartal period, the outcome is particularly dismal, with more than 90% of children dying. In children contracting myocarditis in the first few days to weeks following birth, the outcome is only somewhat better, with perhaps 20% to 30% of children surviving [23]. When myocarditis is contracted in older children and young adults, survival (with or without sustained cardiac dysfunction) is much more likely. Just as myocarditis in children can be devastating clinically, it may be dramatic from a pathologic point of view. The heart depicted in *panels A through D* is from a 10-year-old boy who collapsed suddenly. **A,** A transverse section of the ventricular myocardium reveals edema, mottling, and paleness typical of a markedly infiltrated myocardium. The right ventricular cavity is particularly dilated. Histologically there were numerous areas of heavy mononuclear cell infiltration with associated myocyte destruction. In certain regions of the myocardium where the picture was most dramatic, there was a dense mononuclear cell infiltrate and associated young and mature collagen bundles, indicating a scarring process. **B,** At high power, the lymphocytic nature of the infiltrate can be appreciated (hematoxylin and eosin, × 500). Only a few remaining cardiac myocytes can be appreciated in this field. The etiologic agent for this picture was never identified. *Panels C and D* are taken from the myocardium of a child with influenza A myocarditis. (*continued on next page*)

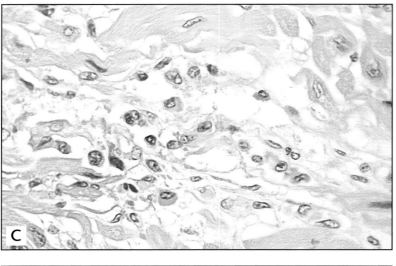

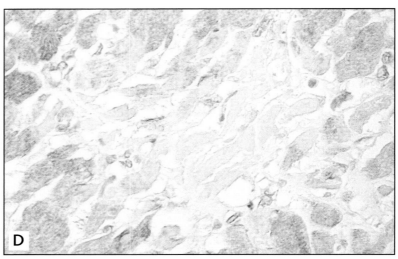

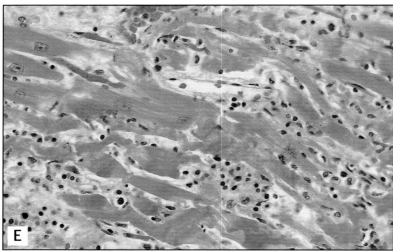

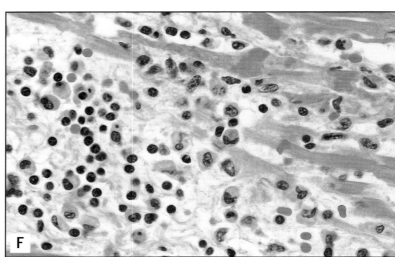

▌**Figure 11-7.** (*continued*)
C, The histologic picture is one of focal myocyte destruction and a polymorphic infiltrate predominated by macrophages. **D,** Based on muscle-specific actin staining (HHF-35 [muscle-specific] antibody), the degree of myocyte loss and the "punched-out" nature of the myocarditic lesions can be appreciated. **E** and **F,** The histopathology of myocardium from an 11-year-old girl with a 4-day illness. The myocardial tissue is striking for the severity of the cell injury and death, the prominence of edema, and the widespread infiltrate (hematoxylin and eosin, × 125 [*panel E*] and ×

500 [*panel F*]). Numerous T cells and macrophages are apparent, and erythrophagocytosis as well as phagocytosis of other cardiac constituents is evident. In situ hybridization and polymerase chain reaction were performed for the genome of several common human cardiotropic viruses. All tests results were negative. This case material represents the enigma of presumed infectious myocarditis that is yet to be linked to an identifiable cause. In younger patients, the establishment of a viral cause for myocarditis is much more readily achieved than in older age groups.

▌**Figure 11-8.**
Histologic field of ventricular myocardium from a patient with active rheumatic carditis. The patient developed subacute progressive heart failure and required heart transplantation [24]. **A,** A perivascular Aschoff lesion (hematoxylin and eosin, × 500). (*continued on next page*)

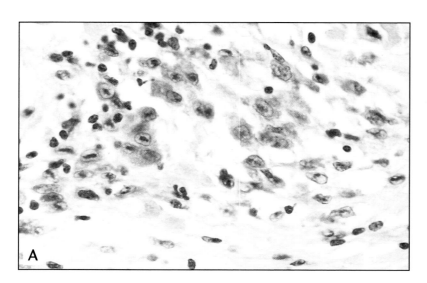

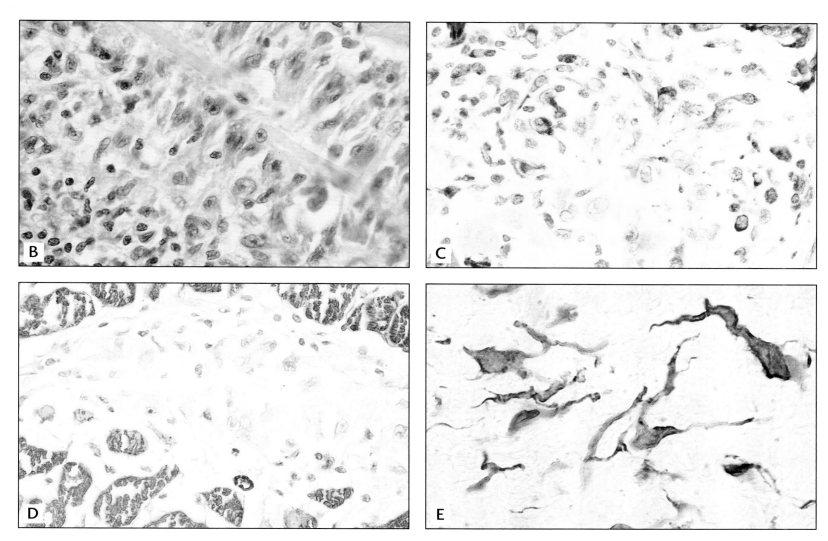

Figure 11-8. (*continued*)
B, On immunohistochemical staining, a number of the cells within the Aschoff lesion are vimentin-positive. **C,** Typically, there are a few T cells in the halo of the Aschoff lesion and numerous macrophage-derived cells centrally. **D,** As illustrated by muscle-specific actin staining, the cells shown are not derived from cardiac muscle. Vimentin staining can also reveal the presence of myofibroblasts in normal and rheumatic heart valve tissue [25] and can illustrate the immunophenotype and tentacular similarity of valvular myofibroblasts in tissue sections (*panel E*) and in tissue culture (*panel F*). Such myofibroblasts are most likely derived from fibroblasts in the valvular interstitium and contribute to the evolving matrix of rheumatic valvulitis.

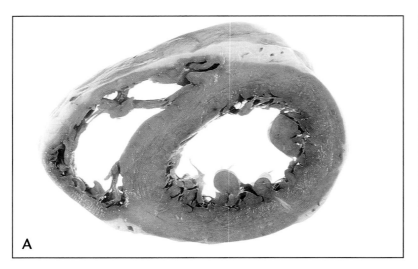

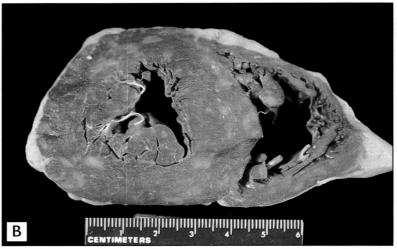

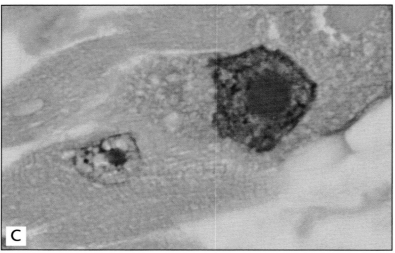

Figure 11-9.

Injured, inflamed, and infected cardiac muscle. These problems are frequent in patients with immune compromise. **A,** A transverse ventricular myocardial section of an autopsy heart with prominent biventricular dilatation is derived from a patient with bone marrow transplantation for non-Hodgkin's lymphoma and subsequent disseminated candidiasis. Epicardial fat is somewhat decreased. The

extent of ventricular failure implied by the dilatation not only reflects the involvement of the myocardium by fungus, but also previous mediastinal irradiation. **B,** At autopsy, cardiac toxoplasmosis may be found to involve the entire myocardium, including both ventricular free walls and the ventricular septum. Multifocal random regions of light coloration are evident in the ventricular myocardium when the heart has been stained fresh with triphenyl tetrazolium chloride (TTC) to highlight viable myocardium as red-brown, and necrotic myocardium as light-staining. The lightly stained areas represent infiltration of inflammatory cells and myocyte necrosis, as well as those myocytes infected directly with toxoplasma. The ventricular cavities are somewhat dilated.

C, Common opportunistic infections may produce myocarditis in the human heart; specifically, cytomegalovirus may directly infect cardiac myocytes, as shown. The infected myocyte is from the heart of an immunosuppressed patient. There is degenerative vacuolization of the cytoplasm in a very large nucleus with a classic magenta, glassy nuclear inclusion. This infected nucleus stands in contrast to the nucleus of an adjacent cardiac muscle cell, which may have a very early infection. In this particular heart, the inclusion was found in a field without other distinct inclusions and without accompanying inflammatory response; however, as noted, the patient was suffering from lymphoma and was immunologically impaired.

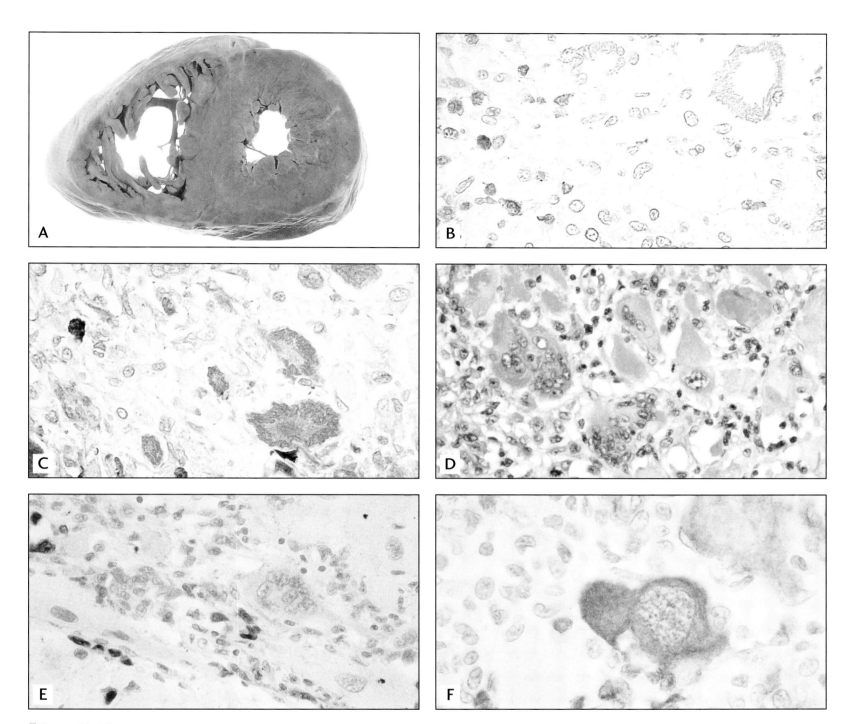

Figure 11-10.

Giant cell myocarditis. Giant cell myocarditis is a particularly injurious form of myocarditis, albeit rare. In a recent overview of the condition, Cooper *et al.* [26] included 63 patients with giant cell myocarditis. Of these, 33 were male and 30 were female patients, and the average age was 42.6 (range, 16 to 69). The rate of death or cardiac transplantation was 89%, with a median survival of 5.5 months from the onset of symptoms to the time of death or transplantation. Given the rapid course of deterioration, the endomyocardial biopsy is an indispensible tool in determining whether heart transplantation should be considered. Although recurrence of giant cell myocarditis has been documented in transplanted donor hearts, the outcome of such transplant recipients has been better than that of patients who do not undergo transplantation. Whether support by a ventricular assist device through the acute illness would alter the outcome following transplantation is unknown. The cause of giant cell myocarditis remains speculative, although a variety of viral causes have been suggested or pursued.

A, A transverse ventricular myocardial section from an autopsy heart affected by giant cell myocarditis. Mottling is widespread and includes gray-tan and darker areas associated with histologic necrosis, cellular infiltration, and edema. The left ventricular free wall and ventricular septum are thickened, and both ventricular chambers are dilated. In this view, the anterior surface of the heart is toward the upper aspect of the figure. **B,** On UCHL-1 staining, the giant cells can be seen to be immunonegative. However, there is a scattering of T lymphocytes throughout the infiltrate. **C,** Staining with MAC387 antibody reveals that at least several of the giant cells are of macrophage origin. **D,** In a different patient with giant cell myocarditis, however, wherein there are equally numerous giant cells and a mixed inflammatory infiltrate (hematoxylin and eosin stain, × 330), immunohistochemistry reveals the giant cells to be macrophage-negative (*panel E*). **F,** Careful examination of the infiltrate reveals certain cardiac muscle cells that are being "transformed" into giant cells, and immunostaining for muscle-specific actin isotypes (α and γ) (HHF-35) reveals certain of the giant cells to be of muscle origin.

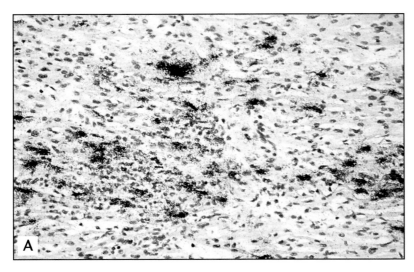

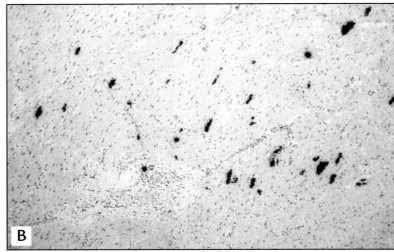

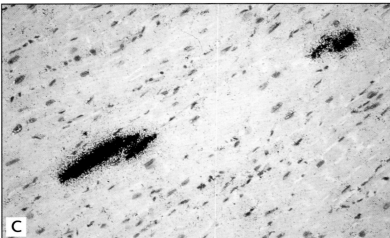

Figure 11-11.

Photomicrographs of myocardium in situ hybridized with a full-length ^{35}S-labeled cDNA probe complementary to the positive strand of coxsackievirus B3m. **A,** In tissue from infants with severe enteroviral myocarditis, multifocal, large-scale injury may be present. Infected zones, including necrotic foci with halos or wavefronts of more recently infected cardiac myocytes, are also visible. Thus, where myocytes have died, the virions have been released and positive- or negative-strand viral RNA are less evident. The active, replicative infection is proceeding in neighboring viable, permissive cells. **B** and **C,** Photomicrographs of ventricular myocardium from adult patients with fatal enteroviral heart disease also illustrate infected cells that are variably associated with areas of advanced myocyte necrosis or an inflammatory infiltrate. Cells with enteroviral genome present are potential sites for viral persistence, as demonstrated previously [12]. The inflammatory infiltrate is rather limited relative to the number of infectious foci, reflecting in part the stage of infection in these hearts, in part the immunologic invisibility of the viral antigens, and in part the nature of myocyte destruction.

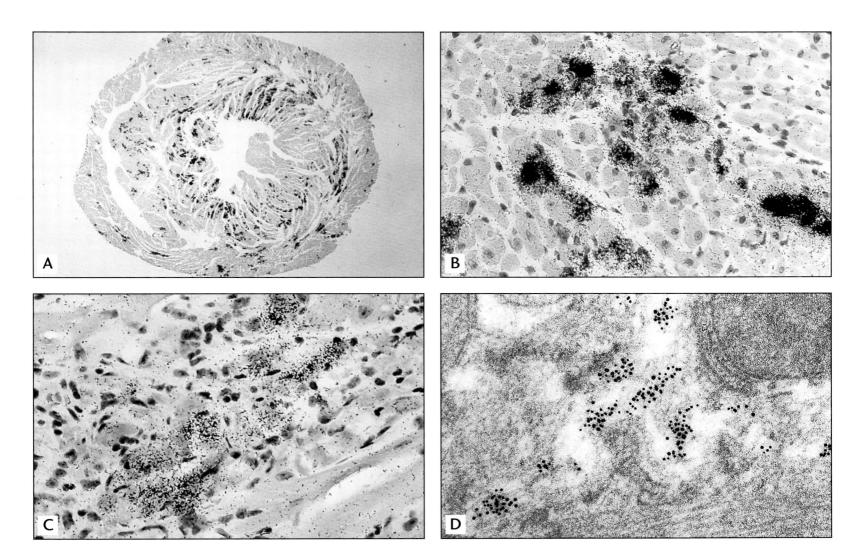

Figure 11-12.

Photomicrographs (**A** through **C**) and electron micrograph (**D**) of in situ hybridization for viral RNA in infected myocardium from male adolescent ACA mice inoculated with 10^5 plaque-forming unit (PFU) coxsackievirus B3 (RK). In permissive murine hosts, the infection is widespread through all aspects of the ventricular walls (*panel A*) and has a pattern of myocyte infection (*panel B*) similar to that observed in human myocardium. As the infectious episode progresses, the infection predominates adjacent to areas of injury and healing, wherein reparative cells appear to be infected (*panel C*). A mild persistent, inflammatory response is most likely driven by residual viral genome or particles, and by healing signals [12]. At the ultrastructural level, viral particles can be localized in myocytes though nonisotopic in situ hybridization with biotinylated CVB3 cDNA (*panel D*). Electron microscopic in situ hybridization also reveals CVB3 RNA associated with the plasma membrane of endothelial cells. The pathophysiologic role of such latter involvement of vascular structures is uncertain but deserves consideration in light of possible microcirculatory effects of coxsackievirus infection [27].

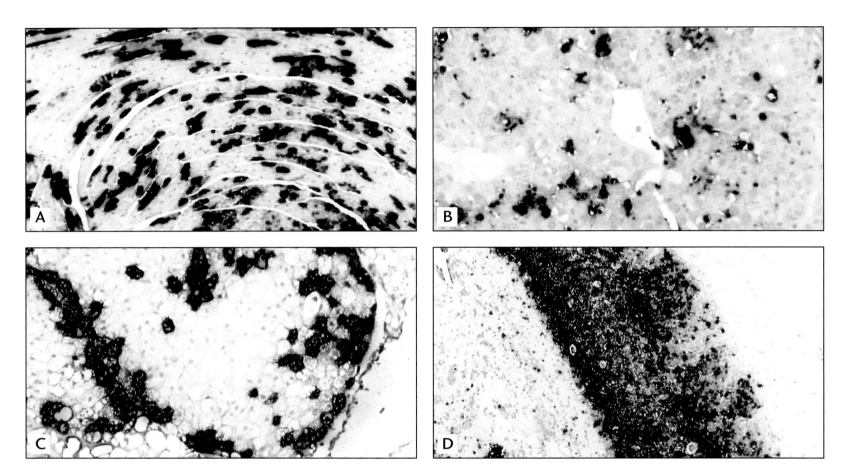

Figure 11-13.

The systemic nature of enteroviral heart disease [13]. These photomicrographs illustrate in situ hybridization positivity for coxsackievirus B3 sense- (positive-) strand viral RNA, based on a digoxigenin-labeled full-length riboprobe, and the extensive organ-based infections in A/J (H-2^a haplotype) mice at day 3 postinfection. **A,** The myocardium has numerous cardiac myocytes that are infected individually or in contiguity. **B,** In the liver, both hepatocytes (large infected cells) and phagocytes along the sinusoids (small infected cells) are involved by the infection. **C,** Adipose tissue is also a prominent site of virus replication, the pattern of infection tending to progress from interstitial or serosal surfaces inward through multiple fat cells. **D,** Localization of virus within the central nervous system involves particular sites.

ACKNOWLEDGMENTS

The authors thank Shelley Wood, Karin Klingel, Stuart Greene, and Parminder Thind
for their assistance in the preparation of figures, graphics, and text for this chapter.

REFERENCES

1. Aretz HT: Myocarditis: the Dallas criteria. *Hum Pathol* 1987, 18:619–624.

2. Parrillo JE, Cunnion RE, Epstein SE, *et al.*: A prospective, randomized, controlled trial of prednisone for dilated cardiomyopathy. *N Engl J Med* 1989, 321:1061–1068.

3. Fuster V, Gersh BJ, Giuliani ER, *et al.*: The natural history of idiopathic dilated cardiomyopathy. *Am J Cardiol* 1981, 47:525–531.

4. Chow LH, Radio SJ, Sears TD, McManus BM: Insensitivity of right ventricular endomyocardial biopsy in the diagnosis of myocarditis. *J Am Coll Cardiol* 1989, 14:915–920.

5. Hauck AJ, Kearney DL, Edwards WD: Evaluation of postmortem endomyocardial biopsy specimens from 38 patients with lymphocytic myocarditis: implications for role of sampling error. *Mayo Clin Proc* 1989, 64:1235–1245.

6. McManus BM, Wood SM: Inflammatory manifestations of toxic and allergic injury to heart and blood vessels. In *Cardiovascular Toxicology*. Edited by Bishop SP, Kerns WD. Oxford, UK: Elsevier; 1997: vol 6.

7. Grist NR, Reid D: Epidemiology of viral infections of the heart. In *Viral Infections of the Heart*. Edited by Banatvala, JE. London, Boston, Melbourne, Auckland: Edward Arnold (a division of Hodder and Stoughton); 1993:23–31.

8. Martino TA, Liu P, Petric M, Sole MJ: Enteroviral myocarditis and dilated cardiomyopathy: a review of clinical and experimental studies. In *Human Enteroviral Infections*. Edited by Rotbart HA. Washington, DC: ASM Press; 1995:291–352.

9. Woodruff JF: Viral myocarditis: a review. *Am J Pathol* 1980, 101:425–484.

10. Figulla HR, Kandolf R, McManus BM: *Idiopathic Dilated Cardiomyopathy*. Berlin: Springer-Verlag.

11. McManus BM, Chow LH, Wilson JE, *et al.*: Direct myocardial injury by enterovirus: a central role in the evolution of murine myocarditis. *Clin Immunol Immunopathol* 1993, 68:159–169.

12. Klingel K, Hohenadl C, Canu A, *et al.*: Ongoing enterovirus-induced myocarditis is associated with persistent heart muscle infection: quantitative analysis of virus replication, tissue damage, and inflammation. *Proc Nat Acad Sci U S A* 1992, 89:314–318.

13. Carthy CM, Yang D, Anderson DR, *et al.*: Myocarditis as a systemic disease: new perspectives on pathogenesis. *Clin Exp Pharmacol Physiol* 1997, 24:997–1003.

14. Edwards WD, Holmes DR, Reeder GS: Diagnosis of active lymphocytic myocarditis by endomyocardial biopsy: quantitative criteria for light microscopy. *Mayo Clin Proc* 1982, 57:419–986.

15. Hauck AJ, Kearney DL, Edwards WD: Evaluation of postmortem endomyocardial biopsy specimens from 38 patients with lymphocytic myocarditis: implications for role of sampling error. *Mayo Clin Proc* 1989, 64:1235–1245.

16. Herskowitz A, Campbell S, Deckers J, *et al.*: Demographic features and prevalence of idiopathic myocarditis in patients undergoing endomyocardial biopsy. *Am J Cardiol* 1993, 71:982–986.

17. McManus BM, Winters GL: Pathology of heart allograft rejection. In *Transplant Pathology*. Edited by Kolbeck PC, Markin RS, and McManus BM. Chicago: ASCP; 1994:197–218.

18. Lieberman EB, Hutchins GM, Herskowitz A, *et al.*: A clinicopathologic description of myocarditis. *J Am Coll Cardiol* 1991, 18:1617–1626.

19. Herskowitz A, Ansari AA: Myocarditis. In *Atlas of Heart Diseases*, vol. II: Cardiomyopathies, Myocarditis, and Pericardial Disease. Edited by Abelmann WH. Philadelphia: Current Medicine; 1995:9.1–9.24.

20. Lustock MJ, Chase J, Lubitz JM: Myocarditis: clinical and pathologic study of 45 cases. *Dis Chest* 1955, 28:243–259.

21. Herskowitz A, Wolfgram LJ, Rose NR, Beisel KW: Coxsackievirus B3 murine myocarditis: a pathologic spectrum of myocarditis in genetically defined inbred strains. *J Am Coll Cardiol* 1987, 9:1311–1319.

22. Swinnen LJ, Costanzo-Nordin MR, Fisher SG, *et al.*: Increased incidence of lymphoproliferative disorder after immunosuppression with the monoclonal antibody OKT3 in cardiac-transplant recipients [see comments]. *N Engl J Med* 1990, 323:1723–1728.

23. Kaplan MH: Coxsackievirus infection in children under three months of age. In *Coxsackieviruses: A General Update*. Edited by Bendinelli M, Friedman H. New York: Plenum Press; 1988:241–252.

24. Gulizia JM, Engel PJ, McManus BM: Acute rheumatic carditis: diagnostic and therapeutic challenges in the era of heart transplantation. *J Heart Lung Transplant* 1993, 12:372–380.

25. Gulizia JM, Cunningham MW, McManus BM: Immunoreactivity of anti-streptococcal monoclonal antibodies to human heart valves: evidence for multiple cross-reactive epitopes. *Am J Pathol* 1991, 138:285–301.

26. Cooper LT Jr, Berry GJ, Shabetai R: Idiopathic giant-cell myocarditis: natural history and treatment. Multicenter Giant Cell Myocarditis Study Group Investigators. *N Engl J Med* 1997, 336:1860–1866.

27. Sole MJ, Liu P: Viral myocarditis: a paradigm for understanding the pathogenesis and treatment of dilated cardiomyopathy. *J Am Coll Cardiol* 1993, 22:99a–105a.43

12

Heart Transplantation: Explant, Biopsy, and Autopsy Characteristics

Gayle L. Winters

Cardiac transplantation is an accepted therapeutic option for patients with end-stage heart failure. The International Society for Heart and Lung Transplantation (ISHLT) Registry has recorded more than 48,000 heart transplants at more than 300 centers worldwide between 1982 and 1998 [1]. Approximately 3000 heart transplants per year are performed worldwide, limited primarily by the availability of donor organs. The success of heart transplantation over the past decade has been attributed to the refinement of candidate selection, use of the endomyocardial biopsy to monitor cardiac allograft rejection, and improvement in immunosuppresssive therapies. Actuarial survival is approximately 80% at 1 year and 65% at 5 years.

Patients with irreversible advanced heart failure are prime candidates for cardiac transplantation. In the United States, nearly 5 million people (1.5% of the population) carry the diagnosis of heart failure, which is the fourth leading cause of hospitalization in adults [2,3]. The upper age limit for cardiac transplantation was traditionally set at 55 years. However, because studies have shown that carefully selected candidates older than 55 years of age may successfully undergo heart transplantation [4], the recipient age limit has been extended into the mid 60s and is often more of an ethical than medical issue. Comorbid conditions that may be exclusionary include systemic illness with poor prognosis; irreversible pulmonary, renal, or hepatic disease; pulmonary hypertension with irreversibly high pulmonary vascular resistence; severe peripheral vascular or cerebrovascular obstructive disease; insulin-dependent diabetes with end-organ damage; active infection; severe obesity; severe osteoporosis; psychosocial instability; and substance abuse.

Donor hearts are procured from individuals with brain death but intact circulation, usually the result of blunt injuries sustained in motor vehicle accidents, penetrating head injuries such as gunshot wounds, or primary central nervous system events. The age of acceptable cardiac donors has gradually increased in efforts to expand the donor pool. Although routine coronary angiograms of donor hearts are logistically impossible, angiography is recommended for male donors older than 45 years of age and female donors older than 50 years of age, especially if cardiac risk factors are identified [5]. Other conditions in donors that may serve as absolute or relative contraindications include HIV infection; hepatitis B or C infection; sepsis; and a history of metastatic cancer, carbon monoxide inhalation, or intravenous drug abuse.

Heart donors and recipients are matched for ABO blood group compatibility and body size. Prospective HLA matching is not routinely performed. Other considerations in allocation of donor hearts include priority on the United Network for Organ Sharing (UNOS) waiting list and distance between donor and recipient centers. The time from harvesting the donor heart until reestablishment of circulation in the recipient (*ie*, ischemic time) is limited to 4 to 5 hours maximum, necessitating close coordination between donor and recipient operating teams.

The contribution of pathology to the discipline of cardiac transplantation is well established. The most visible role is that of the pathologist who interprets endomyocardial biopsies performed to monitor the status of the heart allograft. The diagnosis and grading of acute rejection and assessment of numerous other biopsy findings are important in guiding the clinical management of recipients. Close collaboration between the pathologist and the transplant clinician is essential for the optimal care of these patients. Pathologists may also make important contributions in examining biopsies of the recipient's native heart as part of the evaluation for the cause of cardiac failure, examining explanted recipient hearts, and evaluating failed allografts at explant or autopsy. In addition to providing important diagnostic information, pathologists have the opportunity to add to existing knowledge of the pathobiology of disease processes related to heart failure and transplantation.

PATHOLOGY OF THE EXPLANTED RECIPIENT HEART

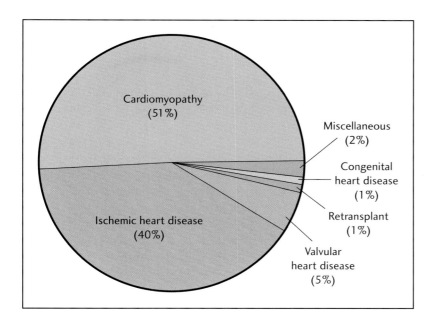

Figure 12-1.

Indications for heart transplantation at Brigham and Women's Hospital. Our 16-year experience at this hospital, in which over 90% of more than 400 adult recipients of cardiac allografts have had end-stage heart failure secondary to cardiomyopathy or ischemic heart disease parallels that reported by the ISHLT Registry, which collects data annually from over 300 transplant centers worldwide [1]. Whereas careful pathologic evaluation of the explanted recipient heart confirms clinical diagnoses and adds to the knowledge of underlying disease states, the discovery of previously undiagnosed conditions or unexpected findings may affect recipient prognosis. In a small percentage of cases, pathologic evaluation of the explanted recipient heart differs from the pretransplant clinical diagnosis. The discrepancy most often involves conditions that mimic the clinical presentation of dilated cardiomyopathy and includes end-stage ischemic heart disease and hypertrophic cardiomyopathy, as well as less common entities such as arrhythmogenic right ventricular cardiomyopathy and congenitally corrected transposition of the great arteries.

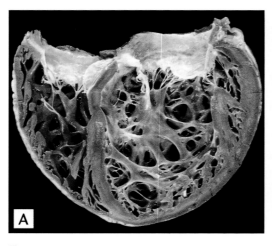 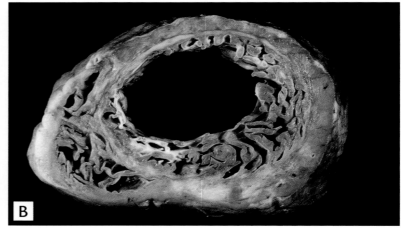

Figure 12-2.

Explanted hearts. **A,** Idiopathic dilated cardiomyopathy, the most common type of cardiomyopathy, is characterized by increased cardiac mass with biventricular dilatation and hypertrophy. No significant ischemic, hypertensive, valvular, or congenital heart disease is present. Although idiopathic, this condition actually represents the end stage of a number of possible insults to the myocardium, including alcohol use, peripartum state, viral myocarditis, and genetic defects. The microscopic changes of myocyte hypertrophy with varying

amounts of myocardial fibrosis are nonspecific and typically do not indicate the cause of the insult. **B,** Chronic ischemic heart disease resulting in cardiac failure is characterized by ventricular dilatation with extensive ventricular scarring, a feature indicating healed myocardial infarctions. Chronic coronary atherosclerosis involving more than one major epicardial coronary artery is usually present; however, acute plaque change is rare.

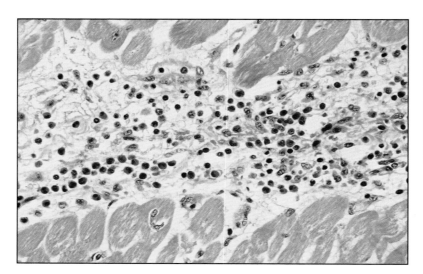

Figure 12-3.

Eosinophilic myocarditis. Eosinophilic, or hypersensitivity, myocarditis has been reported in up to 22% of explanted hearts and has been related to the use of many drugs, specifically to dobutamine in patients with transplants [6–9]. It may occur in association with any form of underlying pathology, including cardiomyopathy, ischemic heart disease, and valvular heart disease. It is characterized by a focal or diffuse inflammatory infiltrate composed of large numbers of eosinophils admixed with lymphocytes and plasma cells. The infiltrate involves both atria and ventricles and is typically located along tissue planes in perivascular spaces. Unlike other forms of myocarditis, little associated myocyte damage generally occurs. This entity is usually an incidental finding in explanted hearts.

DISEASES KNOWN TO RECUR IN ALLOGRAFTS

Amyloidosis
Sarcoidosis
Chagas' disease
Giant cell myocarditis
Melanoma

Figure 12-4.

Diseases known to recur in allografts. The known presence of any of these diseases before transplantation prompts careful consideration of the patient's candidacy. Endomyocardial biopsy of the native recipient heart may be helpful in documenting such conditions. If first diagnosed in the explanted heart, clinicians should be made aware of these findings because recurrence of these diseases after transplantation, often discovered on routine surveillance endomyocardial biopsy [10,11], may produce persistent allograft dysfunction. Patients with sarcoidosis and amyloidosis have undergone successful transplantation; however, progression of the disease may limit the long-term benefits [12,13]. Patients transplanted with active lymphocytic myocarditis have been found to reject the transplanted heart early, at higher frequency, and with increased severity compared with recipients who have other preoperative diagnoses [14].

Pathogenesis, Diagnosis, and Grading of Acute Rejection

ENDOMYOCARDIAL BIOPSY PROTOCOL	
Time	**Biopsy Frequency**
First post transplant year	Weekly × 4
	Biweekly × 2
	Monthly × 6
	Every other month × 2
Second post transplant year	Every 3 months × 2
	Every 6 months
Third (or later) post transplant year	Every 6 months

Figure 12-5.

Endomyocardial biopsy protocol used by Brigham and Women's Hospital. Endomyocardial biopsies are routinely performed after heart transplantation to monitor the status of the heart allograft because histologic findings of rejection usually precede clinical signs and symptoms. Unlike renal or liver transplantation, in which laboratory tests may provide an indication of graft rejection, no laboratory test or noninvasive study has yet proven to be as reliable as the endomyocardial biopsy in the management of heart transplant recipients. Recipients undergo regularly scheduled biopsies according to specific protocols set by each transplant center. In general, biopsies are performed more frequently (*ie*, weekly) during the early posttransplant period. The interval between biopsies becomes longer with increasing time after transplantation, reaching a biopsy frequency of two to four times annually after 1 year. The frequency of endomyocardial biopsies may be increased if there is a change in the clinical status of the recipient or if acute rejection is detected.

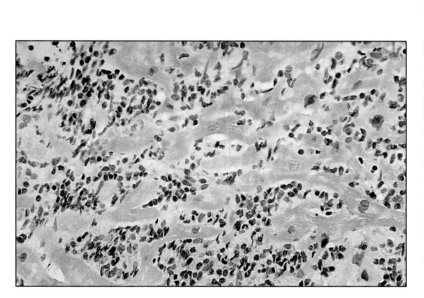

Figure 12-6.

General histologic features of acute rejection. An intermediate grade of rejection is represented and characterized by a dense lymphocytic infiltrate with associated myocyte damage. Damage or injury to the myocardium, originally termed "myocyte necrosis," is an important but sometimes difficult feature to identify. While readily distinguishable cell necrosis may be a feature of more severe forms of rejection, myocyte damage in milder rejection is often characterized by myocyte encroachment by inflammatory cells, resulting in irregular myocyte borders, partial replacement of myocytes, or architectural distortion. The immunologic mechanism by which infiltrating cells induce myocardial cell injury and the type of injury that occurs is not fully understood. Two mechanisms implicated in cell death are necrosis and apoptosis.

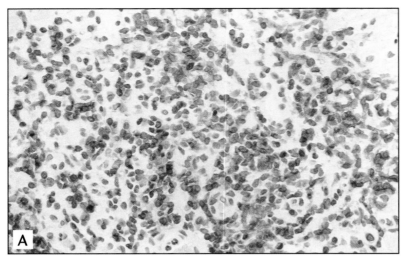
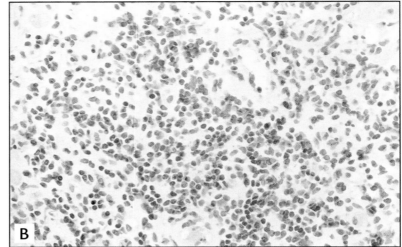

Figure 12-7.

Cellular composition of acute rejection. **A,** The infiltrating cells in a rejecting allograft are predominantly T cells (stained with CD3) that, when subtyped, consist of a mixture of CD4 and CD8 phenotypes. The proportion of CD4 to CD8 cells, however, has not proven useful in the clinical managment of recipients or in predicting clinical outcome. Lymphocyte subtyping, therefore, is not warranted in the routine diagnosis of rejection. **B,** Macrophages (stained with KP1) make up the other major cellular component of rejection.

INTERNATIONAL SOCIETY FOR HEART AND LUNG TRANSPLANTATION STANDARDIZED GRADING FOR CARDIAC BIOPSIES

Rejection Grade	Description
0	No evidence of rejection
1–Mild	
A–Focal	Focal perivascular or interstitial infiltrate without myocyte damage
B–Diffuse	Diffuse infiltrate without myocyte damage
2–Moderate (focal)	One focus of infiltrate with associated myocyte damage
3–Moderate	
A–Multifocal	Multifocal infiltrate with myocyte damage
B–Diffuse	Diffuse infiltrate with myocyte damage
4–Severe	Diffuse polymorphous infiltrate with extensive myocyte damage, with or without edema, hemorrhage, or vasculitis

Non-rejection Biopsy Findings

Quilty effect A and B

Ischemic injury: early (≤ 3 months); late (> 3 months)

Infection

Posttransplant lymphoproliferative disorder

Figure 12-8.

International Society for Heart and Lung Transplantation (ISHLT) grading system for cardiac transplant biopsies [15]. Pathologists use a grading system to consistently communicate biopsy findings to transplant physicians. In general, increasing grades (representing increasing severity) of rejection are defined by increasing numbers of inflammatory cells and foci associated with increasing amounts of myocyte damage. In 1990, the ISHLT grading system for cardiac biopsies was established to allow for comparisons of biopsy results between institutions and to facilitate multi-center clinical trials. It has gained general acceptance worldwide and is the most widely used system in practice today.

ISHLT GRADING SYSTEM CAVEATS

Requires four evaluable pieces of myocardium (each consisting of at least 50% myocardium) examined at three levels through the paraffin block.

Is based on the "worst" histologic area of the biopsy.

Refers to a "multifocal" pattern of rejection to describe discrete foci of rejection with intervening uninvolved myocardium; a "diffuse" pattern involves nearly the entire tissue fragment, and the majority of tissue fragments are usually involved.

Does not use the term "resolving" rejection; any residual rejection should be given a rejection grade, including grade 0 for "resolved" rejection.

Does not routinely require electron microscopy, immunoperoxidase staining, or immunofluorescence.

Is designed for biopsies and not autopsy or explanted hearts.

Is based on histologic findings prior to any treatment except for maintenance immunosuppression.

Provides standardized format for conveying histologic biopsy findings but does not attempt to incorporate clinical parameters or recommend treatment.

Figure 12-9.

Caveats for using the ISHLT (International Society for Heart and Lung Transplantation) grading system. Use of the ISHLT grading system has created a number of issues that have recently been clarified [16]. Optimal care of cardiac transplant recipients requires good communication and close collaboration between pathologists and transplant physicians. Simply reporting a biopsy grade number may not be sufficient in difficult or borderline cases. The diagnostic dilemma should be explained to the clinician, and it may be helpful for the clinician to review the biopsy slides with the pathologist.

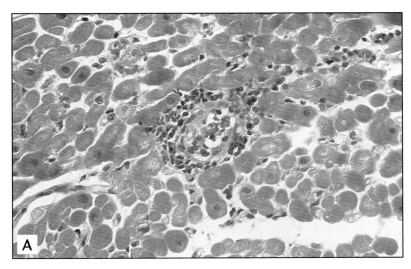

Figure 12-10.

International Society for Heart and Lung Transplantation (ISHLT) grade 1. Grade 1, "mild" rejection, consists of perivascular or interstitial lymphocytic infiltrates without associated myocyte damage that may involve one or more than one of the biopsy fragments. **A,** Grade 1A designates a focal process shown here as a perivascular infiltrate without damage to adjacent myocytes. **B,** Grade 1B designates a diffuse process shown here as an interstitial infiltrate without damage to adjacent myocytes.

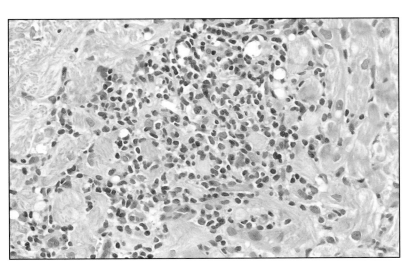

Figure 12-11.

International Society for Heart and Lung Transplantation (ISHLT) grade 2. Grade 2, "focal moderate" rejection, consists of a single focus of lymphocytic infiltration with associated myocyte damage. The area of infiltration is frequently relatively well circumscribed. Additional foci of inflammatory infiltrates (*ie*, grade 1 rejection) may be present elsewhere in the biopsy, but these additional foci should not be associated with myocyte damage.

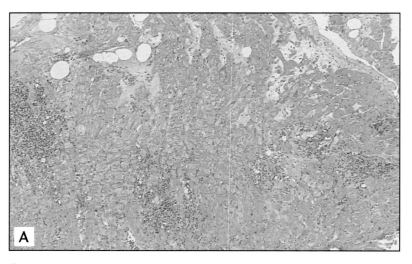

A

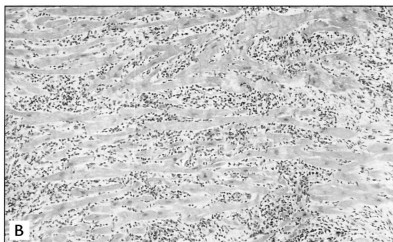

B

Figure 12-12.
International Society for Heart and Lung Transplantation (ISHLT) grade 3. **A,** Grade 3A, "multifocal moderate" rejection, is characterized by multiple (≥ two) inflammatory foci with associated myocyte damage. The foci may be distributed in one or more than one of the biopsy fragments. Intervening areas of uninvolved myocardium are present between the foci of rejection. **B,** Grade 3B, "diffuse moderate" rejection, consists of a diffuse inflammatory process usually involving several of the biopsy fragments. Associated myocyte damage is present in multiple locations.

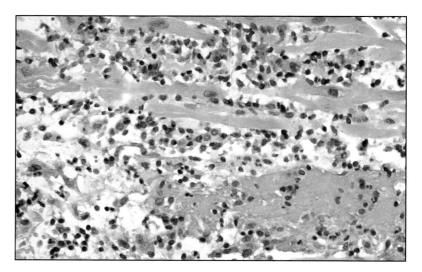

Figure 12-13.
International Society for Heart and Lung Transplantation (ISHLT) grade 4. Grade 4, "severe" rejection, is characterized by a diffuse polymorphous infiltrate consisting of lymphocytes, neutrophils, and eosinophils with multiple areas of associated myocyte damage. Edema and interstitial hemorrhage are usually present, and vasculitis is frequently present. All or nearly all of the biopsy fragments are involved, although the intensity of the infiltrate may vary among fragments. Involvement of the endocardium is common.

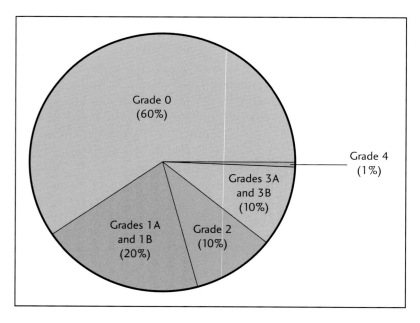

Figure 12-14.
Incidence of rejection grades. Review of over 5000 consecutive biopsies performed at Brigham and Women's Hospital revealed those without evidence of rejection and those with grade 1 rejection to be the most common, accounting for approximately 80% of posttransplant biopsies. Grades 2 and 3 rejection each account for approximately 10% of biopsies and grade 4 rejection is present in less than 1%. The incidence of rejection is highest in the first 3 to 6 months after transplantation.

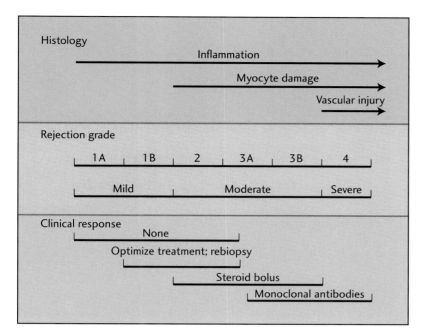

Histology

Inflammation →

Myocyte damage →

Vascular injury →

Rejection grade

| 1A | 1B | 2 | 3A | 3B | 4 |

| Mild | | Moderate | | Severe |

Clinical response

None

Optimize treatment; rebiopsy

Steroid bolus

Monoclonal antibodies

Figure 12-15.

Comparison of biopsy histology, rejection grade, and clinical response. Most heart transplant recipients are maintained on triple immunosuppression consisting of cyclosporine, azathioprine, and prednisone. The exact point in the spectrum of histologic rejection that requires intensification of immunosuppression remains one of the major unresolved issues in the care of cardiac transplant recipients. Immunosuppressive protocols and the threshold for treatment of histologic rejection vary markedly among heart transplant centers [17]. The point at which immunosuppression is intensified ranges from grade 1B to 3A. In general, grades 0 and 1 elicit no change in therapy. The clinical response to grade 2 is the most controversial and treatment options include no change in therapy, maximization of maintenance therapeutic drug levels, cessation of a steroid taper, repeat biopsy earlier than scheduled, or augmentation of immunosuppression. Grades 3 and 4 usually prompt augmentation of immunosuppression, either a steroid bolus or monoclonal antibody therapy such as OKT3 for the most severe forms. Lower grades of rejection (grades 1 and 2) in biopsies from asymptomatic patients have been shown to progress to a higher grade of rejection on the next biopsy in only approximately 15% to 20% of cases [18–23]. The incidence of progression varies inversely with the amount of time after transplantation and drops to less than 5% of biopsies obtained more than 2 years after transplantation.

Other Biopsy Findings After Cardiac Transplantation

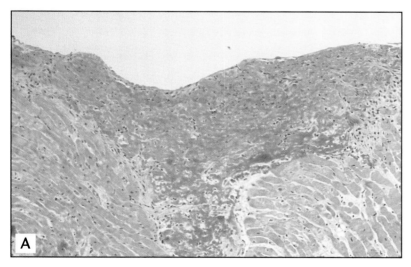

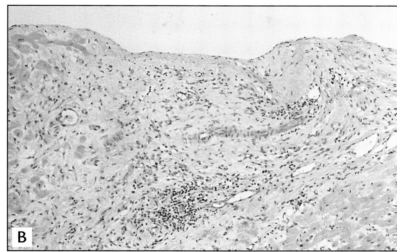

Figure 12-16.

Biopsy site. Obtaining tissue from a previous biopsy site is the most common sampling artifact that may pose difficulties in biopsy interpretation. The average transplant patient undergoes up to 20 biopsies during the first year after transplantation [24]. Because of the rigid structure of the bioptome and constant configuration of the right ventricular trabeculae, the bioptome tends to follow a similar path in any given patient. The histology of the biopsy site reflects the degree of healing that has occurred. Immediately after

a biopsy procedure, fresh thrombus may overlie areas of acute myocyte injury and hemorrhage (*panel A*). Progressive healing results in granulation tissue, often containing a leukocytic infiltrate (*panel B*) that may resemble the inflammatory changes present in acute rejection. The mixed nature of the healing inflammatory infiltrate and the myocyte disarray frequently present at the periphery of the biopsy site may aid in rendering a correct interpretation of the findings.

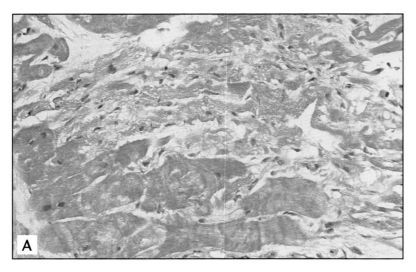

Figure 12-17.

Early ischemic injury. Early ischemic injury is often detected in endomyocardial biopsy specimens obtained 3 months or less after transplantation and arises in the perioperative period during the obligatory ischemic time that accompanies procurement and implantation of a donor heart. It is a frequent finding that has been observed in up to 89% of biopsies obtained during the first 4 weeks after transplantation [25]. **A,** In very early biopsies (*ie*, week 1 to 2 after transplantation), coagulative myocyte necrosis and scattered neutrophils are often the primary findings.

B, Subsequent biopsies (*ie*, weeks 2 to 4 after transplantation) may reveal the healing phase characterized by a mixed

inflammatory infiltrate that may be confused with acute rejection. Additional features that may help to distinguish healing ischemic injury from acute rejection include inflammation predominantly in the interstitium with clear separation from adjacent myocytes, the presence of cellular debris and healing fat necrosis, and mycocyte vacuolization in the adjacent myocardium. Accurate diagnosis of early ischemic injury and distinction from rejection decrease unnecessary immunosuppression and its associated sequelae.

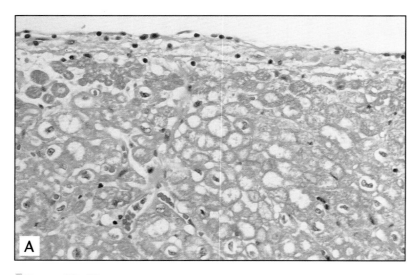

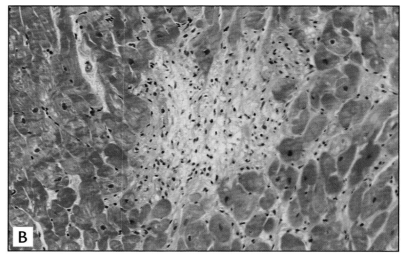

Figure 12-18.

Late ischemic injury. Late ischemic injury detected in endomyocardial biopsies obtained more than 3 months after transplantation results from the perfusion defects caused by graft arteriosclerosis. These pathologic changes are similar to those induced by native coronary atherosclerosis as well as focal lesions secondary to small vessel disease. The changes include subendocardial myocyte vacuolization (*panel A*) indicative of sublethal ischemic injury and microinfarcts (*panel B*), which indicate ischemic necrosis and its

healing (shown here) in a microvascular distribution. A recent review [26] indicated that late ischemic injury detected by endomyocardial biopsy has a positive predictive value of 92% of finding significant graft arteriosclerosis at autopsy but a negative predictive value of only 51%. Therefore, late ischemic injury, when present on endomyocardial biopsies, may provide an early clue to the presence of significant graft arteriosclerosis.

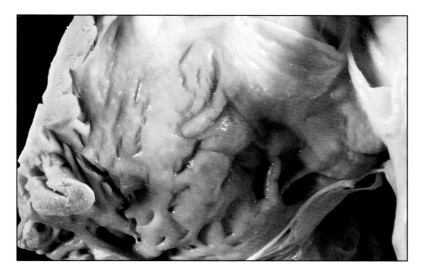

Figure 12-19.

The Quilty effect. The presence of endocardial infiltrates was termed the "Quilty effect" after the first patient in whom they were observed; they correspond to raised cellular nodules arising from the endocardium. They are easily accessible to the bioptome and may be present in 10% to 20% of posttransplant biopsies [27,28]. These lesions may first appear at any time during the posttransplant course and tend to recur in any given patient. The cause of the Quilty effect and its relationship to acute rejection (if any) are unknown. This type of lesion has traditionally been considered distinct from rejection and does not require treatment with intensified immunosuppressive agents. These lesions do not appear to be related to posttransplant lymphoproliferative disorders and do not seem to foretell an adverse clinical outcome.

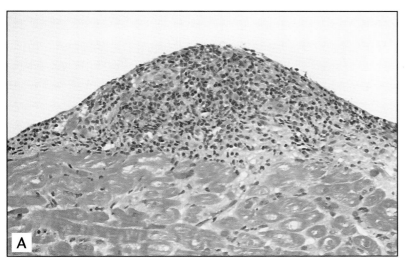

Figure 12-20.

Histologic typing of the Quilty effect. The Quilty effect includes densely cellular endocardial nodules consisting of lymphocytes with occasional macrophages, plasma cells, and numerous small blood vessels. The infiltrates may be confined either to the endocardium (*ie*, Quilty A [*panel A*]) or may extend into the underlying myocardium, where associated myocyte damage may be present (*ie*, Quilty B [*panel B*]). However, histologic typing such as Quilty A and Quilty B does not appear to have any clinical significance [29].

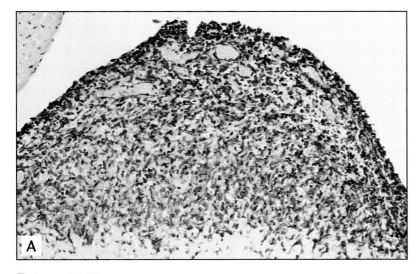

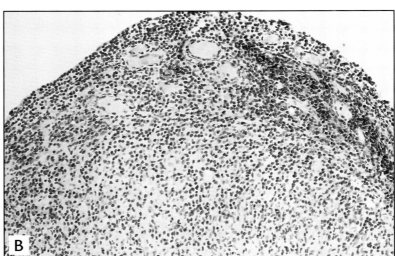

Figure 12-21.

Cellular composition of the Quilty effect. Immunohistochemistry demonstrates that the Quilty effect consists predominantly of T lymphocytes (*panel A*; stained with CD3) with scattered or clusters of B lymphocytes (*panel B*; stained with L26). The presence of B cells, along with the density of the infiltrate and prominent vascularity, may help in differentiating these lesions from acute rejection, particularly in cases in which the lesion extends into the underlying myocardium and no connection to the endocardium is evident.

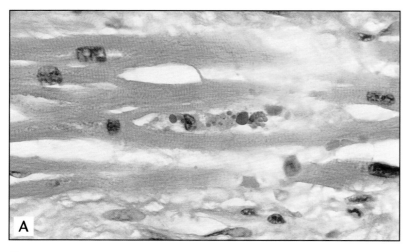

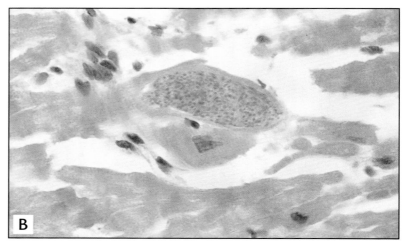

Figure 12-22.

Opportunistic infection. Immunosuppressed cardiac transplant recipients are at increased risk of infection that may involve the heart allograft. The organisms most commonly encountered on endomyocardial biopsy specimens are cytomegalovirus (CMV) (*panel A*) and *Toxoplasma gondii* (*panel B*). These infections may occur as either a primary or reactivated infection. The accompany-

ing

cellular infiltrate is highly variable, and CMV and *Toxoplasma* spp. may incite little or no inflammatory reaction. In suspected cases, immunohistochemistry is used to detect viral antigens and in situ hybridization or polymerase chain reaction is used to detect DNA, all of which may be useful adjuncts to histopathology findings.

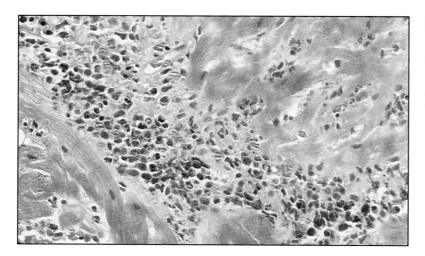

Figure 12-23.

Posttransplant lymphoproliferative disorder (PTLD). PTLD involving the allograft must be differentiated from acute rejection. The lymphocytes are large and atypical with prominent and often multiple nuclei, mitoses, and individual cell necrosis. Most PTLDs are disorders of B-cell origin and are associated with Epstein-Barr virus.

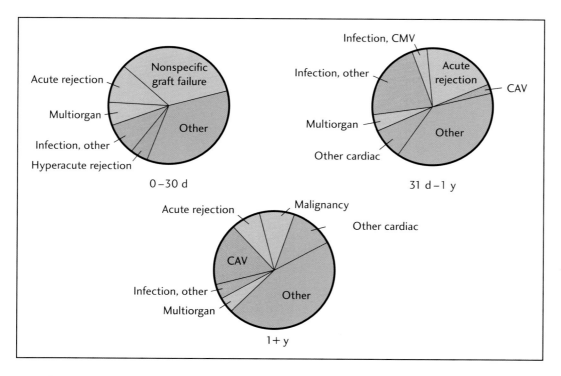

Figure 12-24.

Causes of death after heart transplantion [1]. The predominant cause of death in heart transplant patients varies with the time interval after transplantation. Early after transplantation (0 to 30 days), nonspecific graft failure is the most common cause of death, accounting for almost half of the deaths. In the immediate period (31 days to 1 year), acute rejection and infection are equally represented. Late after transplantation (over 1 year), the single most common cause of death is allograft coronary disease, followed by malignancy and acute rejection. CAV—cardiac allograft vasculopathy. *Adapted from* Hosenpud and coworkers [1].)

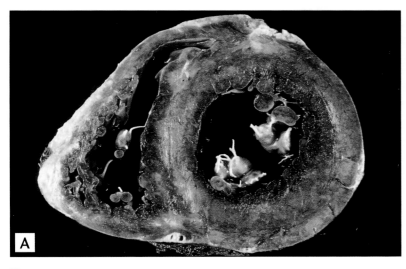

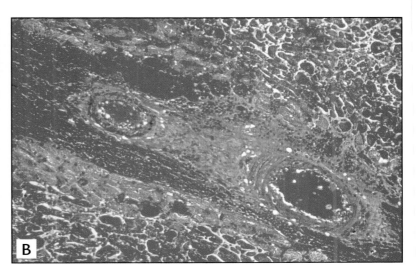

Figure 12-25.

Hyperacute rejection. Hyperacute rejection is a rare event that occurs in less than 1% of cardiac transplant recipients. It occurs immediately or within a few hours of transplantation. **A,** The heart is heavy (550 g) with biventricular dilatation and extensive, diffuse hemorrhagic discoloration of the myocardium. **B,** Histologically, diffuse interstitial hemorrhage and edema are present. Small vessels contain aggregated red cells and fibrin thrombi. Risk factors for hyperacute rejection include prior blood transfusions, repeated pregnancies, multiple cardiac surgeries, and previous transplantation.

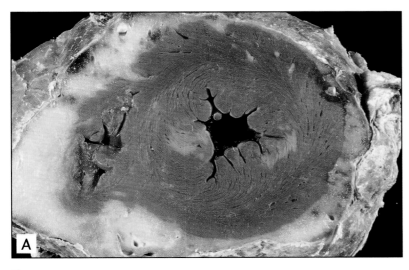

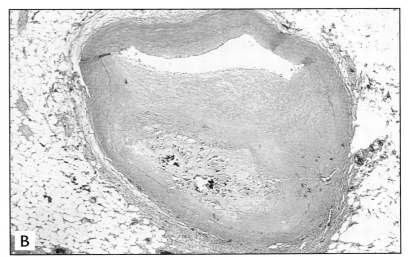

Figure 12-26.

Early graft failure caused by donor heart disease. **A,** Severe cardiomegaly (675 g) with concentric left ventricular hypertrophy. Staining with triphenyltetrazolium chloride (TTC) demonstrates foci of subendocardial infarctions (*pale areas*). **B,** Atherosclerosis was present in all major epicardial coronary arteries with luminal narrowing up to 75%. The donor was a 55-year-old man with several risk factors for coronary artery disease, including hypercholesterolemia. Coronary angiography was, therefore, performed before transplantation, but it failed to detect the severity of disease present in the donor heart.

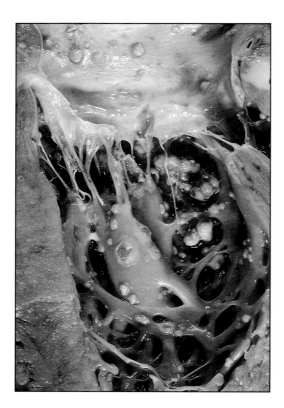

Figure 12-27.

Systemic opportunistic infection involving the allograft. This transplant recipient who died of systemic aspergillosis had extensive involvement of the cardiac allograft. Although infection as a cause of death in heart allograft recipients has decreased during the past decade, it remains a leading cause of morbidity and mortality during the first year after transplantation [1]. Infection in patients surviving at least 1 year after transplantation is less common, and a precipitating event (*ie*, rejection) often requires augmentation of immunosuppression before the development of infection.

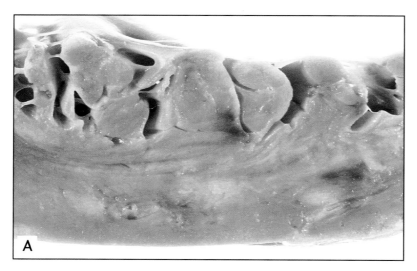

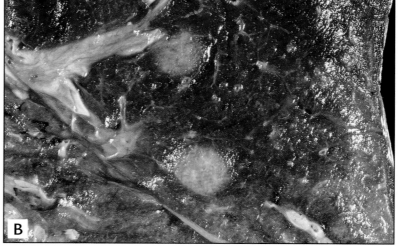

Figure 12-28.

Posttransplant lymphoproliferative disorder (PTLD). PTLD is often an aggressive neoplasm that occurs in approximately 2% of heart transplant recipients and is most likely related to the intensity of the immunosuppressive regimen [30]. It may involve the heart allograft (*panel A*) and frequently involves other extranodal sites, such as the lung (*panel B*), gastrointestinal tract (*panel C*, small bowel), central nervous system, and soft tissues. The mortality exceeds 80%.

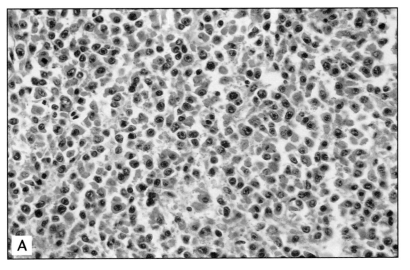

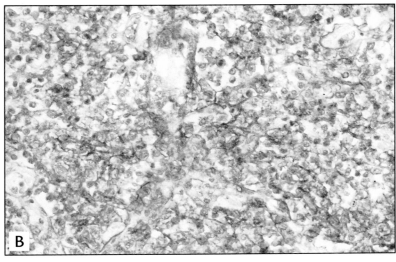

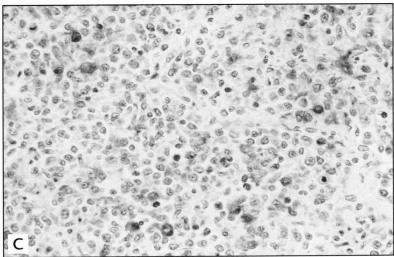

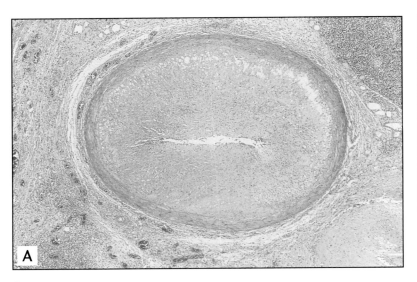

Figure 12-29.

Cellular composition of posttransplant lymphoproliferative disorder (PTLD). **A,** PTLD consists of a monomorphic population of atypical lymphocytes, some with plasmacytoid features.

B, Immunoperoxidase staining (L26) demonstrates a predominant B-cell population. PTLDs are usually disorders of B-cell origin, ranging from benign polyclonal B-cell hyperplasias to monoclonal malignant lymphomas with clonal chromosomal abnormalities.

C, Immunoperoxidase staining (Epstein-Barr virus [EBV]–latent membrane protein) demonstrates cytoplasmic reactivity for EBV antigens. EBV has been strongly associated with PTLDs. It is a herpes virus that selectively infects EBV receptor–positive B lymphocytes resulting in polyclonal activation. Immunosuppressive drugs used to prevent allograft rejection suppress the T-cell responses that would normally keep EBV-induced B-cell proliferations under control [31].

Figure 12-30.

Histology of allograft coronary disease. **A,** Allograft coronary disease consists of concentric intimal thickening that diffusely involves the coronary arteries. The endothelium and internal elastic lamina are essentially intact, and the media is usually of normal thickness or thinned. **B,** The cellularity of the thickened intima varies from minimal to the extensive amount of infiltrate seen here. (*continued on next page*)

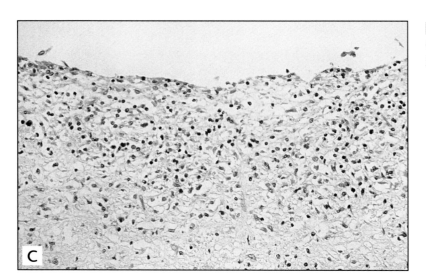

Figure 12-30. (*continued*)
C, The cellular infiltrates are frequently present as superficial bands in the subendothelium and deeper within the intima and media.

CHARACTERISTICS OF ADVANCED ALLOGRAFT CORONARY DISEASE COMPARED WITH NATIVE VESSEL ATHEROSCLEROSIS

Characteristic	Allograft Coronary Disease	Native Vessel Atherosclerosis
Onset	Rapid (months to years)	Slow (years)
Distribution	Generally diffuse	Focal
Lesions	Generally concentric	Eccentric
Calcification	Rare	Common
Cellular infiltrates	Prominent	Variable
Internal elastic lamina	More preserved	Destroyed
Secondary branches and intramural vessels	Affected	Spared

Figure 12-31.
Comparison of allograft coronary disease with native atherosclerosis. In general, allograft coronary disease can be distinguished from native vessel atherosclerosis by the presence of diffuse, generally concentric intimal thickening. Necrosis, calcification, and cholesterol clefts are not prominent in typical early proliferative lesions; however, cholesterol clefts present in a bandlike distribution and lesions resembling typical atheromatous plaques may arise in advanced forms of the disease, particularly after a long posttransplant interval.

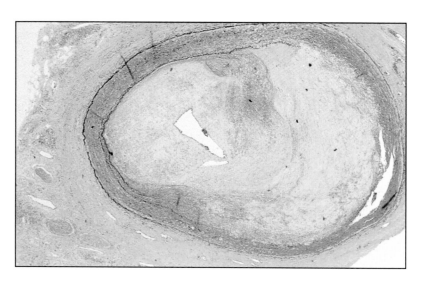

Figure 12-32.
Allograft coronary disease superimposed on native (donor) atherosclerosis (Verhoeff–van Gieson elastic stain). The original atherosclerotic lesion (right portion of vessel) is eccentric, and the internal elastic lamina is destroyed. Allograft coronary disease characterized by concentric intimal thickening surrounds the lumen (left portion of vessel). The internal elastic lamina is intact. (*From* Schoen and Libby [32]; with permission.)

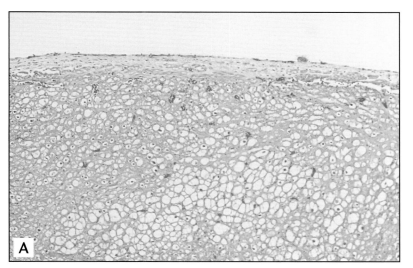

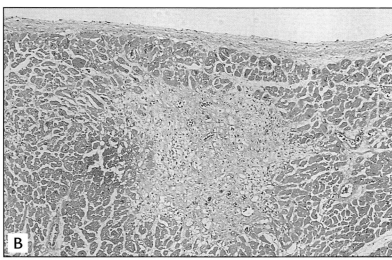

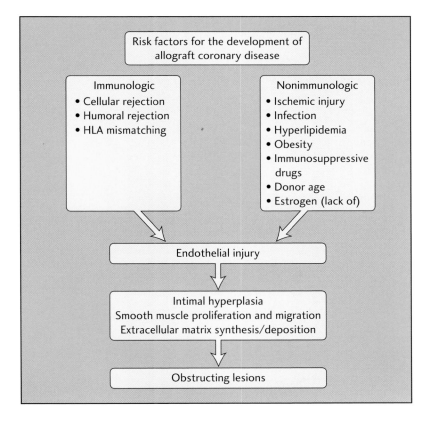

Figure 12-33.

Myocardial pathology secondary to allograft coronary disease. Luminal occlusion by allograft coronary disease results in similar myocardial changes compared with those caused by native vessel atherosclerosis [33]. **A,** Subendocardial myocyte vacuolization is a potentially reversible change suggesting severe but nonlethal chronic ischemia. **B,** Microinfarcts, acute and healing (seen here) tend to be more prevalent in association with allograft coronary disease than in native hearts with typical atherosclerosis suggesting small vessel involvement in allograft coronary disease. **C,** Subendocardial and transmural infarcts resemble those that occur secondary to native vessel atherosclerosis; however, healing is frequently delayed because of the immunosuppressive therapy that the recipients receive.

Figure 12-34.

Risk factors for the development of allograft coronary disease. The pathogenetic mechanisms of initiation and progression of allograft coronary disease are not well defined. The limited involvement of allograft vasculature with sparing of the recipient's native vessels suggests processes that specifically target the allograft resulting in endothelial injury or derangement in the regulation of smooth muscle cell proliferation. Immunologic as well as conventional risk factors have been implicated as having a causal or contributing role. Most likely, the cause is multifactorial. Defining the pathogenetic mechanism responsible for allograft coronary disease may be the key to reducing its incidence and progression so that long-term survival after cardiac transplantation is routinely possible.

REFERENCES

1. Hosenpud JD, Bennett LE, Keck BM, et al.: The registry of the International Society for Heart and Lung Transplantation: sixteenth official report–1999. *J Heart Lung Transplant* 1999, 18:611–626.

2. O'Connell JB, Bristow MR: Economic impact of heart failure in the United States: time for a different approach. *J Heart Lung Transplant* 1994, 13:107–112.

3. Ghali JK, Cooper R, Ford E: Trends in hospitalization for heart failure in the United States, 1973–1986: evidence for increasing population prevalence. *Arch Intern Med* 1990, 150:769–773.

4. Blanche C, Takkenberg JJ, Nessim S, et al.: Heart transplantation in patients 65 years of age and older: a comparative analysis of 40 patients. *Ann Thorac Surg* 1996, 62:1442–1446.

5. Baldwin JC, Anderson JL, Boucek MM, et al.: 24th Bethesda conference: cardiac transplantation: task force 2: donor guidelines. *J Am Coll Cardiol* 1993, 22:15–20.

6. Burke AP, Saenger J, Mullick F, Virmani R: Hypersensitivity myocarditis. *Arch Pathol Lab Med* 1991, 115:754–769.

7. Gravanis MB, Hertzler GL, Franch RH, et al.: Hypersensitivity myocarditis in heart transplant candidates. *J Heart Lung Transplant* 1991, 10:688–697.

8. Lewin D, d'Amati G, Lewis W: Hypersensitivity myocarditis: findings in native and transplanted hearts. *Cardiovasc Pathol* 1992, 1:225–229.

9. Spear G: Eosinophilic explant carditis with eosinophilia: ? hypersensitivity to dobutamine infusion. *J Heart Lung Transplant* 1995, 14:755–760.

10. Gries W, Farkas D, Winters GL, Costanzo-Nordin MR: Giant cell myocarditis: first report of disease recurrrence in the transplanted heart. *J Heart Lung Transplant* 1992, 11:370–374.

11. Oni AA, Hershberger RE, Norman DJ, et al.: Recurrence of sarcoidosis in a cardiac allograft: control with augmented corticosteroids. *J Heart Lung Transplant* 1992, 11:367–369.

12. Valantine HA, Tazelaar HD, Macoviak J, et al.: Cardiac sarcoidosis: response to steroids and transplantation. *J Heart Lung Transplant* 1987, 6:244–250.

13. Hosenpud JD, Uretsky BF, Griffith BP, et al.: Successful intermediate-term outcome for patients with cardiac amyloidosis undergoing heart transplantation: results of multicenter survey. *J Heart Transplant* 1990, 9:346–350.

14. O'Connell JB, Dec GW, Goldenberg IF, et al.: Results of heart transplantation for active lymphocytic myocarditis. *J Heart Transplant* 1990, 9:351–356.

15. Billingham ME, Cary NRB, Hammond EH, et al.: A working formulation for the standardization of nomenclature in the diagnosis of heart and lung rejection: heart rejection study group. *J Heart Transplant* 1990, 9:587–593.

16. Winters GL, Marboe CC, Billingham ME: The International Society for Heart and Lung Transplantion grading system for cardiac transplant biopsies: clarification and commentary. *J Heart Lung Transplant.* 1998, 17:754–760.

17. Miller LW, Schlant RC, Klobashigawa J, et al.: 24th Bethesda conference: cardiac transplantation: task force 5: complications. *J Am Coll Cardiol* 1993, 22:41–54.

18. Laufer G, Laczkovics A, Wollenek G, et al.: The progression of mild acute cardiac rejection evaluated by risk factor analysis: the impact of maintenance steroids and serum creatinine. *Transplantation* 1991, 51:184–189.

19. Yeoh TK, Frist WH, Eastburn TE, Atkinson J: Clinical significance of mild rejection of the cardiac allograft. *Circulation* 1992, 86(suppl II):267–271.

20. Lloveras JJ, Escourrou G, Delisle MB, et al.: Evolution of untreated mild rejection in heart transplant recipients. *J Heart Lung Transplant* 1992, 11:751–756.

21. Winters GL, Loh E, Schoen FJ: Natural history of focal moderate cardiac allograft rejection: is treatment warranted? *Circulation* 1995, 91:1975–1980.

22. Milano A, Caforio ALP, Livi U, et al.: Evolution of focal moderate (International Society for Heart and Lung Transplantation grade 2) rejection of the cardiac allograft. *J Heart Lung Transplant* 1996, 15:456–460.

23. Rizeq MN, Masek MA, Billingham ME: Acute rejection: significance of elapsed time after transplantation. *J Heart Lung Transplant* 1994, 13:862–868.

24. Winters GL: The pathology of heart allograft rejection. *Arch Pathol Lab Med* 1991, 115:266–272.

25. Fyfe B, Loh E, Winters GL, et al.: Heart transplantation-associated perioperative ischemic myocardial injury: morphological features and clinical significance. *Circulation* 1996, 93:1133–1140.

26. Winters GL, Schoen FJ: Graft arteriosclerosis-induced myocardial pathology in heart transplant recipients: predictive value of endomyocardial biopsy. *J Heart Lung Transplant* 1997, 16:985–993.

27. Kottke-Marchant K, Ratliff NB: Endomyocardial lymphocytic infiltrates in cardiac transplant recipients. *Arch Pathol Lab Med* 1989, 113:690–698.

28. Radio SJ, McManus BM, Winters GL, et al.: Preferential endocardial residence of B-cells in the "Quilty effect" of human heart allografts: immunohistochemical distinction from rejection. *Mod Pathol* 1991, 4:654–660.

29. Joshi A, Masek MA, Brown BW, et al.: Quilty revisited: a 10-year perspective. *Hum Pathol* 1995, 26:547–557.

30. Nalesnik MA, Makowka L, Starzl TE: The diagnosis and treatment of posttransplant lymphoproliferative disorders. *Curr Probl Surg* 1988, 25:365–472.

31. Chadburn A, Cesarman E, Knowles DM: Molecular pathology of post-transplantation lymphoproliferative disorders. *Semin Diagn Pathol* 1997, 14:15–26.

32. Schoen FJ, Libby P: Cardiac transplant graft arteriosclerosis. *Trends Cardiovasc Med* 1991, 1:216–223.

33. Neish AS, Loh E, Schoen FJ: Myocardial changes in cardiac transplant-associated coronary arteriosclerosis: potential for timely diagnosis. *J Am Coll Cardiol* 1992, 19:586–592.

13

Native Valvular Heart Disease

Jagdish Butany
Avrum I. Gotlieb

This chapter reviews the major causes of valvular heart disease. Valvular heart disease may be congenital or acquired, and both forms are illustrated. The management of valvular heart disease has improved dramatically in the past 25 years. Among the reasons for this are a better understanding of the pathophysiology of valvular heart disease and relatively easier and more definitive diagnoses with echocardiography, transesophageal echocardiography, CT scans, and magnetic resonance imaging. At the same time, the surgical approach to valvular heart disease has continued to evolve with the introduction of newer and better prosthetic heart valves and the increasing emphasis on repair of diseased heart valves. Valves, like all pathologic specimens, should be examined with the clinical features in mind so the appropriate conclusions may be made. An example of establishing good clinicopathologic correlations is the finding of a "new form" of valvular heart disease associated with the use of an appetite suppressant drug (fenfluramine-phentermine) in a minority of individuals.

The normal human heart valve, although virtually perfect and lasting a lifetime in the majority of individuals, can be involved in infective, inflammatory, infiltrative, and degenerative diseases that result in its malfunction. Perhaps the most commonly affected valve today is the the aortic valve. Aortic stenosis may be valvular (the most common form), subvalvular, or supravalvular. Because of improvements in health care delivery and prevention in industrialized countries, rheumatic heart disease and its sequelae have decreased dramatically. However, with the increased mobility of populations from one part of the world to another, postinflammatory valvular disease continues to be seen worldwide. With its overlay of fibrosis and calcification leading to clinically significant dysfunction, congenital aortic valvular disease now accounts for a large proportion of patients with valvular heart disease. Because of increasing life spans, there is an increased incidence of "senile calcific valvular disease."

The mitral valve, clearly the most complex of the four cardiac valves, is subject to the greatest closing pressures. It is subject to all acquired valvular disease and dysfunction related to ischemic damage. Rupture of one or more chordae tendineae and prolapse of part or all of the mitral leaflet tissue is a fairly common occurrence, resulting in mitral valvular incompetence. A majority of mitral stenoses is related to rheumatic mitral valvular disease, and a minority (most likely less than 0.5%) is related to congenital lesions such as cor triatriatum, endocardial bands, and atrial membranes.

The tricuspid valve, regardless of changes and cause, generally manifests with tricuspid regurgitation. It normally has a large annulus and orifice; therefore, functional stenosis is rare.

Although involvement in congenital cardiac disorders may occur, the common acquired causes are still those related to postinflammatory conditions and those secondary to pulmonary hypertension.

Pulmonary valve involvement is most frequently related to congenital lesions, and survival to adulthood is increasingly seen in these patients. Acquired pulmonary valve disease is rare, which makes it a suitable choice for use in valve "switch" surgery (the Ross procedure) for treating aortic valve disease, especially in young individuals. The pulmonary valve is able to adapt to the higher pressures of the aortic circulation and, at least so far, has been associated with good related results. Acquired pulmonary valve lesions include chronic rheumatic valvular disease, which is very rare in industrialized countries, and the carcinoid syndrome.

Although numerous valvular lesions have been reported and discussed, new and sophisticated diagnostic techniques and advanced prosthetic cardiac valves have made effective treatment and good results a reality, with an increase in life span as well as a significant improvement in quality of life.

VALVE DISEASE

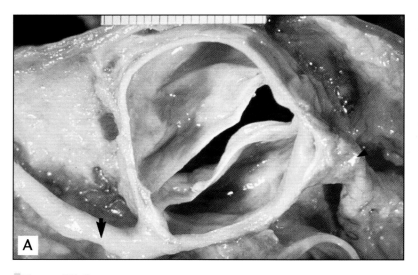 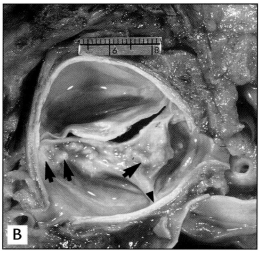

Figure 13-1.

Congenital aortic valve disease. **A,** Congenitally bicuspid aortic valve with mild thickening and no calcification. Two clearly unequal leaflets and two commissures are seen. This 58-year-old patient's valve functioned virtually normally, and there were no clinical symptoms. He died of advanced lung cancer. The commissures may be anterior and posterior or left and right. If anterior and posterior, the coronary ostia, left and right, are usually one in each sinus of Valsalva. If the commissures are left and right, the coronary ostia are usually both in the anterior sinus (*arrowhead* indicates RCA) [1–7].

B, A congenitally bicuspid aortic valve (*arrowhead*) with significant cuspal fibrosis, thickening, and nodular calcification. This congenitally bicuspid and dysplastic valve is from a 24-year-old woman who had undergone aortic commissurotomy 5 years before death. She died suddenly in the hospital while awaiting surgery. The commissures (*long arrows*) are anterior and posterior, the leaflets left and right (*short arrow*). Whereas patients with dysplastic bicuspid valves usually become symptomatic early in life, those with calcified and fibrotic bicuspid valves tend to present in the fifth to seventh decades of life.

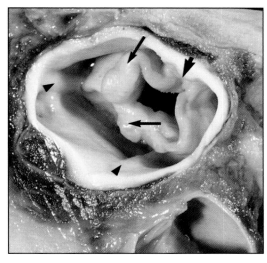

Figure 13-2.

This unicuspid (unicommissural), dysplastic aortic valve is from a 23-year-old woman who died suddenly while dancing. The cusps are thickened (*long arrows*), and the orifice is eccentric (*short arrows*). The orifice is usually linear, looks like an exclamation mark, or is shaped like a key hole, and only one good commissure is identified (*short arrow*). In addition, two raphe-like structures (*arrowheads*) are seen. The patient developed an aortic dissection and died suddenly.

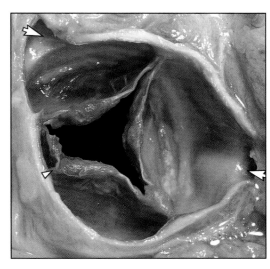

Figure 13-3.

Quadricuspid aortic valve. The patient was a 52-year-old woman on hemodialysis. The four cusps are of variable sizes. The right and left sinuses are normal (*arrows*), but the posterior sinus has two cusps with a smaller left posterior cusp (*arrowhead*). Quadricuspid aortic valves (and quadricuspid pulmonic valves) are exquisitely rare in the general population (< 0.008% to 0.014%). They are more often seen in men than women [4]. This lesion is generally asymptomatic, although calcification and fibrosis of the cusps may occasionally lead to aortic valve dysfunction.

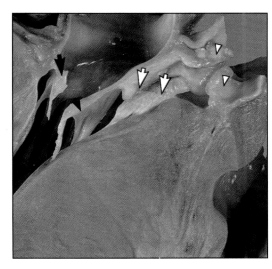

Figure 13-4.

Subaortic stenosis tunnel. Aortic stenosis (AS) is not limited to the valve alone but may involve the subvalvular and the supravalvular structures. Discrete subvalvular AS may be caused by a short or localized fibrous ridge or a circumferential fibrous aortic ring or tunnel [5–7]. Complete fibrous diaphragm may rarely be present. In tunnel subvalvular AS, fibrous thickening (*ie*, endocardial fibrosis) starts close to the aortic valve (AV) and extends downward for 1 to 3 cm (*ie*, the patch of endocardial fibrous thickening is up to 3.0 cm in width). The AV may be normal or show abnormalities. The valve is only mildly incompetent, in most instances. This case is taken from a 12-year-old girl who had a commissurotomy for AS 2 years before she died. One week before she died, a ventricular aortic conduit was placed. The patient died of sepsis in the postoperative period. The dysplastic AV (*white arrowheads*) and the fibrous subaortic ring (*white arrows*) can be seen. *Black arrows* indicate mitral leaflets.

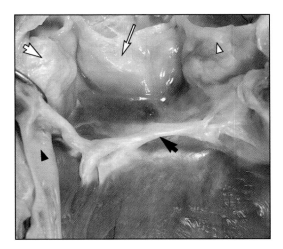

Figure 13-5.

Subaortic stenosis. A fibrous subaortic ridge (*black arrow*) is seen. This discrete band at the top of the interventricular septum was seen in a 15-year-old boy who died suddenly. The aortic valve itself had three dysplastic leaflets (*long arrows, short arrows, arrowhead*). The patient had undergone an open valvuloplasty 10 years earlier. The left ventricle showed marked hypertrophy.

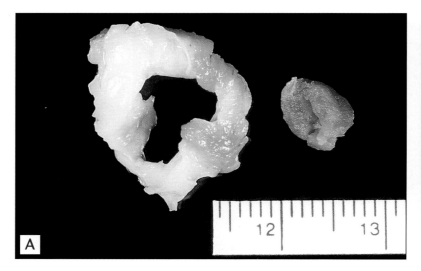

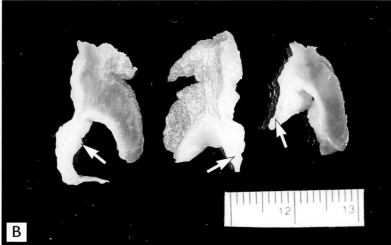

Figure 13-6.

Fibrous subaortic ring. **A,** The surgically excised fibrous subaortic ring shows a ring of thick, dense, white fibroelastic tissue. The deeper surface shows patchy areas of pale yellow-brown muscle and a small myectomy specimen (*right*). The patient had clinical features of aortic stenosis that were found to be related to this

fibrous subaortic ring on echocardiography. **B,** Serial sections of the fibrous subaortic ring with attached muscle show a "hood-like" strip of thickened fibroelastic tissue (*arrows*). The hood-like tissue easily creates significant functional aortic stenosis.

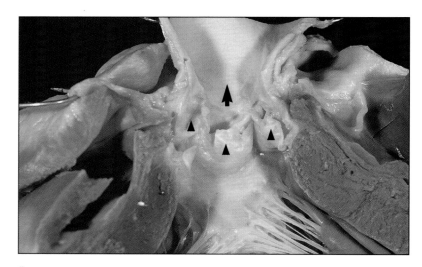

Figure 13-7

Supravalvular aortic stenosis. **A,** An irregular constricted area at the sinotubular junction distal to the aortic valve (*arrow*). The valve has three leaflets that are dysplastic (*arrowheads*). This 14-year-old boy had Williams syndrome and died suddenly.

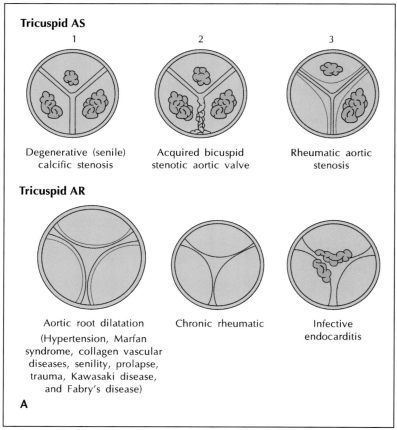

Figure 13-8.

Aortic valve (AV) disease. Shown is the incidence of different forms of AV disease at surgery. **A,** Types of acquired tricuspid AV disease. (*continued on next page*)

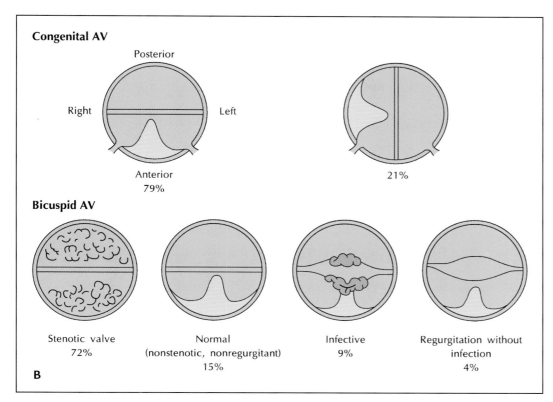

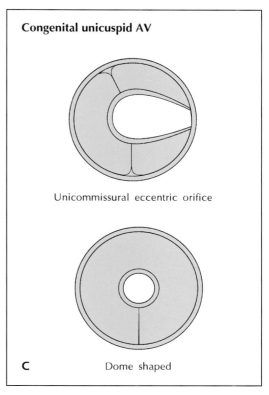

Congenital AV

Posterior

Right — Left

Anterior
79%

21%

Bicuspid AV

Stenotic valve
72%

Normal
(nonstenotic, nonregurgitant)
15%

Infective
9%

Regurgitation without
infection
4%

B

Congenital unicuspid AV

Unicommissural eccentric orifice

C Dome shaped

Figure 13-8. (*continued*)
B, Congenitally bicuspid (nondysplastic) AV. **C,** Unicuspid AV. (*Adapted from* Dare and coworkers [10]; with permission.)

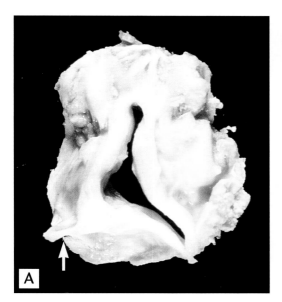

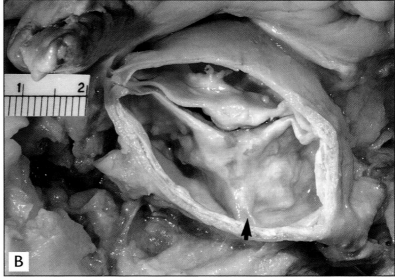

A **B**

Figure 13-9.
Bicuspid aortic valve (AV). Congenitally bicuspid and acquired bicuspid AVs [11]. **A,** Congenital bicuspid AV surgically excised from a 66-year-old man. This shows fibrotic thickening of cusps and raphe (*arrow*). Extensive nodular calcification of the cusps and raphe is evident. The leaflets are anterior and posterior. In congenitally bicuspid AVs, the raphe is usually rudimentary and stops short of the free margin of the cusp, although the raphe may occasionally be larger, thicker, and reach nearly to the free margin of the cusp, necessitating a much closer examination before a definitive diagnosis can be made. (Transverse sections through the region of the raphe may be helpful in deciding between a commissure and a raphe.) In surgically excised specimens, especially those removed in pieces, a definitive morphologic diagnosis can be very difficult. **B,** Acquired bicuspid and stenotic AV [12]. Specimen from a 65-year-old man who died suddenly while awaiting heart valve replacement. Three commissures are seen (*arrows*). Two are easily identified, but the third necessitates closer examination. In addition, the commissures are equidistant, and their upper margins are at the same level. (*continued on next page*)

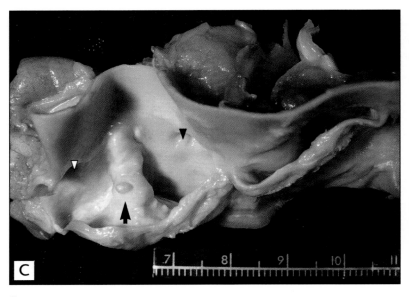

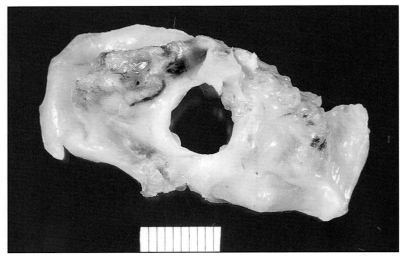

Figure 13-9. (*continued*)

C, The left ventricular outflow tract has been opened, and the view from the aortic end shows two functional leaflets with a prominent raphe (*white arrowhead*) and a normal commissure (two normal commissures) (*black arrowhead*). In acquired AV stenosis, the cause of the lesion is hard to determine and may be related to a previous, healed endocarditis or rheumatic valve disease restricted to two cusps and one intervening commissure.

Figure 13-10.
Congenitally acommissural aortic valve. This sheetlike valve from an 11-year-old boy with severe aortic stenosis and incompetence has a central circular orifice. The "cuspal" tissue is thickened and calcified over much of its extent.

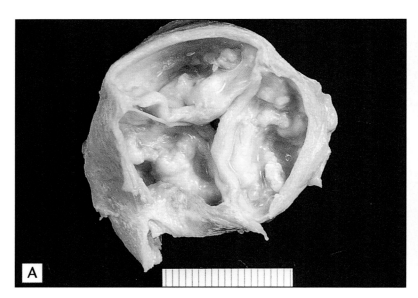

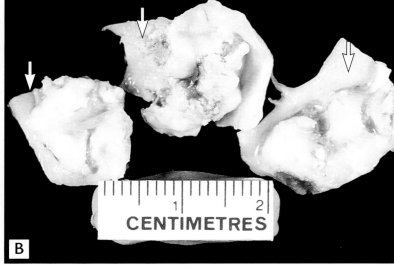

Figure 13-11.
Degenerative aortic valve (AV) disease. **A,** Seen in significantly older individuals, usually in the late seventh and eighth decades, the valve has three cusps and three commissures, which must have been morphologically and functionally unremarkable for a long time. The cusps show fibrotic thickening and nodular calcification and a stenotic orifice. Nodular calcific masses are seen on the flow as well as the nonflow surfaces. The commissural regions are usually easily identifiable.

B, Surgically excised, three cuspid AVs. The three cusps are clearly identified. Each (for variable degrees) shows large, heavily calcified, nodular masses in the body of the cusp. The lunular region, although thickened because of fibrosis, shows relatively little calcification (*arrow*). (*continued on next page*)

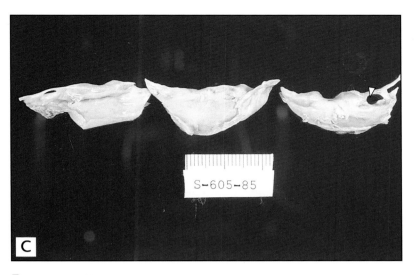

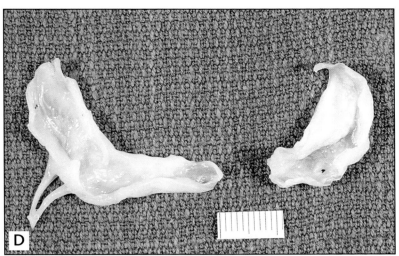

Figure 13-11. (*continued*)

C, Degenerative AV disease. The degree of cusp thickening and calcification is often variable. This three-cuspid valve removed from a 78-year-old woman shows relatively mild cusp thickening and relatively mild calcification. One of the cusps shows large fenestrations (*arrowhead*). Nevertheless, the valve was dysfunctional and the patient did well postoperatively.

D, Congenitally bicuspid AV with AV incompetenece. This surgically excised AV from a 21-year-old man shows two unequal cusps. The larger cusp (*left*) shows the raphe, and the cuspal tissue itself shows mild to moderate myxomatous change. There was no evidence of calcification.

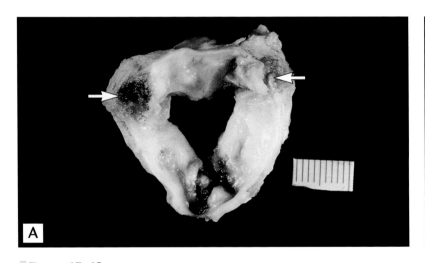

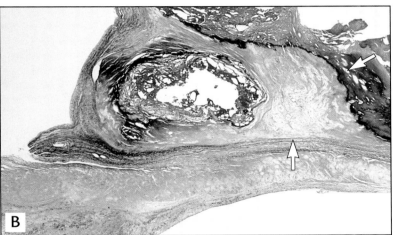

Figure 13-12.

Rheumatic aortic valve (AV). **A,** Surgically excised AV showing three commissural regions, three nearly equal-sized cusps. All three commissural regions, as well as cusps, show marked fibrosis, fusion of the commissures, and extensive calcification (*arrows*).

B, Histologic section through a fused commissure showing cusp fibrosis and commissural fusion with calcification. The elastic plate of both cusps is seen and extends to the commissure (*arrows*).

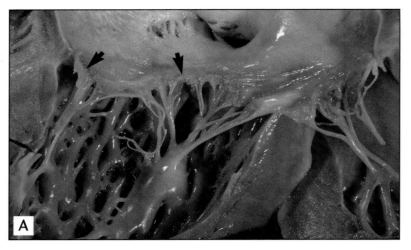

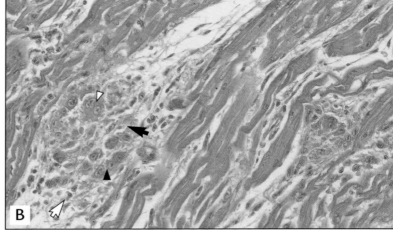

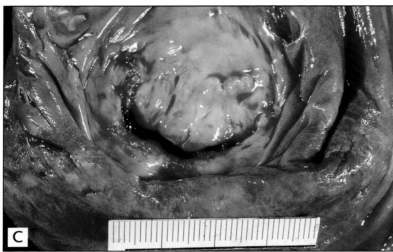

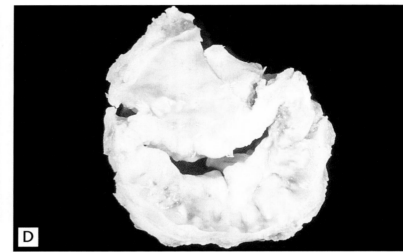

Figure 13-13.

Mitral valve (MV) disease. Acute rheumatic MV disease occurs with acute rheumatic heart disease [13]. Migratory polyarthritis (ie, large joints), pancarditis, subcutaneous nodules, edema marginatum of the skin, and chorea are present. Grossly, the heart is usually mildly enlarged and appears flabby with a fibrinous ("bread-and-butter") pericarditis. The valves (acute phase), one or more, show verrucal lesions, most frequently on the left side of the heart.

In Western countries, chronic rheumatic valvulitis manifests after a long latent period ranging from 5 to 30 years with a mean of 19 years. However, in southeast Asia, most likely because of recurrent streptococcal infection and lack of treatment, severe MV disease may manifest in the early teens with massive cardiomegaly and congestive heart failure [14].) The risk of chronic rheumatic valvulitis after an episode of acute rheumatic fever is 18% to 65% and is highest in patients with rheumatic carditis, which results in congestive heart failure. In the Western world, the incidence of rheumatic fever has declined dramatically, although there have been occasional reports of a resurgence in young military recruits and civilian populations in recent years [15,16]. In military recruits, the occurrence is believed to be related to the close quarters in military barracks. The MV alone is affected in one third of patients, and both left-sided valves are involved in one third. The tricuspid valve is very occasionally involved, and pulmonary valve involvement is very rare (although it is seen occasionally in developing countries).

A, MV showing small verrucous (1- to 2-mm diameter), reddish pink, friable vegetations along the line of closure (*arrows*). This 18-year-old mentally retarded man suffered a cardiac arrest and had a recent history of fever and diarrhea of unknown duration. The endocardium showed mixed acute and chronic inflammatory infiltrates as well as occasional macrophages and Aschoff bodies.

B, Aschoff nodules are small areas of fibrinoid necrosis and are usually perivascular. Lymphocytes, macrophages, and occasional plasma cells are seen surrounding an area of fibrinoid change or collagen degeneration. Anitchow cells have a round or ovoid nucleus with chromatin condensed at the nuclear periphery and along the center, which results in the classic owl-eyed and caterpillar appearance. Aschoff giant cells are multinucleate cells formed by the fusion of Anitchkow histiocytes.

C, Specimen from a 58-year-old man showing a severely dilated left atrium (walls are folded over to be accommodated in this picture) and markedly thickened anterior and posterior leaflets. The orifice is "fish mouth" or "C" shaped. The leaflet tissue is much less mobile than usual and adds to the degree of stenosis.

D, Surgically excised mitral valve from a 55-year-old woman showing a markedly thickened, fibrotic, and extensively calcified anterior and posterior leaflet. The commissures are fused and calcified. Both leaflets were stiffened, and the orifice was severely stenosed. (*continued on next page*)

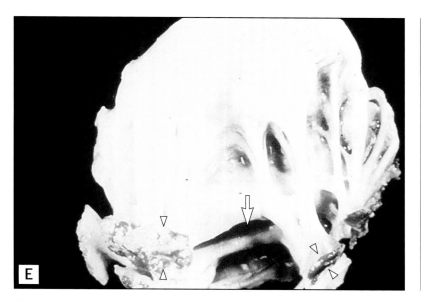

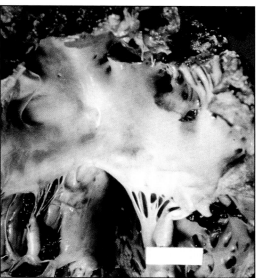

Figure 13-13. (*continued*)

E, Surgically excised MV (ventricular view). The orifice of this valve (*arrow*) is severely stenosed. Although the leaflets are thickened, fibrotic, and fused, the chordae tendineae are also markedly thickened, extensively fused, and form a prominent subvalvular component to the MV stenosis. The cut end of the chordae tendineae often shows bits of myocardium from the papillary muscles (*arrowheads*). Although the dominant lesion in these valves is stenosis, a degree of incompetence is invariably present because of the stiffening of the cusps.

Figure 13-14.

Rheumatic tricuspid valve disease. Right side of heart showing a dilated right atrium from a 54-year-old woman who died of other causes. The tricuspid valve is one virtually continuous sheet of tissue. No commissures are identified. The leaflet tissue is thickened, and the chordae tendineae show mild thickening. The commissures are fused. (Clinically, the patient had tricuspid regurgitation and an enlarged, tender liver.)

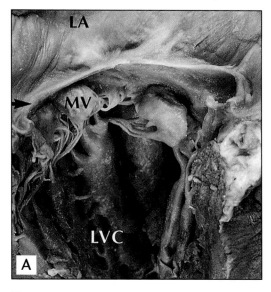

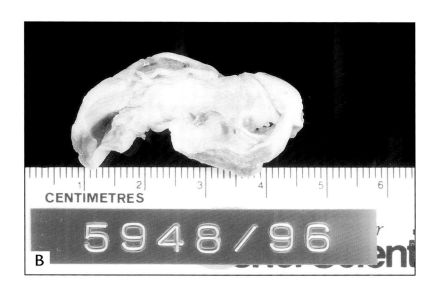

Figure 13-15.

Mitral valve (MV) stenosis. MV stenosis may be very rarely caused by congenital causes such as a supravalvular ring and cor triatriatum. **A,** A supravalvular ring (*arrows*). A circumferentially running, shelflike strip of endocardium situated above the MV from a child with double inlet left ventricle and ventricular septal defect. **B,** Cor triatriatum. A membrane in the left atrium divides the chamber into a large upper and small lower one with one or many perforations resulting in variable degrees of functional MV stenosis.

Aschoff nodules are foci of fibrinoid necrosis (*black arrow*), lymphocytes (*white arrow*), macrophages, and occasional plasma cells. The macrophages are of two specific types. The Anitschkow cell (*black arrowhead*, or Aschoff cell) has round to ovoid nuclei with chromatin condensation at the nuclear periphery and in the center; this feature has resulted in the designations "owl-eyed" and "caterpillar cell." Aschoff giant cells (*white arrowhead*) are multinucleated cells formed from Anitschkow's histiocytes.

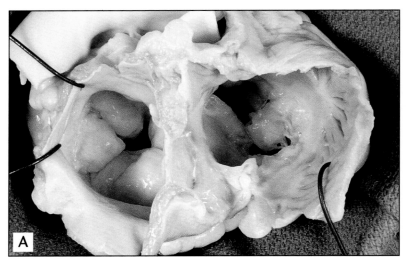

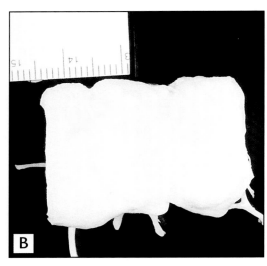

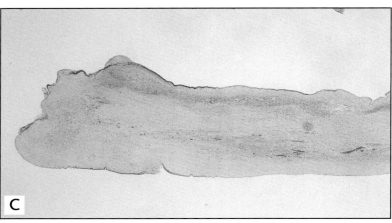

Figure 13-16.
Mitral valve prolapse (MVP). MVP is a common finding in the general population: the incidence ranges from 3% to 5% and is significantly higher in women. However, the majority of symptomatic patients who need therapeutic management are men. Ten percent to 15% of patients have symptomatic mitral regurgitation (MR). Severe MVP can occasionally be associated with sudden, unexpected death [17].

A, This mitral valve (MV) is from a 34-year-old man who died suddenly while waiting to enter his workplace. He had no previous cardiac history. The MV is markedly enlarged, and both leaflets show areas of significant "billowing" or prolapse. The chordae tendineae are thin and elongated. The ventricular aspect of the valve often appears to have a markedly increased number of chordae tendineae. Valvular tissue is pearly white and soft and the cut margins look edematous.

B, Surgical specimen showing a resected segment of mitral leaflet tissue (from the posterior mitral leaflet, usually one scallop) [18,19]. The pearly white piece of mitral leaflet has cut edges that appear markedly thickened and edematous. Ruptured chordae tendineae with chordal tapering and pointed tips tapering to a fine threadlike appearance or a drumstick-like appearance of an old ruptured chorda tendina are seen; the appearance is consistent with a ruptured chordae tendineae. These are different than the transverse surgically cut ends.

C, Histologically, the MV (on Movat staining) leaflets show significantly widened zona spongiosa with increased amounts of acid mucopolysaccharides (green on most Movat stains). Valvular interstitial cells are most likely involved in mucopolysaccharide metabolism because they regulate cardiac valve structure and function [20].

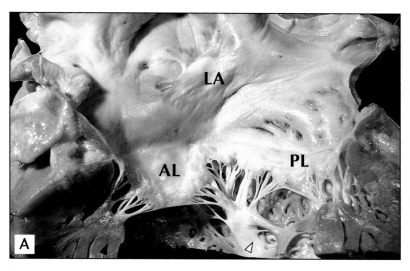

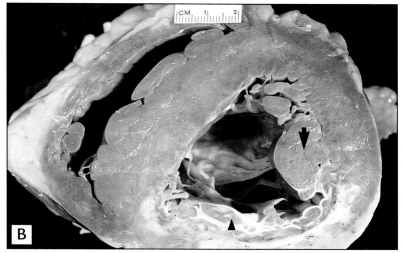

Figure 13-17.

Ischemic mitral regurgitation. Myocardial ischemic damage involving the papillary muscle or its base (*ie*, the left ventricle underlying it) often leads to mitral regurgitation (MR) because of papillary muscle dysfunction. In the presence of papillary muscle rupture, MR occurs acutely and is more severe than with ischemic damage alone, which leads to regurgitation a lot more gradually.

A, The posterior papillary muscle (PPM) shows fibrosis and loss of muscle bulk in a patient who had severe coronary artery disease involving the right coronary artery and the circumflex coronary artery. This 60-year-old man had a healed myocardial infarct

involving the left ventricle. Clinically, he was in significant congestive heart failure and had mitral regurgitation. Note scarred and thinned PPM (*white arrowhead*) whereas the APM is hypertrophied (*black arrowhead*). Note dilated left atrium (LA).

B, Anterior papillary muscle (APM). The papillary muscle shows scarring (*arrowhead*) and is flat, firm, and fibrotic, whereas the APM is "plump" and hypertrophied (*arrow*). The left atrium is dilated, and closer inspection often shows wrinkling of the posterior wall of the endocardium. AL—anterior leaflet; PL—posterior leaflet.

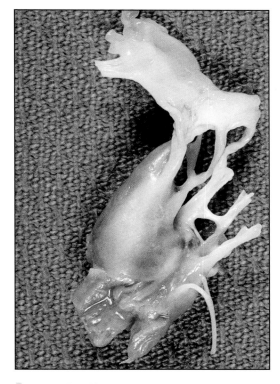

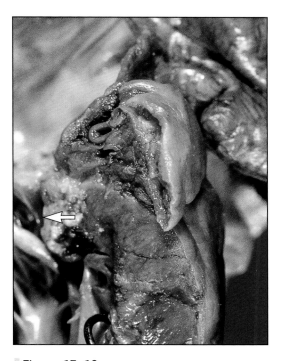

Figure 13-18

Papillary muscle rupture. The infarct may be subendocardial and often involves the rupture of one head of a left ventricular papillary muscle.

Figure 13-19.

Mitral annular calcification (MAC). Usually seen in older individuals, women more often than men, older than 70 years of age. MAC may be very minimal or massive, when the atrioventricular groove and the adherent annulus have a diameter of more than 1 cm extending all around the posterior mitral leaflet (PML). The basal portion or more of the PML gets adhesed to this annular calcific mass and leads to mitral regurgitation (MR) [21]. This 82-year-old woman had mitral valvular incompetence. The mitral annulus showed extensive calcification, and much of the anterior mitral leaflet was adherent to this calcific mass.

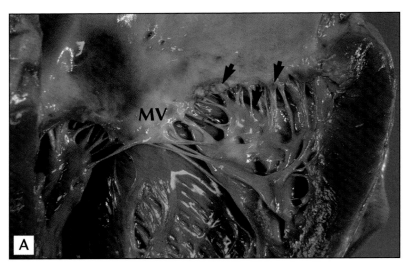

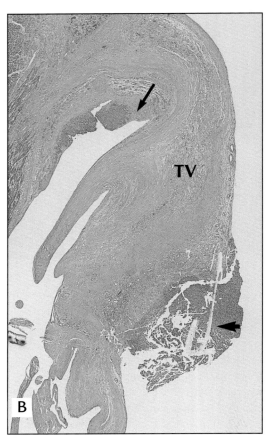

Figure 13-20.

Connective tissue diseases. Connective tissue diseases such as systemic lupus erythematosus (SLE) can involve the heart and valves. The mitral valve, especially the ventricular aspect, is most frequently involved and shows small nodules or verrucous vegetations of Libman-Sacs endocarditis. **A,** This 21-year-old woman with SLE diagnosed 2 years before death developed systemic hypertension and renal failure. The opened left heart shows the verrucous vegetations of Libman-Sacs endocarditis (*arrows*) [22–24]. Vegetations are seen in the medial and lateral scallop in this photograph. A common finding in these diseases is a nonspecific pericarditis [25]. Similar lesions can be seen in the antiphospholipid antibody syndrome. **B,** The tricuspid valve from the heart shown in *panel A* shows vegetations on the atrial (*short arrow*) and ventricular (*long arrow*) surfaces. The most typical location for the vegetations of SLE is the ventricular surface at the base of the valve. This case shows lesions on both surfaces. TV—tricuspid valve.

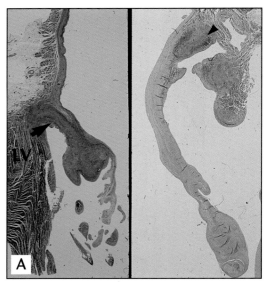

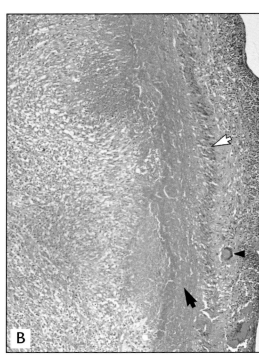

Figure 13-21.

Rheumatoid aortic valve (AV) disease. Five percent of patients with rheumatoid disease develop cardiac involvement [26]. These granulomatous rheumatoid lesions can be seen in the pericardium, myocardium, endocardium, and valve tissue. This involvement is proportionate to the degree of severity of the systemic disease, and the AV and mitral valves (MV) are most frequently involved. Clinical evidence of valvular involvement is rare; when manifest, it is usually regurgitation.

Specimen from a 56-year-old woman with a 10-year history of severe rheumatoid arthritis. **A,** The MV shows thickening and the presence of rheumatoid nodules in the valve leaflet and the left ventricular endocardium (*arrow*). The AML contains a rheumatoid nodule (*arrowhead*) at its basal attachment. **B,** A histologic section of endocardium near the valve insertion shows a rheumatoid nodule (*black arrow*) with central necrosis, surrounding palisading histiocytes (*white arrow*) and giant cells (*arrowhead*) and extensive chronic inflammation.

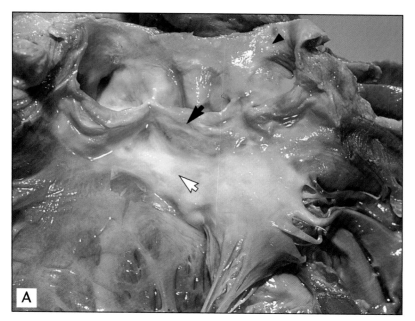

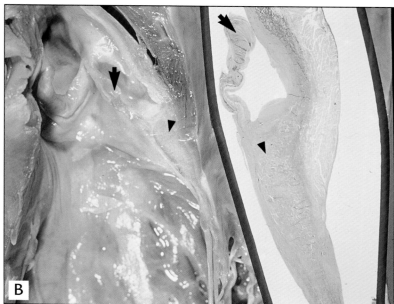

Figure 13-22

Ankylosing spondylitis. **A,** Cardiac involvement in ankylosing spondylitis is seen in 3.5% to 10.0% of patients with duration of disease from 10 to 30 years [27]. Aortic annular dilatation, as well as fibrosis and inflammation of aortic wall (*arrowhead*) and valve cusps, are seen. Mitral insufficiency is rare. This gross photograph of an aortic valve demonstrates thickening of the leaflets (*black arrow*) and a dot on the anterior leaflet of the mitral valve (*white arrow*).

B, Inflammation and scarring extend below the aortic valve to include the anterior mitral leaflet, resulting in a bump on the anterior leaflet (*arrowheads*). The gross heart (*left side of panel*) shows cut surface of the bump with corresponding histologic sections (*right side of panel*). *Arrows* show left aortic cusp. (*Courtesy of* William C. Roberts, Dallas, Texas.)

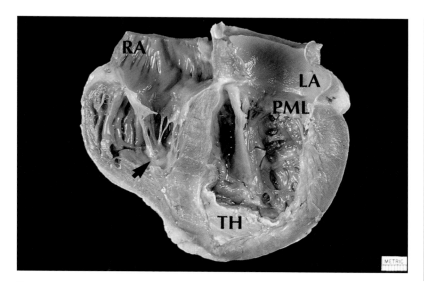

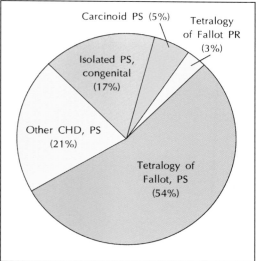

Figure 13-23.

Hypereosinophilic syndrome. This syndrome is associated with significant eosinophilia (> 1500 eosinophils per mm^3), thromboembolic phenomena, and generalized arteritis. The syndrome typically occurs in middle-aged men, and cardiac changes are associated with high morbidity and mortality. In the acute phase, cardiomegaly with apical and in-flow biventricular mural thrombi on the ventricular surfaces of atrioventricular valves is present. Eosinophils are seen within thrombi and may involve small intramural coronary arteries, and eosinophilic myocarditis may be evident.

Shown is a heart from a 9-year-old boy with eosinophilic leukemia of 9 months' duration showing biventricular dilatation and hypertrophy (four-chamber view). *Arrows* denote typical endocardial fibrosis in the right ventricle and left atrium. PML—posterior mitral leaflet; RA—right atrium; TH—thrombus.

Figure 13-24.

Pathologic findings in surgically excised pulmonary valve (PV) replacement. PV disease is more often congenital than acquired. Pulmonary stenosis can occur as an isolated congenital anomaly, and the stenosis may be valvular, infundibular, and supravalvular. CHD—congenital heart disease; PH—pulmonary hypertension; PR—pulmonary regurgitation; PS—pulmonary stenosis; TR—tricuspid regurgitation; TS—tricuspid stenosis.

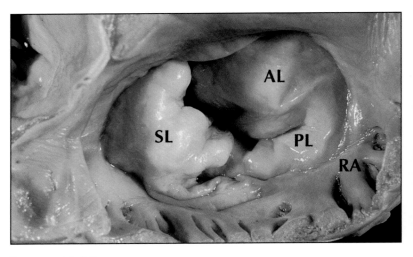

Figure 13-25.

Tricuspid valve (TV) disease. TV prolapse alone is rare and is seen in about 0.1% to 5.5% of the population and in about 22% of patients with mitral valve prolapse. Tricuspid regurgitation is generally mild and does not correlate with the morphologic severity of the prolapse. TV prolapse involves mainly the septal leaflet (SL) alone or both the septal and the anterior leaflets (AL). The right atrium is usually of normal size. PL—posterior leaflet; RA— right atrium.

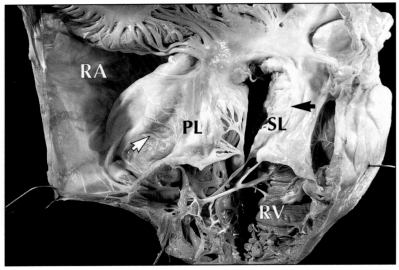

Figure 13-26.

Ebstein's anomaly. This is an uncommon form of congenital heart disease associated with tricuspid regurgitation and very rarely tricuspid stenosis [28]. The tricuspid valve is displaced downward so the right atrium is markedly enlarged and the right ventricle smaller. The anterior tricuspid leaflet (ATL) is large and sail-like (typically called the "sail anterior leaflet"), with opposition of the leaflet against the right ventricular (RV) wall.

The free edge of the anterior leaflet (AL) may attach directly into the RV wall or have abnormal papillary muscles; its attachment to the crista supra ventricularis is always directly chordal. The proximal chamber may be large or small depending on the extent of downward displacement of the TV. The endocardium of the atrialized RV is fibrotic with poorly developed trabeculae carnae. The distal chamber is located behind the ATL. LA—left atrium, LV—left ventricle, PV—pulmonary valve.

ENDOCARDITIS

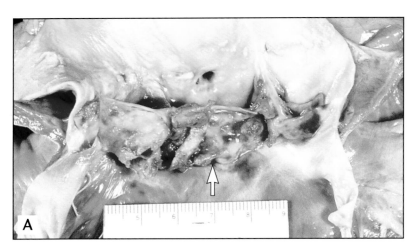

Figure 13-27.

Infective endocarditis (IE). IE was commonly seen on morphologically abnormal valves (congenital or acquired). Today, fewer than 50% of valves with IE have any underlying morphologic abnormality. IE is also often seen in intravenous drug abusers (increased incidence on right-sided valves) and immunoincompetent individuals [29]. IE-associated complications include destruction of valvular tissue, spread to adjacent valves (*eg*, aortic to mitral), sinus of Valsalva rupture, fistulae into the right atrium and right ventricle, bundle block, rupture into the pericardial sac, and septic emboli.

A, Aortic valve (AV) showing vegetations of IE (*arrow*) caused by *Staphylococcus aureus* infection in a 60-year-old woman with an otherwise normal three-cuspid valve. The *arrow* shows an area of leaflet destruction and perforation. (*continued on next page*)

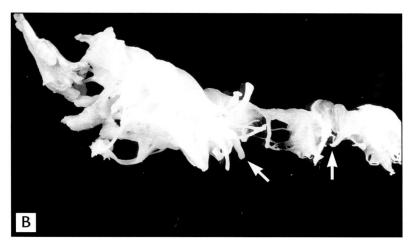

Figure 13-27. (*continued*)
B, Surgically excised mitral valve (MV) showing MV prolapse (MVP) in a patient with superimposed bacterial endocarditis. The mitral regurgitation had worsened. Some of the chordae tendineae are ruptured (*arrows*). Today, MVP is the common underlying condition in patients with infective endocarditis (54% of cases).

REFERENCES

1. Dare AJ, Vinot JP, Edwards WE, *et al.*: New observations on the etiology of aortic valve disease: a surgical pathology study of 236 cases from 1990. *Hum Pathol* 1993, 24:1330–1338.

2. Davies MJ: Pathology of cardiac valves. *Post-graduate Pathology Series,* 1980.

3. Edwards JE: The congenital bicuspid aortic valve [editorial]. *Circulation* 1961, 23:485–486.

4. Fischler D, Fitzmaurice M, Ratcliffe NB Jr: Quadricuspid aortic valve. *Am J Cardiovasc Pathol* 1990, 3:91–94.

5. Katz NM, Buckley NJ, Liberthson RR: Discrete membranous subaortic stenosis: report of 31 patients, review of the literature and delineation of management. *Circulation* 1977, 56:1034–1039.

6. Kelly DT, Wulfsberg E, Rowe RD: Discrete subaortic stenosis. *Circulation* 1972, 46:309–322.

7. Maron BJ, Redwood DR, Roberts WC, *et al.*: Tunnel subaortic stenosis: left ventricular out-flow tract obstruction produced by fibromuscular tubular narrowing. *Circulation* 1976, 54:404–416.

8. Pansegrau DG, Kioshos JM, Durnin RE, Kroetz FW: Supravalvular aortic stenosis in adults. *Am J Cardiol* 1973, 31:635–641.

9. Peterson TA, Todd DB, Edwards JE: Supravalvular aortic stenosis. *J Thorac Cardiovas Surg* 1965, 50:734–741.

10. Dare AJ, Veinot JP, Edwards WE, *et al.*: Evaluation of surgically excised mitral valves: revised recommendations based on changing operative procedures in the 1990s. *Hum Pathol* 1993, 24:1286–1293.

11. Roberts WC: The congenitally bicuspid aortic valve: a study of 85 autopsy cases. *Am J Cardiol* 1970, 26:72–83.

12. Waller VF, Carter JB, William HJ Jr, *et al*: Bicuspid aortic valve: comparison of congenital and acquired types. *Circulation* 1973, 48:1140–1150.

13. Besterman E: The changing face of acute rheumatic fever. *Br Heart J* 1970, 32:579–582.

14. Angelini A, Ho SY, Anderson, RH, *et al.*: The morphology of the normal aortic valve as compared with the aortic valve having two leaflets. *J Thorac Cardiovas Surg* 1989, 98:362–378.

15. Feuer J, Spiera H: Acute rheumatic fever in adults: resurgence in the Hasidic Jewish Community. *J Rhematol* 1997, 24:337–340.

16. Da Silva NA, Periera BA: Acute rheumatic fever: still a challenge. *Rheumat Dis Clin North Am* 1997, 23:545–568.

17. Lane CD: Sudden unexpected death in young adults due to right ventricular dysplasia. *J Forens Sci* 1997, 42:148–150.

18. Dare AJ, Harrity PJ, Tazellar HD, *et al.*: Evaluation of surgically excised mitral valves: revised recommendations based on changing operative procedures in the 1990's. *Hum Pathol* 1993, 24:1286–1293.

19. Nakano K, Eishi K, Kobayashi J, *et al.*: Surgical treatment for prolapse of the anterior mitral leaflet. *J Heart Valve Dis* 1997, 6:470–474.

20. Mulholland DL, Gotlieb AI: Valvular interstitial cells: regulator of the cardiac valve structure and function. *Cardiovasc Pathol* 1997, 6:167–174.

21. Roberts WC: Morphologic features of normal and abnormal mitral valve. *Am J Cardiol* 1983, 51:1005–1028.

22. Bulkley BH, Roberts WC: Systemic lupus erythematosus as a cause of severe mitral regurgitation: new problem in an old disease. *Am J Cardiol* 1975, 305–308.

23. Musial J: Valvular heart disease in SLE: another symptom of the disease or a hallmark of secondary antiphospholipid syndrome [letter]? *Eur Heart J* 1997, 18:1836–1837.

24. Edwards JE: Lesions causing or simulating aortic insufficiency. *Cardiovasc Clin* 1973, 5:127–148.

25. Lockshin MD: Pathogenesis of the antiphospholipid antibody syndrome. *Lupus* 1996, 5:404–408.

26. Bulkley BH, Roberts WC: Ankylosing spondylitis and aortic regurgitation. *Circulation* 1973, 48:1014–1020.

27. Bulkley BH, Ridolfi RL, Salyer WR, *et al.*: Myocardial lesions of progressive systematic sclerosis: a cause of cardiac dysfunction. *Circulation* 1976, 53:483–489.

28. Daliento L, Angelini A, Ho SY, *et al.*: Angiographic and morphologic features of the left ventricle in Ebstein's malformation. *Am J Cardiol* 1997, 80:1051–1059.

29. Connolly HM, Crary JL, McGoon MD, *et al.*: Valvular heart disease associated with fenfluramine-phentermine. *N Engl J Med* 1997, 337:581–588.

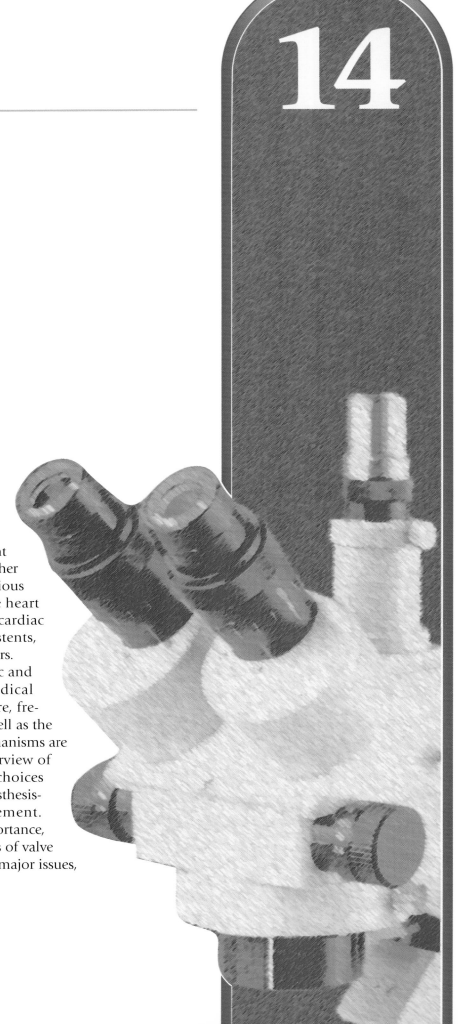

Prosthetics

Frederick J. Schoen

Data from the National Center for Health Statistics and the American Heart Association indicate that 5.4 million major cardiovascular operations (including catheterization procedures) were performed in the United States in 1997, including 700,000 open heart surgeries and 145,000 pacemaker insertions. Concurrent with and enabling the broad application of these and other surgical and interventional procedures is the use of various prostheses and medical devices, including substitute heart valves, aortocoronary and peripheral vascular grafts, cardiac assist devices (and potentially total artificial hearts), stents, umbrellas, patches, pacemakers and their leads, and others.

Despite the importance for cardiologists and cardiac and vascular surgeons of cardiovascular prostheses, medical devices, and their constituent biomaterials, the nature, frequency, and pathologic anatomy of complications as well as the responsible blood–tissue–biomaterials interaction mechanisms are not widely known. This chapter provides a visual overview of these considerations intended to facilitate informed choices among therapeutic options, enhance recognition of prosthesis-associated problems, and optimize patient management. Owing to the extensive and long-term use, clinical importance, and availability of relevant data on many different types of valve prostheses [1], as well as the fact that they illustrate the major issues, these devices are emphasized in this chapter.

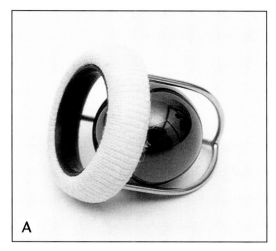

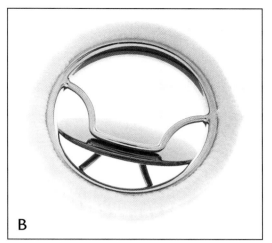

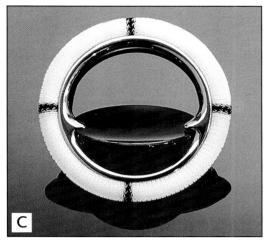

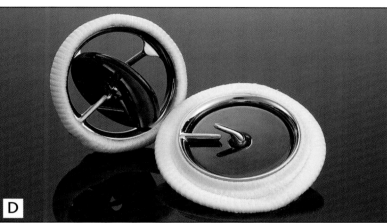

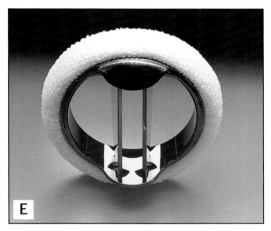

Figure 14-1.

Mechanical heart valve prostheses. Dozens of mechanical valves have been implanted in humans; five are shown here. **A,** Starr-Edwards caged-ball valve (Baxter Cardiovascular Corp., Irvine, CA). Starr-Edwards valves claim the longest continuous clinical use (since 1960). The one-piece cage consists of a circular orifice and three (aortic) or four (mitral) thin struts joined at the apex. The poppet is molded from silicone rubber and impregnated with barium to render it radiopaque. The extensive and well-documented clinical results with these prostheses serve as a benchmark for the clinical results with mechanical valves [2]. **B,** Bjork-Shiley tilting disk valve (previously manufactured by Shiley, Inc., Irvine, CA). This was the first widely used valve with an occluder fabricated from pyrolytic carbon. The Bjork-Shiley convexoconcave modification was also an extremely popular valve but is no longer in use because of problems with strut fractures (see Fig. 14-10A). The Bjork-Shiley Monostrut prosthesis (not shown) has recently been approved by the Food and Drug Administration for general use. **C,** The OmniScience valve (Medical, Inc., Minneapolis, MN), a successor to the discontinued Lillehei-Kaster pivoting disk valve, has a smoothly curved pyrolytic carbon disk and a one-piece titanium cage with short struts. The disk opens to 80°. The OmniCarbon valve (Medical, Inc., Minneapolis, MN) is similar to the OmniScience valve but is completely coated with pyrolytic carbon (not shown).

D, The Medtronic-Hall valve (Medtronic Inc., Minneapolis, MN) has a polytef sewing ring, a titanium housing machined from a solid cylinder and a carbon-coated disk with flat parallel sides. The disk, which opens to 75° in the aortic model and 70° in the mitral model, is retained by an S-shaped guide strut that protrudes through a hole in the center of the disk. **E,** The most popular mechanical valve in use today, the St. Jude bileaflet tilting disk valve

(St. Jude Medical, Inc., St. Paul, MN) is composed entirely of pyrolytic carbon; the leaflets open to 85°. The St. Jude valve was the first clinically successful bileaflet valve and has been used in more than 500,000 patients since its first implant in 1977. Its occluding mechanism consists of two semicircular leaflets that swing apart during opening, resulting in three separate flow areas. The housing of the valve is a cylindrically shaped piece of pyrolytic carbon with two rounded tabs called *pivot guards* that project up from the inflow side. The inside surfaces of these tabs are flat and contain two butterfly-shaped indentations that retain the leaflets. Small "ears" at the end of each diameter of the thinned semicircle leaflets fit into these indentations, which secure the leaflets in the housing and define their limits of travel.

Other bileaflet valves are available. The Baxter (formerly Edwards lifesciences, Santa Ana, CA) TEKNA valve has curved leaflets that move slightly downstream as they open. This valve experienced some fractures of the leaflets and housing and was taken off the market while it was thoroughly restudied and revised. It has been reintroduced in Europe after several slight modifications that were incorporated into a new design to reduce stresses on the valve during closing and thereby reduce cavitation, a problem of microbubble formation and implosion that was thought to induce the mechanical damage. The Carbomedics bileaflet valve (Sulzer Carbomedics, Austin, TX) has flat leaflets and a solid pyrolytic carbon housing with a titanium ring for stiffening and radiopacity. The cavities in the housing that contain the pivot recesses are located in the main body of the housing. (*Part A courtesy of* Edwards Lifesciences, Santa Ana, CA; *part B courtesy of* Shiley Inc., Irvine, CA; *part C courtesy of* Medical, Inc., Inver Grove Heights, Minneapolis, MN; *part D courtesy of* Medtronic Inc., Minneapolis, MN; *part E courtesy of* St. Jude Medical, Inc., St. Paul, MN).

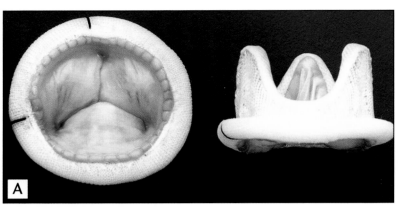

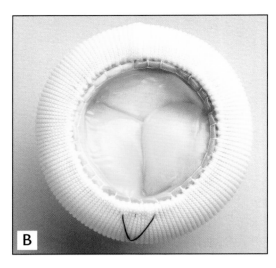

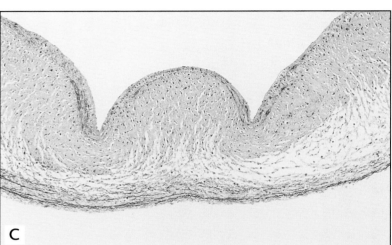

Figure 14-2.

Stented porcine bioprosthetic valves. **A,** Carpentier-Edwards porcine standard valve (Baxter Cardiovascular Corp., Irvine, CA). The rim of the valve is a flexible wire stent made of metal, intended to reduce stresses on the leaflets and orifice. A flexible Mylar cylinder surrounds and supports the metal mesh frame. The annulus is asymmetrically shaped to obliterate the muscle shelf of the porcine right coronary cusp. **B,** Hancock porcine bioprosthesis (Medtronic, Inc., Minneapolis, MN), aortic view. This valve was introduced by Hancock Laboratories in 1970 as the first commercial tissue valve. The stents are circular and composed of a flexible polypropylene cylinder with a radiopaque metallic ring added for rigidity. Porcine bioprostheses are fabricated from an aortic valve harvested from a pig and preserved using the glutaraldehyde treatment method developed by Carpentier and coworkers (described by Schoen [3]). **C,** The layered histologic appearance of a porcine aortic valve in Movat stain. Elastin is black and collagen yellow in the Movat stain [4].

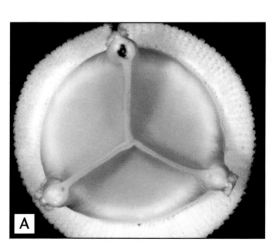

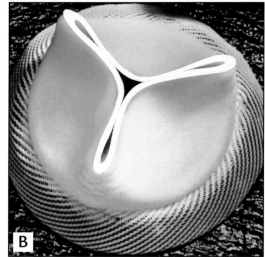

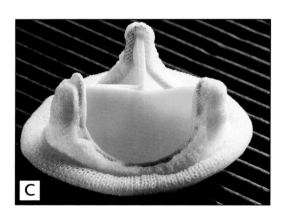

Figure 14-3.

Bovine pericardial bioprosthetic valves. These tissue valves are fabricated from parietal pericardium harvested from a cow. In the Ionescu-Shiley valve (Shiley Inc., Irvine, CA) (*panel A*), the first commercially available pericardial valve, and the Mitroflow pericardial valve (Mitroflow International, Inc., Richmond, British Columbia, Canada) (*panel B*), three individual pieces of pericardium are applied to the outside of the stent. In these two designs, failures because of tearing were prominent (see Fig.

14-13). The Carpentier-Edwards pericardial bioprosthesis valves (Edwards Lifesciences, Santa Ana, CA, formerly Baxter HealthCare, Inc., Irvine, CA) (*panel C*) received Food and Drug Administration approval in 1991; in this valve, the leaflets are supported on the inside of the stent posts. Results have been superior to those of the earlier pericardial valves [5]. The major potential advantage of pericardial valves is a more complete and symmetric opening for better hemodynamics.

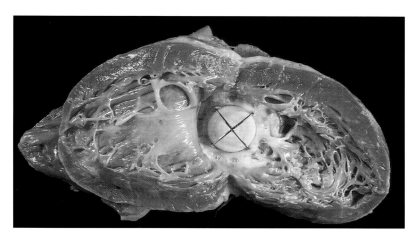

Figure 14-4.
Myocardial limitations to the success of cardiac valve replacement surgery. Specimen explanted at cardiac transplantation of a patient 28 years after Harken disk mitral valve replacement and in whom the myocardium deteriorated insidiously after valve surgery. Valvular heart disease induces substantial changes in myocardial configuration and composition that may regress only partly, if at all, after surgery and may lead to late cardiac failure. (*From* Schoen [6]; with permission.)

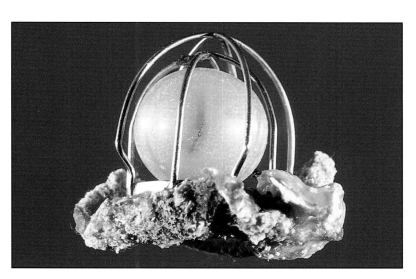

Figure 14-5.
Harken caged-ball aortic valve removed for prosthetic valve endocarditis 22 years after implantation. The poppet of this valve has a superficial crack that was probably not functionally significant. Both this valve and that shown in Figure 14-10 emphasize that patients may survive extended intervals despite having valves that would be today considered obsolete. Such patients (and their valves) may be encountered by both clinicians and pathologists. (*From* Schoen [7]; with permission.)

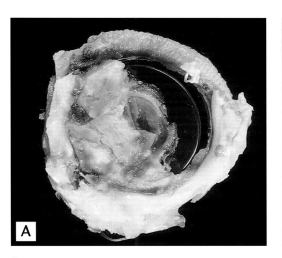 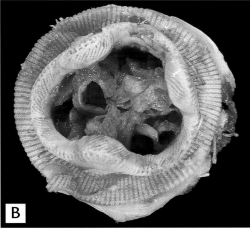

Figure 14-6.
Valve thrombosis. **A,** Thrombotic occlusion of Bjork-Shiley tilting disk prosthesis (previously manufactured by Shiley, Inc., Irvine, CA). The thrombus was initiated in the region of stasis immediately downstream of the minor orifice of the fully opened disk.
B, Thrombotic occlusion of a porcine bioprosthesis; nodular thrombus fills the prosthetic sinuses of Valsalva. Contemporary prostheses generally have thromboembolic rates of 2% to 4% per patient year [8,9]. The risk factors for prosthetic heart valve thromboembolism include mechanical versus bioprosthetic valves, valve designs with focally static flow (mitral versus aortic site), and patients with multiple versus isolated valves, those with inadequate anticoagulation control or none at all, those with atrial fibrillation with or without left atrial enlargement or thrombus, and at early postoperative intervals (to several months) [10]. As in the cardiovascular system in general, Virchow's triad (*ie*, surface thrombogenicity, hypercoagulability, and locally static blood flow) largely predicts the relative propensity toward thrombus formation and the location of thrombotic deposits with specific valve prostheses. Platelet survival measurements and assays of circulating platelet-release products indicate that platelets are activated by prosthetic heart valves. Although administration of platelet-suppressive drugs largely normalizes indices of platelet formation and partially reduces the frequency of thromboembolic complications in patients with mechanical prosthetic valves, such therapy alone does not confer adequate protection against thromboembolism. Because prosthetic valve thrombi organize slowly if at all, thrombolytic therapy has been used with some success in valve thrombosis [11].

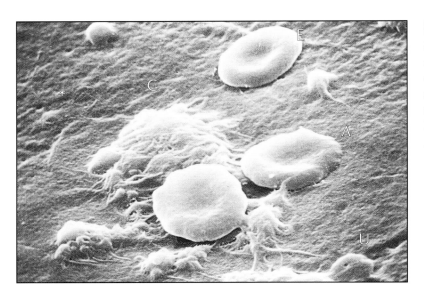

Figure 14-7.

Scanning electron photomicrograph of early thrombotic deposits on heart valve material exposed to blood. There is a background of protein absorption (*asterisk*) with numerous platelets in various stages of adhesion, ranging from relatively unaffected (U) to adherent to activated (A) forms, some aggregated in clumps (C). Erythrocytes (E) are probably passive bystanders in thrombus formation. (*From* Schoen [12]; with permission.)

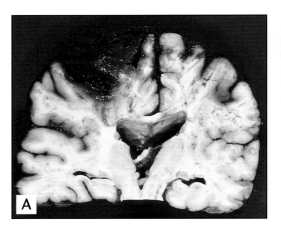

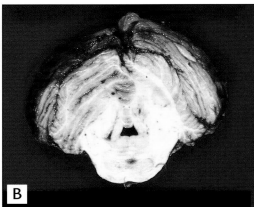

Figure 14-8.

Anticoagulation-related fatal cerebrovascular accident. **A,** Cerebral hemisphere. **B,** Cerebellum. The chronic anticoagulation required in many patients receiving prosthetic valves induces a risk of hemorrhage, particularly retroperitoneal, gastrointestinal, and cerebral, at a frequency approximately 4% per patient year; as many as 25% of such events are fatal [13]. The adequacy of warfarin anticoagulation (as assessed by INR) is the most important factor affecting not only thrombotic but also bleeding complications in patients with mechanical valves.

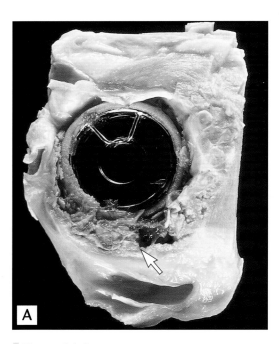

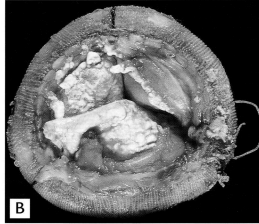

sewing ring, with secondary tissue destruction around the prostheses, causing a ring abscess. The consequences of prosthetic valve endocarditis include sepsis, embolization of vegetations, congestive heart failure secondary to obstruction or regurgitation caused by bulky vegetations, or ring abscess causing paraprosthetic leak, cardiac rupture, or heart block caused by conduction system damage. Such infections respond infrequently to antibiotic therapy and have a high mortality rate (≥ 60%). Although bioprosthetic valve endocarditis is often localized to the prosthesis sewing ring and complicated by ring abscess and its sequelae, such infections may involve and indeed are occasionally limited to the cuspal tissue. Cuspal involvement may cause obstruction or secondary cuspal tearing or perforation with valve incompetence. Prosthetic valve endocarditis has a high frequency of staphylococcal infection (especially *Staphylococcus epidermidis*), particularly in early prosthetic valve endocarditis. (*Part A from* Schoen [12]; with permission.)

Figure 14-9.

Prosthetic valve endocarditis. **A,** Mechanical valve. **B,** Bioprosthetic valve. Infective endocarditis occurs in 1% to 6% of patients with valve prostheses [14]. Because synthetic biomaterials used in mechanical prostheses generally cannot support bacterial or fungal growth, prosthetic valve infections are almost always localized to the prosthesis–tissue junction at the

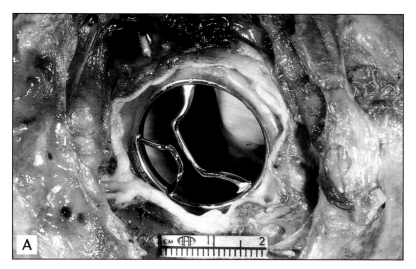 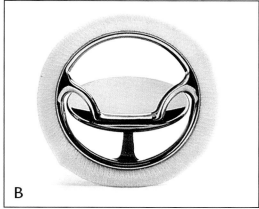

Figure 14-10.

Mechanical valve durability failure (structural deterioration). **A,** Strut fracture in Bjork-Shiley convexo-concave valve (previously manufactured by Shiley, Inc., Irvine, CA). **B,** Unimplanted Bjork-Shiley convexoconcava (C-C) valve for comparison. Durability failures of many valve types have been widely discussed in the literature [15–17] . The silicone elastomeric ball occluders of early caged-ball prosthesis absorbed blood lipids leading to swelling, distortion, grooving, cracking, embolization of poppet material, or abnormal poppet movement (ball variance), especially in aortic valve replacement. Mitral ball variance was distinctly less common than aortic. Changes in elastomer fabrication in 1964 virtually eliminated lipid-related ball variance in subsequently implanted valves. Caged-disk valves with plastic disks frequently developed disk wear with notching, reduction in diameter, and resultant valve incompetence. Valves with plastic-coated struts often have wear concentrated on this coating. Cloth-covered caged-ball valves (intended to lower thromboembolic risks through tissue ingrowth into the fabric, yielding a favorable biologic surface) have suffered problems related to cloth abrasion and fragmentation by the occluder, in some cases leading to poppet escape. Such problems have been overwhelmingly more common with valves in the aortic than the mitral position. Contemporary tilting disk valves designed with pyrolytic carbon occluders with or without carbon cage components have favorable durability. Pyrolytic carbon (deposited in a fluidized bed as a coating of dense carbon deposited on a graphite substrate machined in the configuration of the valve parts) has high strength and high wear and fatigue resistance [18]. Its widespread use as an occluder and strut-covering material for mechanical valve prostheses eliminated abrasive wear as a prominent long-term complication of cardiac valve replacement. Fractures of metallic or carbon components of disk valves occur rarely. However, in a small cohort of Edwards-Duromedics valves (Edwards Lifesciences, formerly Baxter Healthcare, Inc., Santa Ana, CA), either the disk or the housing suffered critical fractures [19]. An unusually large cluster of frequently fatal complication of the widely used Bjork-Shiley C-C heart valve occurred in which the welded outlet strut fractured because of metal fatigue and separated from the valve leading to disk escape [20], as shown in *panel A.*

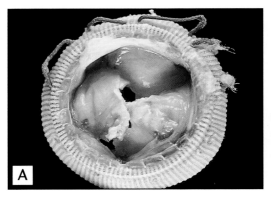

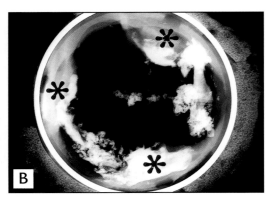

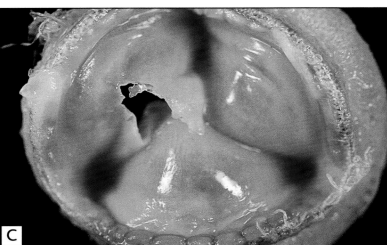

Porcine bioprosthetic valve failure caused by calcification. **A,** Valve with calcification and cuspal tearing. **B,** Radiograph of heavily calcified porcine valve (commissures denoted by *asterisks*). The major cause of dysfunction of cardiac valve bioprostheses is sterile tissue degeneration (primary tissue failure), especially that related to cuspal mineralization [21,22]. Regurgitation through tears secondary to calcification is the most frequent clinical pathologic failure mode of porcine valve (at least 75% of degenerative failures). Pure stenosis caused by calcific cuspal stiffening and cuspal tears or perforations unrelated to either calcification or endocarditis occur less frequently.

C, Noncalcific porcine valve tear. The clinical presentation of bioprosthetic valve failure is heterogeneous; most patients have insidious development of cardiac dysfunction, but approximately 5% deteriorate rapidly.

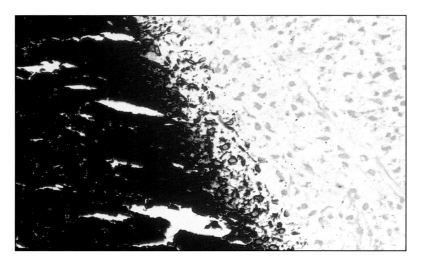

Figure 14-12.
Pathogenesis and effects of bioprosthetic valve calcification, as delineated by clinical and experimental investigations. Calcific deposits in bioprosthetic tissue occur initially in the residual connective tissue cells of the bioprosthetic tissue [23]. Calcification of collagen and other extracellular matrix occurs later. Experimental investigation has delineated host and implant factors in calcification and has shown that dynamic mechanical stress and strain promote calcification of bioprosthetic valve tissue, but immunologic factors probably play no role. The most critical determinants of the propensity of bioprosthetic tissue to calcify probably relate to the tissue preparation method used—glutaraldehyde fixation potentiates mineral deposition. Considerable academic and industrial research and developmental efforts designed to interrupt critical events in valve calcification are underway [3,24,25].

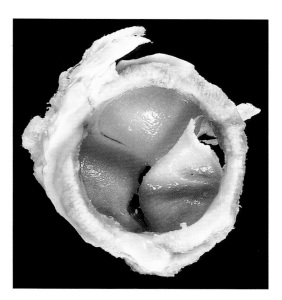

Figure 14-13.

Failure of an Ionescu bovine pericardial bioprosthetic valve (Shiley Inc., Irvine, CA) with extensive cuspal tear and resultant incompetence but no calcification. The first-generation bovine pericardial bioprostheses had a greater propensity for late calcific and noncalcific primary tissue failure than their porcine valve counterparts. Cuspal defects in pericardial valves are most frequently commissural and basal and are largely related to the continuous trauma of the tissue against the bare Dacron (AI du Pont de Nemours & Co., Inc., Wilmington, DE) cloth [26,27]. Despite favorable clinical results with a second-generation model, the Carpentier-Edwards pericardial valve (Edward Lifesciences, Santa Ana, CA, formerly Baxter Cardiovascular Corp., Irvine, CA) failures noted with this model are similar to those observed with earlier pericardial valves. (*From* Schoen [12]; with permission.)

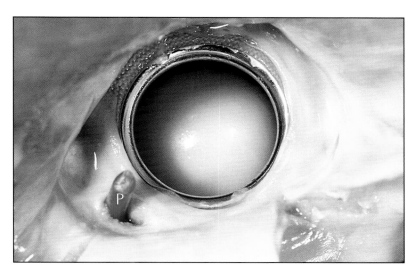

Figure 14-14.

Paravalvular leak. Small paravalvular leak viewed from the left ventricle demonstrated by a probe (P). Early paravalvular leak is usually the result of either suture knot failure, inadequate suture placement or separation from sutures from a pathologic annulus with endocarditis complicated by ring abscess, myxomatous valvular degeneration (floppy mitral valve), or calcified valvular annulus. It is fostered by a continuous rather than interrupted suture line. Late small paravalvular leaks are usually caused by anomalous tissue retraction from the sewing ring between sutures during healing. Paravalvular leaks may be clinically inconsequential, may aggravate hemolysis, or may cause heart failure through regurgitation.

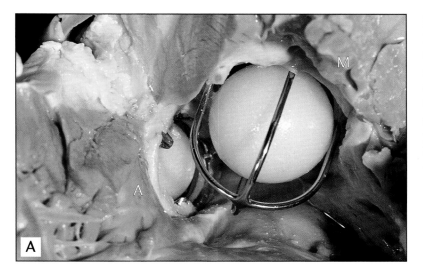

Figure 14-15.

Prosthetic disproportion and extrinsic factors. **A,** Size disproportion of Starr-Edwards valve (Edwards Lifesciences, Santa Ana, formerly Baxter Cardiovascular Corp., Irvine, CA) in the mitral (M) and aortic (A) valve positions. Valves with a high profile, such as Starr-Edwards valves, are generally not used for mitral valve replacement in patients with a small ventricular cavity, where prosthetic disproportion owing to placement of an inappropriately large valve may result in septal irritation, interference to left ventricular emptying, or decreased occluder motion. (*continued on next page*)

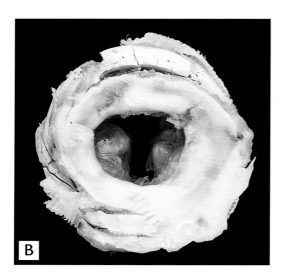

Figure 14-15. (*continued*)

B, Excessive pannus formation extending over a sewing ring and occluding approximately 50% of the orifice area of this valve that was removed from a right ventricular outflow tract conduit in a child. Exuberant overgrowth of fibrous tissue may instead prevent full mechanical valve occluder excursion or cause stenosis of a bioprosthesis. Other factors extrinsic to a valve prostheses that may promote stenosis or regurgitation of a properly selected and sized-valve substitute include 1) a large mitral annular calcific nodule or septal hypertrophy that may prevent full excursion of a tilting disk valve occluder; 2) interference with tilting disk valve occluder motion by valve remnants (such as a retained posterior mitral leaflet) or unraveled or long sutures or knots; 3) restriction of cuspal motion by sutures looped around bioprosthetic valve stents, particularly pericardial bioprostheses; or 4) perforation of a bioprosthetic valve cusp by suture ends cut too long or unraveled. Although intermittent sticking of otherwise intact bileaflet tilting disk prostheses has been recognized, some such valves appear to function normally when removed, and the source of the in vivo malfunction is unclear.

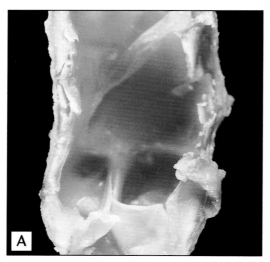

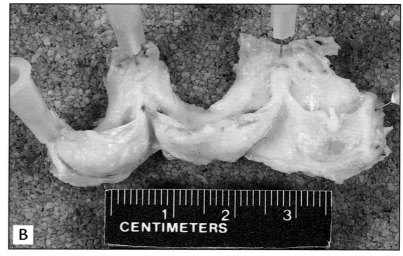

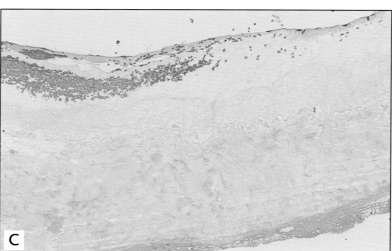

Figure 14-16.

Valvular homografts. **A,** Pulmonary valvular homograft and pulmonary artery, conduit used as a right ventricular outflow tract in a child, removed because of growth and calcification-related stenosis. The valve cusps are free of calcification, but the aortic wall has dense mineralization with stiffening. **B,** Aortic valve homograft removed from an adult showing marked sagging of aortic valve cusps causing valvular insufficiency. **C,** Histologic features of typical long-term aortic valve homograft demonstrating bland hyalinized structure without originally transplanted cuspal interstitial or endothelial cells or inflammatory cells. There is a cuspal hematoma in the *upper left-hand corner*. Allografts are valves transplanted from one person to another. Irradiation, harsh chemical preservatives, and high concentrations of antibiotics used in the 1960s led to a high rate of valve degeneration [28]. Cryopreservation techniques developed in the 1970s have led to a resurgence in their use, now largely limited by supply. Allograft valves are the preferred substitute for aortic valve replacement because they have excellent hemodynamics, require no anticoagulation, and have low thrombogenicity. Pulmonary homografts have also been used to replace the aortic or pulmonic valves. Homografts are used in the semilunar position in children, in adults for re-implantation of an infected prosthetic aortic valve, and as a possible alternative to mechanical valves in aortic valve replacement in adults younger than 50 years of age.

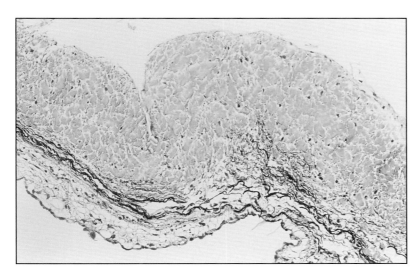

Figure 14-17.
Pulmonary autograft aortic valve replacement (Ross procedure). First reported in 1967, this procedure is gaining popularity. It consists of an autotransplant of the pulmonary valve to the aortic position with the coronary arteries reimplanted into the new root [29]. The pulmonary valve is then replaced by an aortic or pulmonary homograft. This photomicrograph shows a pulmonary autograft valve cusp removed after 6 years demonstrating near-normal trilayered aortic architecture, approximately normal complement of aortic valve interstitial cells, and intact valvular corrugations.

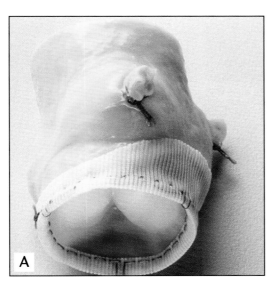

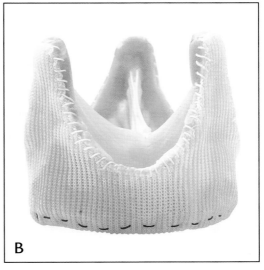

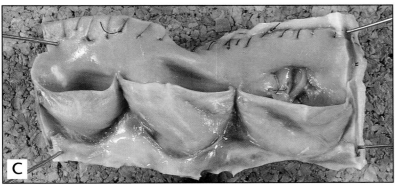

Figure 14-18.
Stentless porcine valves. **A,** Medtronic FreeStyle (Medtronic, Inc., Minneapolis, MN). **B,** St. Jude Toronto SPV (St. Jude Medical, Inc., St. Paul, MN). **C,** Medtronic FreeStyle valve removed at autopsy after non–valve-related death 4 years postoperatively. To achieve some of the perceived benefits of homograft valves but with an easily available commercial product, stentless porcine valves have been developed. Both the FreeStyle and the Toronto SPV were approved for general use by the Food and Drug Administration in 1997. The potential benefit is achieved at the expense of a more difficult implant technique compared with a stented porcine valve. Stentless porcine valves are used in one of three ways: 1) as a conventional valve replacement with the excised valve sewn into the subcoronary position in the host's aorta, 2) as a mini-root replacement, with the donor aortic root inserted inside the host aorta (inclusion technique), and 3) as a complete root replacement. The Medtronic FreeStyle valve can be implanted using any of the three techniques, but the St. Jude Medical Toronto SPV is used only as subcoronary valve replacement [30]. Additional nonstented valves are currently undergoing clinical testing. (*From* Fyfe and Schoen [31]; with permission.)

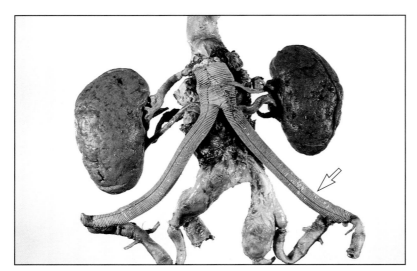

Figure 14-19.

Uncomplicated aortobifemoral graft (*arrow*) removal at autopsy. (*Courtesy of* Bruce McManus, St. Paul's Hospital, Vancouver, Canada).

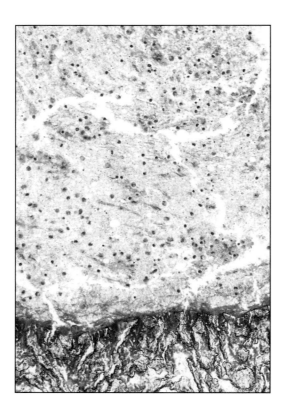

Figure 14-20.

Vascular graft infection. Histology of infected expanded polytetrafluoroethylene graft showing wall inflammation and vegetations at the blood-contacting surface. Despite the use of prophylactic systemic antibiotic agents during surgery, infection of implanted vascular prostheses occurs in up to 6% of patients and has a high mortality rate. Because the anastomotic suture line is almost invariably involved in the septic process, an infected vascular graft is usually associated with a mycotic false aneurysm, and rupture with hemorrhage at the graft site may be the presenting sign. Infection early after surgery is most often initiated by intraoperative contamination or wound complications in the groin. In contrast, as with prosthetic valves, hematogenous seeding after a transient bacteremia is usually responsible for late infections.

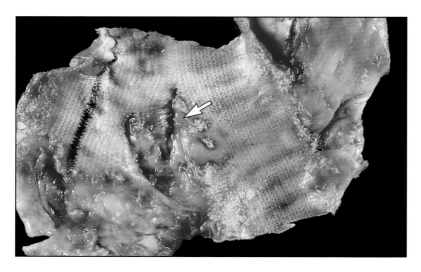

Figure 14-21.

Fragmentation of a Dacron (AI du Pont de Nemours & Co., Inc., Wilmington, DE) graft in the iliac artery causing false aneurysm. Area of defect is designated by the *arrow*. Progressive deterioration of a prosthesis can cause mechanical failure at the anastomotic site or in the body of the prosthesis leading to formation of an aneurysm or of a false aneurysm caused by rupture. The causes of delayed failure of a synthetic prosthesis include chemical, thermal, or mechanical damage to polymeric yarn materials during manufacture, fabric defect induced during manufacture or during insertion, and postoperative biodegradation of the graft material. (*From* Schoen [16]; with permission.)

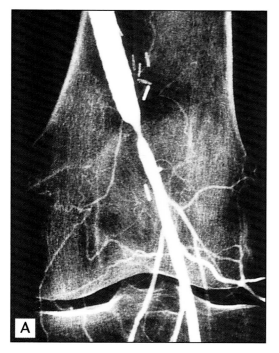

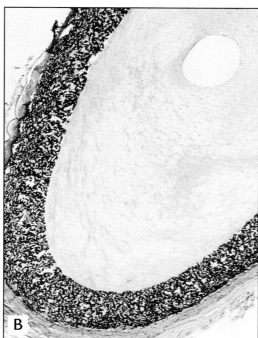

Figure 14-22.

Anastomotic intimal hyperplasia of the distal anastomosis of a Gore-Tex (WL Gore & Associates, Inc., Medical Products DI, Flagstaff, AZ) expanded polytetrafluoroethylene graft causing failure. **A,** Angiogram. **B,** Photomicrograph demonstrating luminal occlusive material. Late failure of clinical and experimental vascular grafts, especially those smaller than 8 mm in diameter, is frequently caused by fibrous thickening of the inner capsule. Intimal hyperplasia has been observed in virtually all types of synthetic and biological grafts. In vein grafts, it is often diffuse, leading to progressive luminal reduction of the entire graft, but in synthetic vascular prostheses, intimal hyperplasia is predominantly at or near the anastomoses. Intimal fibrous hyperplasia is an exaggeration of the normal arterial response to healing. (*From* Schoen [32]; with permission.)

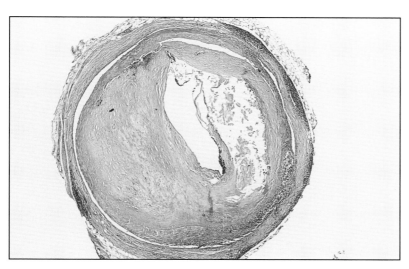

Figure 14-23.

Atherosclerosis of saphenous vein bypass graft. Such lesions typically show an attenuated fibrous cap situated between a necrotic

core and the lumen. The primary pathologic processes responsible for occlusion of saphenous vein bypass grafts in either the aorto-coronary or peripheral locations are thrombosis (usually early closure), intimal fibroproliferative hyperplasia (a few months to years in a process similar to that which occurs in the synthetic vascular graft, [see Fig. 14-23B]), and atherosclerosis (overwhelmingly the most frequent cause of graft occlusion after several years or more) [33]. The potential for disruption and embolization of atherosclerotic lesions in vein grafts is probably greater than that for native atherosclerotic lesions in the coronary arteries. In graft disease, plaques often have poorly developed fibrous caps. Atherosclerosis may cause late graft aneurysms. In contrast to the approximately 60% patency rate beyond 10 years for saphenous vein bypass grafts in the coronary circulation, the autologous internal mammary artery has a patency rate of approximately 90% after 10 years, greatly exceeding that of saphenous vein grafts [34,35,]. A low frequency of significant postoperative pathologic changes, including atherosclerosis, is associated with this substantial late patency rate.

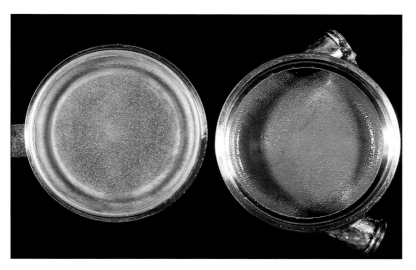

Figure 14-24.

Generalized thrombotic accumulation on textured bladder of the fibrillar pump surface of the ThermoCardio Systems (TCI, Woburn, MA) fibrillar pump surface. This textured (fibrillar) elastomeric polyurethane surface represents one approach to the development of a nonthrombogenic blood-contacting surface, essential for the success of a clinically useful temporary or permanent cardiac assist device or artificial heart [36]. Although smooth surfaces often accumulate small, focal microscopic thrombotic deposits with embolic potential, the textured surfaces accumulate a platelet or fibrin pseudointimal membrane, associated with a low frequency of clinically significant embolic sequela.

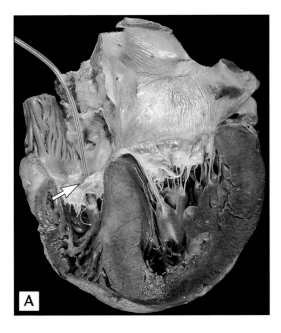

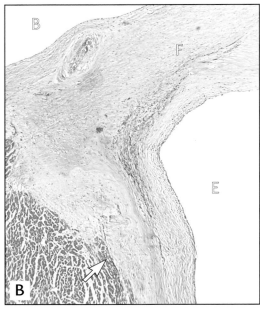

Figure 14-25.
Pacemaker. **A,** Long-standing transvenous pacer properly positioned in the right ventricular apex (*arrow*). Note that the pacer is intertwined with and fibrosed to the tricuspid valve. Removal of such a lead could cause damage to the valve. **B,** Fibrous capsule surrounding pacemaker electrode at the right ventricular apex. This low-power photomicrograph demonstrates the site of the electrode (E), fibrous capsule (F) separating the electrode from blood (B) in the right ventricular chamber and the fibrous capsule (*arrow*) separating electrode from the surrounding mural myocardium (M). The fibrous capsule on the myocardial side separates the electrode from excitable myocardium and contributes to the electrical threshold.

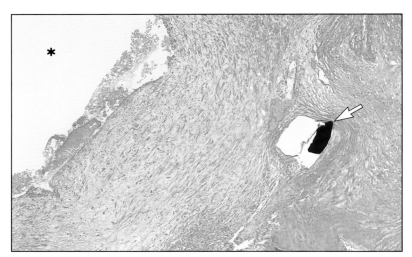

Figure 14-26.
Photomicrograph of metallic coronary arterial stent in-situ with mild intimal thickening, separating the artery wall from the lumen (*asterisk*). One stent wire is seen (*arrow*).

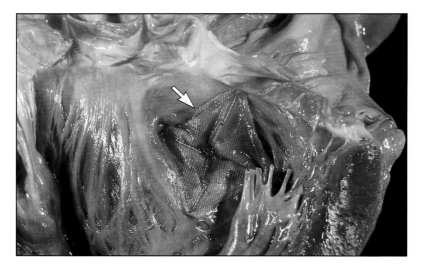

Figure 14-27.
Acute myocardial infarction–associated ventricular septal defect partially closed by "clam shell" occluder device. Such devices represent (*arrow*) an interventional approach to closing an intracardiac shunt [37].

REFERENCES

1. Vongpatanasin W, Hillis LD, Lange RA: Prosthetic heart valves. *N Engl J Med* 1996, 335:407–416.

2. Orsulak TA, Schaff HV, Puga FJ, *et al.*: Event status of the Starr-Edwards aortic valve to 20 years: a benchmark for comparison. *Ann Thorac Surg* 1996, 63:620–626.

3. Schoen FJ, Levy RJ: Tissue heart valves: current challenges and future research perspectives. *J Biomed Mater Res* 1999, 47:439–465.

4. Ferans VJ, Spray TL, Billingham ME, *et al.*: Structural changes in glutaraldehyde-treated porcine heterografts used as substitute cardiac valves: transmission and scanning electron microscopic observations in 12 patients. *Am J Cardiol* 1978, 41:1159–1184.

5. Cosgrove DM, Lytle BW, Taylor PC, *et al.*: The Carpentier-Edwards pericardial aortic valve: ten-year results. *J Thorac Cardiovasc Surg* 1995, 110:651–662.

6. Schoen FJ: Pathologic considerations in the surgery of adult heart disease. In *Cardiac Surgery in the Adult*. Edited by Edmunds LH. New York: McGraw Hill; 1997:85–144.

7. Schoen FJ: Pathology of cardiac valve replacement. In *Guide to Prosthetic Cardiac Valves*. Edited by Morse D, Steiner RM, Fernandez J. New York: Springer-Verlag; 1985:209–238.

8. Grunkemeier GL, Rahimtoola SH: Artificial heart valves. *Ann Rev Med* 1990, 41:251–263.

9. Atkins CW: Results with mechanical cardiac valvular prostheses. *Ann Thorac Surg* 1995, 60:1836–1844.

10. Edmunds LH Jr: Thrombotic and bleeding complications of prosthetic heart valves. *Ann Thorac Surg* 1987, 44:430–445.

11. Hurrell DG, Schaff HV, Tajik AJ: Thrombolytic therapy for obstruction of mechanical prosthetic valves. *Mayo Clinic Proc* 1996, 71:605–613.

12. Schoen FJ: Cardiac valve prostheses, pathological and bioengineering considerations. *J Cardiac Surg* 1987, 2:65–108.

13. Levine MN, Raskob G, Landefeld S, *et al.*: Hemorrhagic complications of anticoagulant treatment. *Chest* 1995, 108 (suppl):276–295.

14. Vlessis AA, Khaki A, Grunkemeier GL, *et al.*: Risk, diagnosis and management of prosthetic valve endocarditis: a review. *J Heart Valve Dis* 1997, 6:443–465.

15. Roberts WC: Complications of cardiac valve replacement: characteristic abnormalities of prostheses pertaining to any or specific site. *Am Heart J* 1982, 103:113–122.

16. Schoen FJ: *Interventional and Surgical Cardiovascular Pathology: Clinical Correlations and Basic Principles*. Philadelphia: WB Saunders; 1989.

17. Schoen FJ: Approach to the analysis of cardiac valve prostheses as surgical pathology or autopsy specimens. *Cardiovasc Pathol* 1995, 4:241–255.

18. Cao H: Mechanical performance of pyrolytic carbon in prosthetic heart valve applications. *J Heart Valve Dis* 1996, 5(suppl I):32–49.

19. Klepetko W, Moritz A, Mlczoch J, *et al.*: Leaflet fracture in Edwards-Duramedics bileaflet valves. *J Thorac Cardiovasc Surg* 1989, 97:90–94.

20. Erichsen A, Lindblom D, Semb G, *et al.*: Strut fracture with Bjork-Shiley 70° Convexo-Concave valve: an international multi-institutional follow-up study. *Eur J Cardiothorac Surg* 1992, 6:339–346.

21. Schoen FJ, Kujovich JL, Webb CL, *et al.*: Chemically determined mineral content of explanted porcine aortic valve bioprostheses: correlation with radiographic assessment of calcification and clinical data. *Circulation* 1987, 76:1061–1066.

22. Turina J, Hess OM, Turina M, *et al.*: Cardiac bioprostheses in the 1990s. *Circulation* 1993, 88:775–781.

23. Schoen FJ, Hirsch D, Bianco RW, *et al.*: Onset and progression of calcification in porcine aortic bioprosthetic valves implanted as orthotopic mitral valve replacements in juvenile sheep. *J Thorac Cardiovasc Surg* 1994, 108:880–887.

24. Vyavahare NR, Chen Weiliam, Joshi RR, *et al.*: Current progress in anticalcification for bioprosthetic and polymeric heart valves. *Cardiovasc Pathol* 1997, 6:219–229.

25. Schoen FJ, Levy RJ, Nelson AC, *et al.*: Onset and progression of experimental bioprosthetic heart valve calcification. *Lab Invest* 1985, 52:523–532.

26. Walley VM, Keon WJ: Patterns of failure in Ionescu-Shiley bovine pericardial bioprosthetic valves. *J Thorac Cardiovasc Surg* 1987, 93:925–933.

27. McGonagle Wolff K, Schoen FJ: Morphologic findings in explanted mitroflow pericardial bioprosthetic valves. *Am J Cardiol* 1992, 70:263–264.

28. Grunkemeier GL, Bodnar E: Comparison of structural valve failure among different "models" of homograft valves. *J Heart Valve Dis* 1994, 3:556–560.

29. Kouchoukos NT, Davilla-Roman VG, Spray TL, *et al.*: Replacement of the aortic root with a pulmonary autograft in children and young adults with aortic valve disease. *N Engl J Med* 1994, 330:1–6.

30. Del Rizzo DF, Goldman BS, David TE, *et al.*: Aortic valve replacement with a stentless porcine bioprosthesis: multicentre trial. *Can J Cardiol* 1995, 11:597–603.

31. Fyfe BS, Schoen FJ: Pathological analysis of nonstneted Freestyle aortic root bioprosthese treated with amino oleic acid. *Sem Thorac Cardiovasc Surg* 1999, 11:151–156.

32. Schoen FJ: Blood vessels. In *Pathologic Basis of Disease*, edn 6. Edited by Cotran RS, Kumar V, Collins T. Philadelphia: WB Saunders; 1999: 493–541.

33. Nwasokwa ON: Coronary artery bypass graft disease. *Ann Intern Med* 1995, 123:528–545.

34. Lytle BW, Cosgrove DM: Coronary artery bypass surgery. *Curr Probl Surg* 1992, 29:733–807.

35. Bourassa MG: Long-term vein graft patency. *Curr Opin Cardiol* 1994, 9:685–691.

36. Slater JP, Rose EA, Levin HR, *et al.*: Low thromboembolic risk without anticoagulation using advanced-design left ventricular assist devices. *Ann Thorac Surg* 1996, 62:1321–1328.

37. Ruygrok PN, Serruys, PW: Intracoronary stenting from concept to custom. *Circulation* 1996, 94:882–890.

15

Primary and Secondary Tumors of the Cardiovascular System

Allen Burke
Renu Virmani

Cardiac tumors that give rise to clinical symptoms are rare. Primary tumors of the heart are found at autopsy at an incidence of only 0.02 % [1]. Of these, the cardiac myxoma is the most common primary heart tumor, followed by primary cardiac sarcomas and a host of mostly benign lesions. The age at presentation is an important clue to the type of cardiac tumor that may be encountered. In the fetus, newborn, and infant, cardiac teratomas and rhabdomyomas represent virtually all solid cardiac masses. In young children and adolescents, the cardiac fibroma is the most common heart tumor. In adults, myxomas and sarcomas represent the vast majority of heart tumors, each with a mean age at presentation of about 50 years.

Several tumors are unique to the heart (having no histologic counterpart elsewhere in the body). These include the myxoma and rhabdomyoma. In addition, papillary fibroelastoma, a peculiar endocardial growth that partly recapitulates the structure of a heart valve, and lipomatous hypertrophy of the atrial septum, composed of brown fat and hypertrophied cardiac myocytes, occur only within the heart.

Symptoms attributable to cardiac tumors are legion, and occur as a result of mass effect, obstruction to blood flow, embolic phenomena, interference with electrical conduction, pericardial constriction, and metastatic disease. The capacity of the cardiac myxoma to confound the attending physician is well known, and has earned the title of the "great mimicker" among heart tumors. With the widespread use of echocardiography, CT, and magnetic resonance imaging, the clinical diagnosis of cardiac tumors has become relatively straightforward and commonplace; however, a definitive diagnosis is still dependent on histologic evaluation.

A variety of conditions may produce cardiac masses that are not true tumors. The common mural cardiac mass is the thrombus, which may mimic cardiac myxoma, especially if calcified. Unlike myxoma, mural thrombi generally occur only if there is underlying obstruction to blood flow, poorly contractile ventricles or atria (organic heart disease) or coagulopathy. Two forms of cardiomyopathy may form tumor-like masses: histiocytoid and hypertrophic cardiomyopathy. Histiocytoid cardiomyopathy is characterized by multiple collections of oncocytic myocytes, and results in cardiac arrhythmias in infants and children. In the surgical literature, these small tumors are called "hamartomas" or Purkinje cell hamartomas. Hypertrophic cardiomyopathy is characterized by asymmetric hypertrophy of the ventricular septum. Although originally considered a type of hamartoma, it is now well recognized that hypertrophic cardiomyopathy is best characterized as a disease of heart muscle secondary to a genetic defect; the mass of hypertrophic myocytes rarely if ever forms a discrete mass.

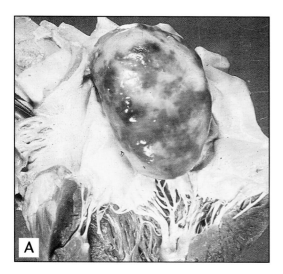

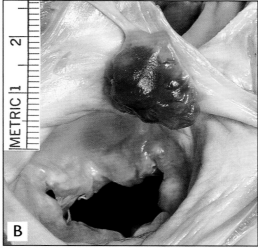

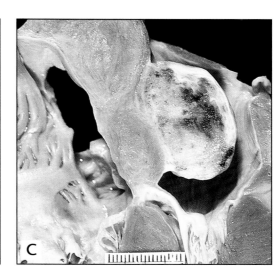

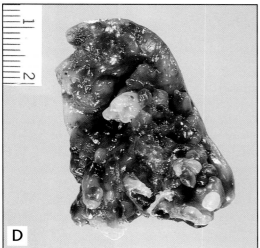

Figure 15-1.

Gross appearance of cardiac myxoma. The gross appearance of cardiac myxoma may be varied. **A,** There is a large, smooth-surfaced tumor in the left atrium. Echocardiographic studies during life may show prolapse of the tumor through the valve orifice during diastole. Smooth-surfaced myxomas tend to present with symptoms of heart failure and rarely cause embolic showers. **B,** In the fresh state, the tumor surface may appear quite hemorrhagic, resembling an organized thrombus. The site of tumor attachment at the fossa ovalis, however, is typical of myxoma. Thrombi tend to occur in other areas of the atria, especially appendages. **C,** The cut surface of this atrial myxoma demonstrates myxomatous areas interspersed with areas of hemorrhage, the typical location at the level of the fossa ovalis, and the relationship of the tumor to the inflow of the left ventricle. **D,** This surgically resected tumor demonstrates the friable, irregular surface with focal fibrin thrombus that embolic cardiac myxomas possess.

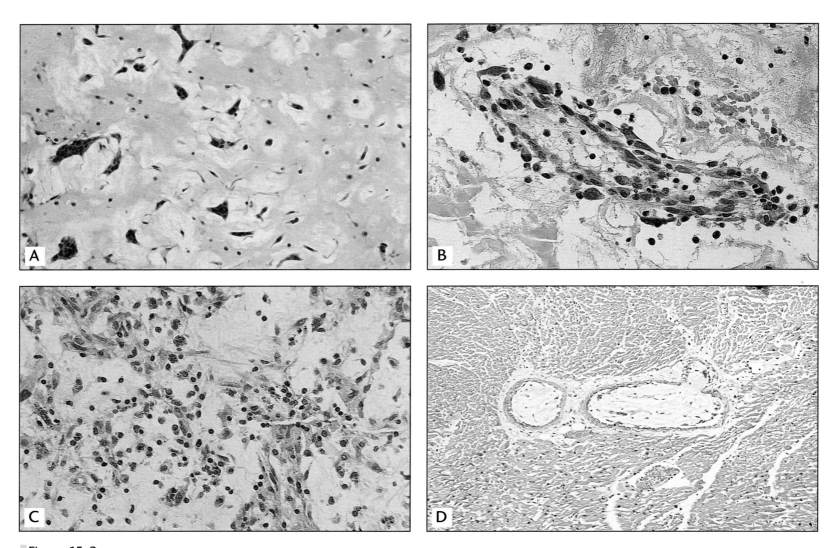

Figure 15-2.

Histologic findings in cardiac myxoma. **A,** The histologic hallmark of the cardiac myxoma is the finding of syncytia of cells floating in a stroma rich in proteoglycans. **B,** Myxoma cells appear, at times, to derive from capillaries, often forming ring structures infiltrated by inflammatory cells. **C,** The myxoma-vascular structures are almost invariably accompanied by large numbers of hemosiderin-laden macrophages, which is indicative of ongoing hemorrhage. The hemorrhage may result in areas of organized thrombi, as well as gamma bodies similar to those seen in shrunken spleens of

patients with sickle cell disease. Other degenerative changes typical of myxoma include fibrosis, calcification (more often right-sided tumors), and ossification. These changes result in a heterogeneous appearance, both grossly and microscopically, to the tumor, which may be partly hemorrhage, partly fibrotic, and partly calcified. In many cases, the myxoid background of the lesion may be almost entirely lacking, due to secondary changes, and diagnostic myxoma structures may be hard to locate. **D,** Myxoma may embolize into small arteries within the heart, resulting in myocardial infarction or sudden death.

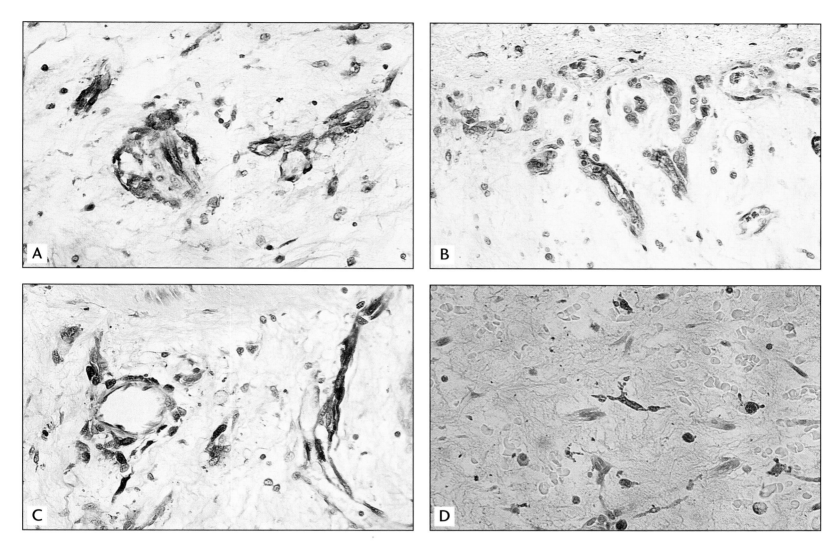

Figure 15-3.

Immunohistochemical findings in cardiac myxoma. The immuno-histochemical features of cardiac myxoma are varied, because there are multiple cell types, and because of the pluripotentiality of the myxoma cell. The precise nature of the myxoma cell is debated, but it is believed to derive from a primitive endocardial cushion cell. **A,** The myxoma cell expresses a variety of antigens, including CD31, and other endothelial markers. **B,** CD34 may be only weakly expressed; in this example, staining is limited to the capillaries. **C,** S-100 expression is typical, indicating that there may be neural differentiation in cardiac myxomas. Other neural markers are, however, generally negative. The stroma of the cardiac myxoma is rich in inflammatory cells. **D,** A recently described cell in the cardiac myxoma is that of the factor XIIIa-positive dendritic cell, a cell found in a variety of vascular tumors.

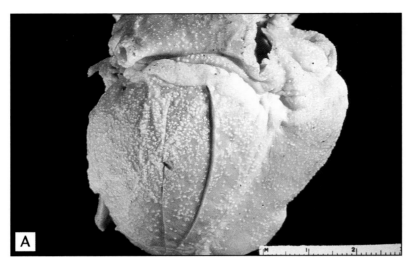

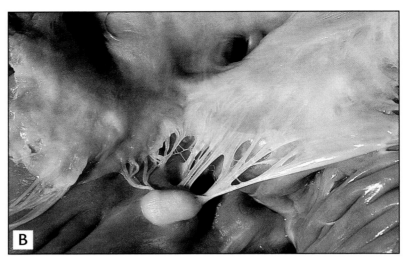

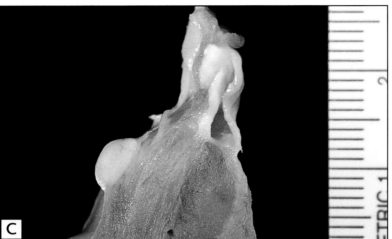

Figure 15-4.

Gross findings in cardiac rhabdomyoma. Cardiac rhabdomyomas may occur anywhere in the myocardium. The vast majority of rhabdomyomas occur in the ventricles; atrial rhabdomyomas account for only 1% of tumors. The ventricular location is more likely the free wall than the ventricular septum by a ratio of 2:1, and tumors are often located near the atrioventricular valves. The tumors are almost always multiple in patients with tuberous sclerosis, but they may be single, especially sporadic tumors. **A,** The innumerable tiny tumors on the epicardial surface are known as "rhabdomyomatosis." The tumors are well circumscribed, are yellow-tan, and are easily distinguished from surrounding myocardium, as seen in the single rhabdomyoma in *panels B and C.* They are often near the endocardium, and, when a large size is attained, the tumors may result in valvular obstruction. Although the majority of tumors are asymptomatic, they may result in heart murmurs, congestive heart failure, sudden death, and arrhythmias. Conduction disturbances related to cardiac rhabdomyoma include Wolff-Parkinson-White syndrome, ventricular and supraventricular tachycardias, and tachyarrhythmias.

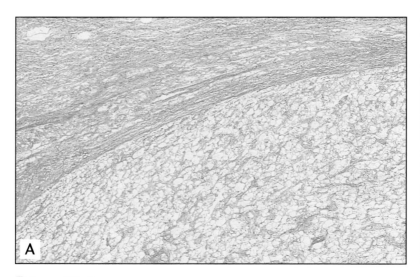

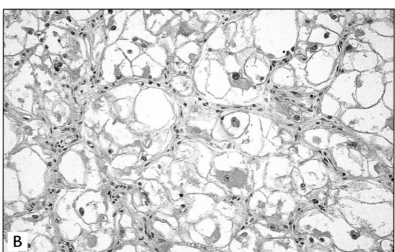

Figure 15-5.

Cardiac rhabdomyoma, histologic findings, and comparison to histiocytoid cardiomyopathy. The characteristic histologic findings of cardiac rhabdomyoma are a discrete border with surrounding myocardium, vacuolization of myocytes, and enlargement of the tumor cell nuclei and cytoplasm. **A,** Low-magnification image of a

circumscribed rhabdomyoma. The cause of the vacuolization of rhabdomyoma cells is the accumulation of glycogen and disordered myofilaments. **B,** On high magnification, characteristic "spider" cells are seen, with artifactual retraction of cytoplasm from the centrally placed nuclei. (*continued on next page*)

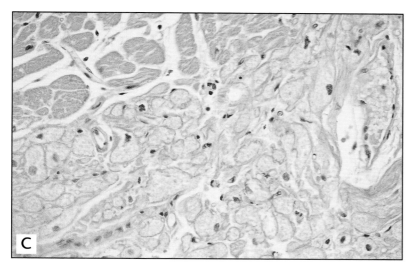

C

Figure 15-5. (*continued*)

The differential diagnosis of cardiac rhabdomyoma includes glycogen storage disease and Purkinje cell hamartoma (histiocytoid cardiomyopathy). In contrast to rhabdomyoma, glycogen storage disease is a diffuse process. **C,** Histiocytoid cardiomyopathy is characterized by bubbly, minimally hypertrophied cells that ultrastructurally are oncocytic, containing abundant mitochondria.

Ultrastructural and immunohistochemical studies of cardiac rhabdomyoma document that the tumor cells are of cardiac myocyte origin. They possess abundant glycogen, small and sparse mitochondria, and cellular junctions resembling intercalated disks surround the periphery of the cell. Conversely, the intercalated disks of differentiated myocytes are located exclusively at the poles of the cell. The distribution of the intercalated disks resembles that of cardiac myoblasts. Immunohistochemically, cardiac rhabdomyoma cells express desmin, actin, and myoglobin, which are localized to the cytoskeleton and myofilaments visible on light and electron microscopy.

CARDIAC FIBROMA

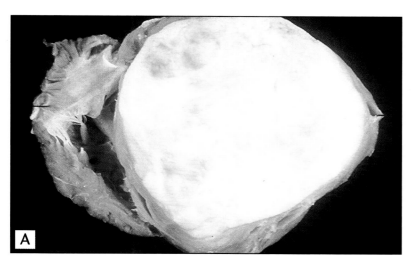

A

B

Figure 15-6.

Gross findings in cardiac fibroma. Cardiac fibromas occur almost exclusively in the ventricles as single lesions. The differential diagnosis of cardiac tumors in children includes rhabdomyomas and fibromas. The latter is favored if there is calcification, if the tumor is single, and if there is no evidence of tuberous sclerosis. Cardiac fibromas are occasionally a manifestation of the Gorlin-Goltz syndrome (basal cell nevus syndrome), but the association is far weaker than that between tuberous sclerosis and rhabdomyoma. The basal cell nevus syndrome has recently been mapped to chromosome 9q22 [2].

The gross features of fibroma include apparent circumscription, and a bulging, whorled appearance somewhat similar to leiomyomas. They occasionally achieve massive proportions, replacing much of the myocardial mass (*panels A and B*). The gross differential diagnosis includes healed infarction and rhabdomyoma. In contrast

to healed infarction, there is a bulging tumor rather than thinning of the ventricular free wall. In contrast to rhabdomyoma, the tumor is fibrous, single, dense, white, and may contain calcifications; rhabdomyomas are softer and more yellow. In general, fibromas are larger than rhabdomyomas, although size is not a reliable differentiating criterion.

Cardiac fibroma may present as a mass lesion or as cardiac arrhythmias. Presenting symptoms include sudden death [3], obstruction of blood flow [4], arrhythmias or heart murmurs [5], and obstruction of left ventricular outflow simulating hypertrophic cardiomyopathy [6]. Surgical excision may be curative [7]. Some tumors are so large that heart transplantation may be the only treatment option [8]. Rarely, fibromas may be diagnosed in utero [9], although the most commonly diagnosed fetal heart tumor is the rhabdomyoma; less commonly diagnosed is the teratoma.

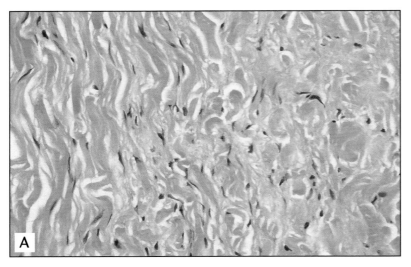

Figure 15-7.
Microscopic findings in cardiac fibroma. Cardiac fibromas are composed of fibroblasts, collagen, elastic fibers, and, often, calcific areas. The proportion of fibroblasts decreases with age, with an increase in the amount of acellular fibrous tissue [7]. **A,** In children and young adults, a typical cardiac fibroma contains scattered fibroblasts, dense collagen bundles, and less mature collagen. **B,** Elastic fibers are present in over 50% of cases and may be helpful in the diagnosis, especially if there is little tissue sample (elastic stain). The margins of the tumors, despite the gross circumscription, are infiltrative. Despite the histologic infiltrating pattern and difficulty in complete excision in many patients, there is little evidence that cardiac fibroma is an aggressive, expanding tumor akin to soft tissue fibromatoses.

The differential diagnosis of the histologic appearance of cardiac fibroma includes fibrosarcoma and scar. The former is rare in children, in whom fibromas may be cellular and histologically quite similar to fibrosarcoma. In children and adults, fibromas are invariably heavily collagenized. The histologic distinction between fibroma and scar may be impossible, and depends on gross findings and clinical history.

LIPOMATOUS HYPERTROPHY OF THE ATRIAL SEPTUM

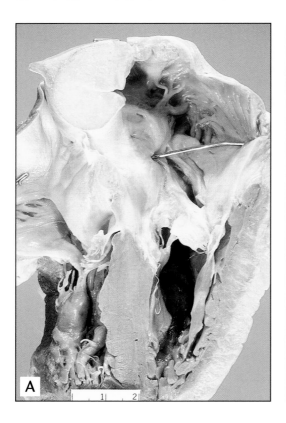

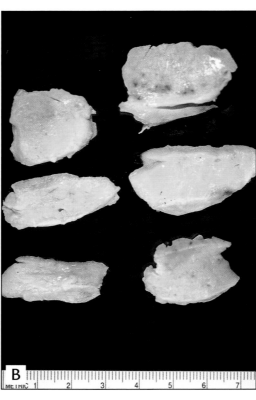

Figure 15-8.
Gross findings in lipomatous hypertrophy of the atrial septum. Lipomatous hypertrophy is a relatively common condition at autopsy, but only rarely causes clinical symptoms. Symptoms attributable to lipomatous hypertrophy include arrhythmias, especially supraventricular tachycardias, and obstruction to right atrial blood flow. **A,** Grossly, lipomatous hypertrophy results in a nearly spherical mass that projects into the right atrium at the level of the oval fossa. By ultrasound, the differential diagnosis includes mural thrombus and right atrial myxoma; magnetic resonance and CT scans are able to determine fat density and arrive at a specific diagnosis [10,11]. Occasionally, severe atrial arrhythmias or superior vena cava obstruction may necessitate tumor removal.
B, Surgically resected tumors have the gross appearance of fat. The size of the tumor may exceed 10 cm on rare occasion, and prompt the incorrect clinical diagnosis of a liposarcoma. However, liposarcomas of the atrium are extremely rare, and should be diagnosed only with histologic confirmation.

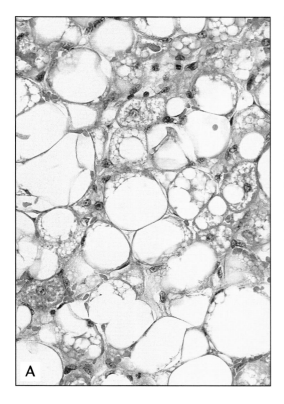

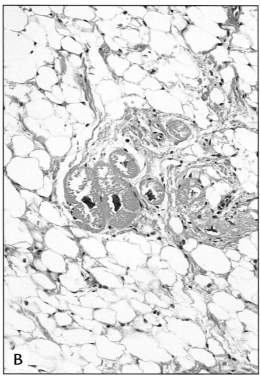

Figure 15-9.
Histologic findings in lipomatous hypertrophy of the atrial septum. The histologic triad of lipomatous hypertrophy includes normal fat, brown fat, and hypertrophied myocytes (*panels A and B*). There may be a degree of fibrosis and patches of chronic inflammation as well. The histologic features are not significantly different from the normal atrial septum, with the exception of enlarged, bizarre myocytes. These often mislead the pathologist to a false diagnosis of malignancy [12], but the presence of brown fat is nearly pathognomonic for this lesion. Occasionally, brown fat cells are mistaken for lipoblasts. However, in contrast to liposarcoma, there is no "chicken-wire" vascular background of a myxoid liposarcoma, and nuclear atypia and deformity of lipoblasts are not seen.

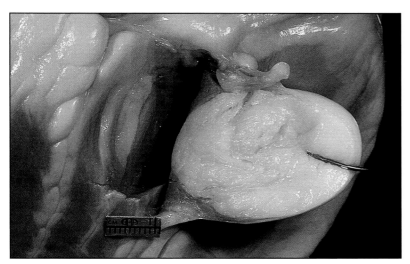

Figure 15-10.
Cardiac lipoma. Rarely, a true lipoma may occur in the heart. Although these are most commonly located on the epicardial surface, as in this example, virtually any area in the heart by be involved, including the atria, ventricles, ventricular septum, and endocardium.

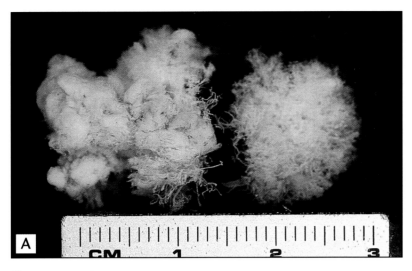

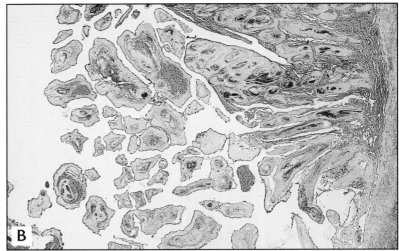

Figure 15-11.

Pathologic features in papillary fibroelastoma. Papillary fibroelastoma, or fibroelastic papilloma, is a peculiar growth that resembles a large Lambl's excrescence. The latter is a filiform papillary growth that occurs at the lines of closure of any valve, predominately the aortic valve in the central portion (location of the nodules of Aranti), and are composed of avascular fronds of tissue similar to chordae tendineae. There is some evidence that papillary fibroelastomas and Lambl's excrescences are caused in part by abnormal flow around the valve, and that they grow by organized thrombus. Unlike Lambl's excrescences, papillary fibroelastomas may occur anywhere on the endocardium, be larger than 1 cm, and result in symptoms.

A, Grossly, the papillary fibroelastoma resembles a "sea anemone," best appreciated by immersion in water. In our experience, papillary fibroelastomas occur on the endocardium remote from valves (36%), aortic valve (28%), mitral valve (18%), tricuspid valve (8%), pulmonary valve (5%), and multiple valves (5%). Once

diagnosed generally as incidental findings at autopsy, papillary fibroelastomas are now routinely being surgically resected. The incidence of left-sided tumors is therefore increasing, as well as tumors in unusual endocardial sites that may be removed for diagnostic or therapeutic purposes. These lesions may cause transient ischemic attacks, myocardial ischemia, and even sudden death [13–15]. Because of the possibility of significant complications, excision is recommended, often with sparing of the underlying valve [16]. Most patients with papillary fibroelastoma are adults, although a tumor in a 3-year-old child was reported recently [17].

B, Histologically, there is a proliferation of vascular fronds and papillae, lined by a single layer of endothelium. The cores of the papillary fronds are rich in proteoglycans, smooth muscle cells, and elastic fibers. Immunohistochemical studies have demonstrated that the surface cells are endothelial, with collagen type IV multilayered linear staining beneath the surface. Unlike myxoma, muscle-specific actin is absent in the stellate cells of the stroma [15].

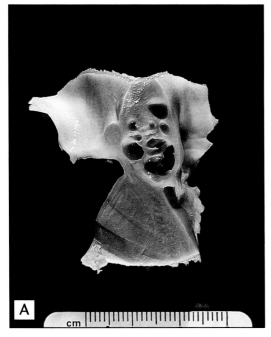

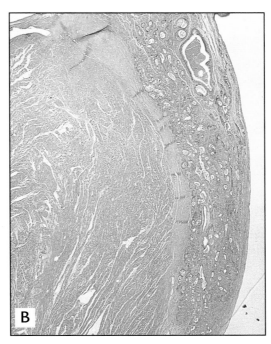

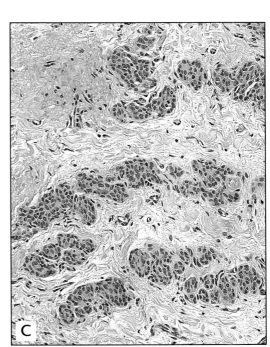

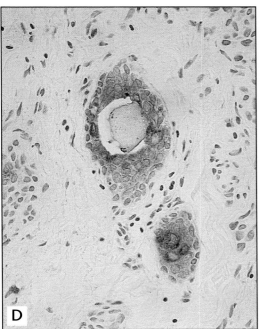

Figure 15-12.

Pathologic features in the atrioventricular nodal tumor. Once described as the smallest tumor that can cause sudden death, the atrioventricular nodal tumor is a developmental rest of endodermal cysts that arises exclusively in the atrioventricular nodal region. The antiquated term *mesothelioma* should be avoided because any evidence for mesothelial differentiation has been soundly refuted [18]. Most patients with this "tumor" have congenital heart block, although rare patients without conduction system disturbances have been described. Several extracardiac abnormalities have been documented in patients with atrioventricular nodal tumors, especially endocrine [19,20]. **A,** The gross appearance may demonstrate cystic structures; in as many examples, the tumor is not detected grossly, and only appreciated at histologic examination. The cystic glands occur exclusively in the region of the atrioventricular node and atrial approaches to the atrioventricular node (*panel B*); there is no encroachment on or involvement of the central fibrous body or ventricular septum. Microscopically, the rests are composed of cysts that are lined by cuboidal, stratified squamous, transitional, or combined epithelium. They are often compressed without visible lumina (*panel C*). The rests may contain mucin-producing cells and there is often expression of carcinoembryonic antigen (*panel D*), B72.3 antigen and other glandular markers. There may be a fibrotic stroma, but inflammation and granulation tissue is not generally present in reaction to the tumor.

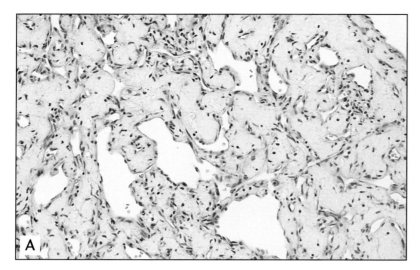

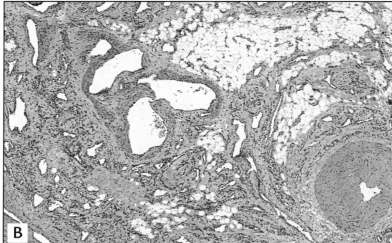

Figure 15-13.

Histopathologic features of cardiac hemangioma. Cardiac hemangiomas are rare tumors that may occur at any age. Although usually sporadic, they may be associated with hemangiomas of the gastrointestinal tract or skin, and result in a consumptive coagulopathy, Kasabach-Merritt syndrome, if large [21]. Characteristic features of cardiac hemangiomas have been imaged by CT and magnetic resonance [22].

Cardiac hemangiomas are of two basic pathologic types. **A,** Circumscribed hemangiomas are histologically uniform and composed of cavernous vascular spaces, often with a myxoid background. They may be easily excised at surgery and are often endocardial-based masses that project into the lumen, but they may occur in the pericardium. The lesions are occasionally misdiagnosed pathologically as myxomas because of their vascularity and myxoid stroma. Infiltrating cardiac hemangiomas are more likely to cause symptoms than circumscribed hemangiomas, and often result in cardiac arrhythmias because of their intramural location. **B,** In contrast to circumscribed cardiac hemangiomas, dysplastic arteries infiltrate the myocardium. In addition, there are often areas of capillary hemangioma and fat infiltrates, resulting in considerable histologic heterogeneity. These hemangiomas bear many histologic similarities to intramuscular hemangiomas of skeletal muscle.

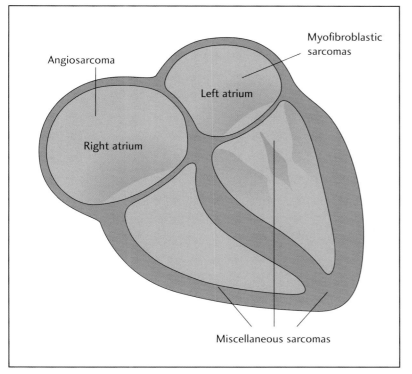

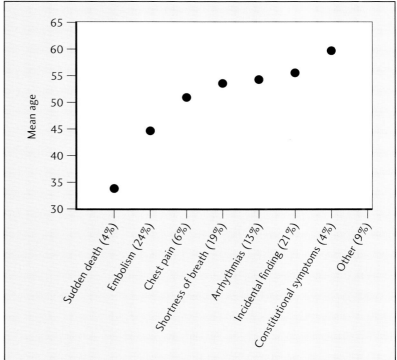

Figure 15-14.

Intracardiac locations of cardiac sarcomas. This figure demonstrates the most likely histologic type of cardiac sarcoma based on intracardiac location. However, any histologic type may occur anywhere in the heart. The most common location of cardiac sarcoma is the left atrium, accounting for 50% to 75% of cases [23,24]. Left atrial sarcomas are usually of myofibroblastic derivation, with various degrees of differentiation into leiomyosarcomatous or fibrosarcomatous differentiation. These tumors likely arise from the intima, because they have histologic similarities to aortic intimal sarcomas and are generally endocardial-based lesions projecting into the atrial cavity. The most common phenotype is malignant fibrous histiocytoma, and malignant osteoid or chondrosarcoma is present in about 10% of cases. Left atrial sarcomas are often clinically diagnosed as myxomas. For unknown reasons, angiosarcomas, the second most common type of cardiac sarcoma, occur most frequently in the right atrium, often with extension onto the pericardial surfaces [25,26]. Unusual types of cardiac sarcomas include rhabdomyosarcomas, synovial sarcomas, liposarcomas and neurofibrosarcomas, although generalizations are difficult to make regarding these subtypes of sarcoma. Rhabdomyosarcomas are often found within the ventricular walls, synovial sarcomas on the epicardial surface, liposarcomas near the atria, and neurofibrosarcomas at the base of the heart. There is no predicting, however, what the morphology of the sarcoma will be in an individual case, based on cardiac location.

Figure 15-15.

Histologic types of cardiac sarcomas and mean age at presentation. Cardiac sarcomas are represented by a large variety of morphologic subtypes. This figure portrays our collection of 184 cardiac sarcomas, which is biased toward undifferentiated tumors and those difficult to classify. In published series, angiosarcomas are the single largest group.

Among this group of 184 cardiac sarcomas, the mean age of presentation is approximately 45 years—slightly younger than cardiac myxoma. Certain tumors (*eg*, rhabdomyosarcoma) appear to occur in younger individuals. The overall survival of cardiac sarcomas is poor, regardless of histologic subtype, and is usually measured in months. There is no clear association between histologic type and prognosis. Tumor necrosis, mitotic rate, and metastases at the time of surgery are adverse prognostic factors. Treatment for cardiac sarcomas includes radiation therapy, chemotherapy, and cardiac transplantation.

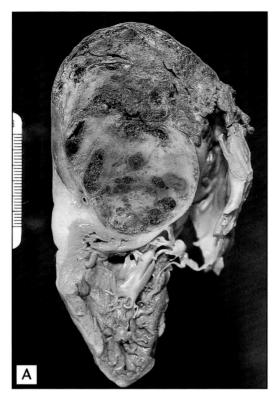

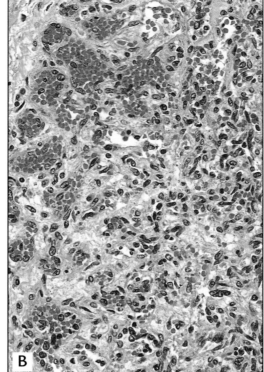

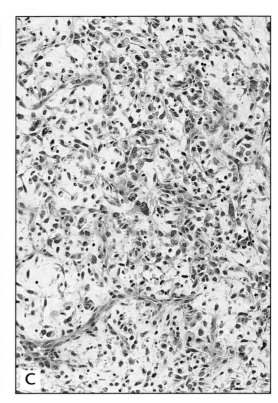

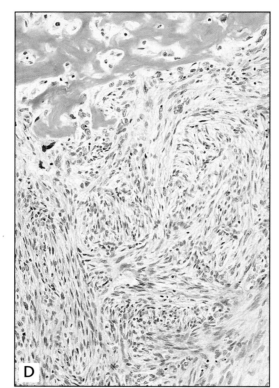

Figure 15-16.

Pathologic features of cardiac sarcoma. The most common histologic type with a specific phenotype is the angiosarcoma. **A,** Grossly, these are bulky, infiltrating, hemorrhagic tumors that often occur in the right atrium. **B,** Histologically, angiosarcomas are formed by atypical endothelial cells forming vascular lumina. **C,** Left atrial tumors are generally a mixed variety with leio- or fibrosarcomatous areas; many of the tumors are termed *malignant fibrous histiocytoma*. **D,** Occasionally, areas of osteosarcoma or chondrosarcoma may be present.

CARDIAC LYMPHOMA

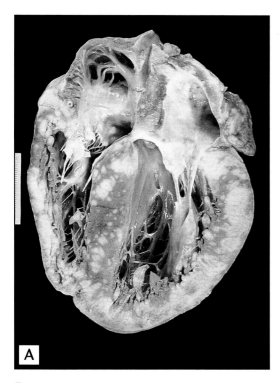

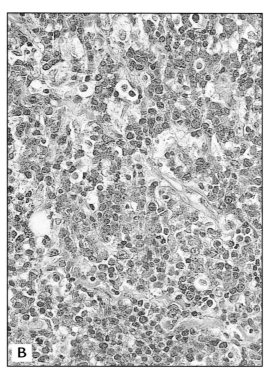

Cardiac lymphomas are almost exclusively B cell, and include small noncleaved follicular center cell, intermediate lymphoma, B-immunoblastic, large cell undifferentiated, large cell noncleaved, Burkitt's (*panel B*), and centroblastic-centrocytic (cleaved follicular center cell) lymphoma. At the periphery of tumor nodules, there is infiltration of the myocardium. The differential diagnosis includes other small round cell tumors, such as embryonal rhabdomyosarcoma, metastatic small cell carcinoma, and undifferentiated sarcoma.

Although extranodal lymphoma is being frequently reported in AIDS patients, less than 5% of lymphomas of AIDS patients involve the heart or pericardium. Over 50% of cardiac lymphomas that are reported currently occur in patients with no known immunosuppression. Therefore, a particular association between lymphomas in immunocompromised patients and cardiac location is lacking, and most cases are reported as entities in single patients. Cardiac lymphomas seen in immunocompromised patients are usually high-grade, B-cell neoplasms; the most frequent histologic types are immunoblastic, small noncleaved cell and diffuse large cell [27,28].

Cardiac involvement occurs in 10% to 25% of autopsied patients with disseminated lymphoma. Secondary involvement of the myocardium by lymphoma is far more common than primary lesions.

Figure 15-17.

Pathologic features of cardiac lymphoma. Lymphomas located entirely within the pericardial sac are rare. The mean age at presentation is approximately 60 years, and the most common presenting symptoms are related to congestive heart failure, pleural effusions, conduction system disturbances, and chest pain. Localization of tumor and assessment of response to treatment is facilitated by transesophageal echocardiography, magnetic resonance imaging, and CT.

A, Grossly, primary cardiac lymphoma is characterized by multiple masses of firm, white nodules characteristic of extracardiac lymphoma. The heart is usually enlarged. The sites of the heart most often affected are the right atrium, followed by the right ventricle, left ventricle, left atrium, atrial septum, and ventricular septum.

REFERENCES

1. Reynen K: Frequency of primary tumors of the heart. *Am J Cardiol* 1996, 77:107.

2. Unden AB, Stahle-Backdahl M, Holmberg E, *et al.*: Fine mapping of the locus for nevoid basal cell carcinoma syndrome on chromosome 9q. *Acta Derm Venereol* 1997, 77:4–9.

3. Mohammed W, Murphy A: Cardiac fibroma presenting as sudden death in a six-month-old infant. *West Indian Med J* 1997, 46:28–29.

4. Bapat VN, Varma GG, Hordikar AA, *et al.*: Right-ventricular fibroma presenting as tricuspid stenosis: a case report. *Thorac Cardiovasc Surg* 1996, 44:152–154.

5. Busch U, Kampmann C, Meyer R, *et al.*: Removal of a giant cardiac fibroma from a 4-year-old child. *Tex Heart Inst J* 1995, 22:261–264.

6. Veinot JP, O'Murchu B, Tazelaar HD, *et al.*: Cardiac fibroma mimicking apical hypertrophic cardiomyopathy: a case report and differential diagnosis. *J Am Soc Echocardiogr* 1996, 9:94–99.

7. Burke AP, Rosado-de-Christenson M, Templeton PA, Virmani R: Cardiac fibroma: clinicopathologic correlates and surgical treatment. *J Thorac Cardiovasc Surg* 1994, 108:862–870.

8. Michler RE, Goldstein DJ: Treatment of cardiac tumors by orthotopic cardiac transplantation. *Semin Oncol* 1997, 24:534–539.

9. Munoz H, Sherer DM, Romero R, *et al.*: Prenatal sonographic findings of a large fetal cardiac fibroma. *J Ultrasound Med* 1995, 14:479–481.

10. Lynch M, Clements SD, Shanewise JS, *et al.*: Right-sided cardiac tumors detected by transesophageal echocardiography and its usefulness in differentiating the benign from the malignant ones. *Am J Cardiol* 1997, 79:781–784.

11. Meaney JF, Kazerooni EA, Jamadar DA, Korobkin M: CT appearance of lipomatous hypertrophy of the interatrial septum. *AJR Am J Roentgenol* 1997, 168:1081–1084.

12. Burke AP, Litovsky S, Virmani R: Lipomatous hypertrophy of the atrial septum presenting as a right atrial mass. *Am J Surg Pathol* 1996, 20:678–685.

13. Brown RD Jr, Khandheria BK, Edwards WD: Cardiac papillary fibroelastoma: a treatable cause of transient ischemic attack and ischemic stroke detected by transesophageal echocardiography. *Mayo Clin Proc* 1995, 70:863–868.

14. Colucci V, Alberti A, Bonacina E, Gordini V: Papillary fibroelastoma of the mitral valve: a rare cause of embolic events. *Tex Heart Inst J* 1995, 22:327–231.

15. Rubin MA, Snell JA, Tazelaar HD, *et al.*: Cardiac papillary fibroelastoma: an immunohistochemical investigation and unusual clinical manifestations. *Mod Pathol* 1995, 8:402–407.

16. Minatoya K, Okabayashi H, Yokota T, Hoover EL: Cardiac papillary fibroelastomas: rationale for excision. *Ann Thorac Surg* 1996, 62:1519–1521.

17. de Menezes IC, Fragata J, Martins FM: Papillary fibroelastoma of the mitral valve in a 3-year-old child: case report. *Pediatr Cardiol* 1996, 17:194–195.

18. Burke AP, Anderson PG, Virmani R, *et al.*: Tumor of the atrioventricular nodal region: a clinical and immunohistochemical study. *Arch Pathol Lab Med* 1990, 114:1057–1062.

19. Strom EH, Skjorten F, Stokke ES: Polycystic tumor of the atrioventricular nodal region in a man with Emery-Dreifuss muscular dystrophy. *Pathol Res Pract* 1993, 189:960–967.

20. Declich P, Sironi M, Isimbaldi G, Bana R: Atrio-ventricular nodal tumor associated with polyendocrine anomalies. *Pathol Res Pract* 1996, 192:54–61.

21. Burke A, Johns JP, Virmani R: Hemangiomas of the heart: a clinicopathologic study of ten cases. *Am J Cardiovasc Pathol* 1990, 3:283–290.

22. Kemp JL, Kessler RM, Raizada V, Williamson MR: MR and CT appearance of cardiac hemangioma [case report]. *J Comput Assist Tomogr* 1996, 20:482–483.

23. Putnam JB Jr, Sweeney MS, Colon R, *et al.*: Primary cardiac sarcomas. *Ann Thorac Surg* 1991, 51:906–910.

24. Burke AP, Cowan D, Virmani R: Primary sarcomas of the heart. *Cancer* 1992, 69:387–395.

25. Ohtahara A, Hattori K, Fukuki M, *et al.*: Cardiac angiosarcoma. *Intern Med* 1996, 35:795–798.

26. Burke A, Virmani R: Primary cardiac sarcomas. In *Atlas of Tumor Pathology: Tumors of the Cardiovascular System*. Washington, DC: Armed Forces Institute of Pathology; 1996.

27. Chim CS, Chan AC, Kwong YL, Liang R: Primary cardiac lymphoma. *Am J Hematol* 1997, 54:79–83.

28. Sommers KE, Edmundowicz D, Katz WE, Hattler BG: Primary cardiac lymphoma: echocardiographic characterization and successful resection. *Ann Thorac Surg* 1996, 61:1001–1003.

16

Pathology of Cardiac Arrhythmias

Jeffrey E. Saffitz
Frank Zimmerman
Bruce D. Lindsay

Arrhythmias are a leading cause of morbidity and mortality in the United States and other economically developed societies. Lethal ventricular arrhythmias typically arise in a setting of acute or chronic ischemic heart disease or congestive heart failure in which considerable pathologic changes in heart muscle have occurred. However, many other clinically important and potentially deadly arrhythmias may arise in hearts that show subtle or no obvious pathology. Pathologists are often confronted with autopsies of patients who died of documented or suspected arrhythmias and face the daunting task of analyzing the gross and microscopic pathologic anatomy of sudden cardiac death. Pathologists are also frequently asked to study the hearts of individuals with specific syndromes in which arrhythmias are a prominent feature or in whom clinical electrophysiologic procedures, devices, or drugs had been used previously. Too often, pathologists are uncertain about how to approach these problems and how to regard and interpret the significance of pathologic findings in the context of clinical electrophysiologic events. The goal of this chapter is to provide practicing pathologists with a conceptual framework for analyzing the hearts of patients with known or suspected arrhythmias. The authors believe that this goal can best be met if the pathologist has a basic appreciation of electrophysiologic mechanisms underlying each major type of arrhythmia. This mechanistic approach helps to focus the pathologist's attention on specific anatomic regions or tissues of the heart and conduction system and provides a rational basis for the interpretation of pathologic anatomy. In most cases of clinically significant arrhythmias, pathologic changes are nonspecific and do not by themselves establish that a particular type of arrhythmia occurred during life. However, the pathologist will be in a stronger position to judge the potential functional significance of pathologic findings in arrhythmogenesis when equipped with a basic understanding of arrhythmia circuits, knowledge of specific features of trigger mechanisms, and a sense of the structural alterations in heart muscle (*ie*, anatomic substrates) associated with different types of cardiac arrhythmias.

This chapter consists of a brief introductory section on basic structure-function relationships in cardiac electrophysiology followed by separate sections organized according to major types of arrhythmias. In each section, basic mechanisms are illustrated and, when possible, a few specific examples of associated pathologic features are shown. Neither the arrhythmia categories nor the examples of pathologic changes causing or contributing to each arrhythmia are in any way exhaustive. Rather, we have focused on the most common, clinically important arrhythmias and some special topics in which recent advances have elucidated basic mechanisms.

STRUCTURE–FUNCTION RELATIONSHIPS IN CARDIAC ELECTROPHYSIOLOGY: AUTOMATICITY, CONDUCTION, AND REENTRY

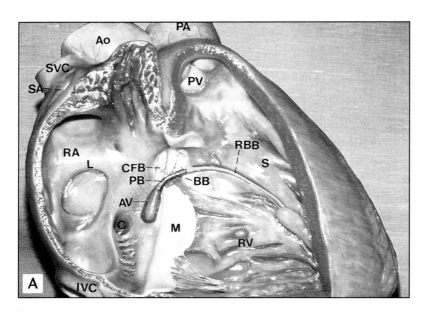

Figure 16-1.

The cardiac conduction system seen from the right (*panel A*) and left (*panel B*) sides of the heart. The specialized conduction system of the heart includes the sinoatrial (SA) node, atrioventricular (AV) node, His bundle, right and left bundle branches, and the Purkinjë network. The electrical impulse that initiates the heart beat is formed in the SA node, a crescent-shaped "region" of pacemaker cells located in the general vicinity of the epicardial groove of the

sulcus terminalis at the junction of the superior vena cava and the right atrium (*panel A*). The impulse generated in the SA node activates the atria, which conduct the impulse to the AV node, a subendocardial structure located on the floor of the right atrium at the apex of the triangle of Koch (delineated by the tendon of Todaro, the annulus of the septal tricuspid valve leaflet, and the os of the coronary sinus) (*panel A*). Conduction through the AV node, which normally provides the sole electrical connection between atrial muscle and the ventricular conduction system, is very slow. This creates a delay in ventricular activation that facilitates transport of blood from the atria to the ventricles before the ventricular muscle is electrically activated and ventricular contraction is initiated. The AV node is divided into three regions: the compact node, the transitional zone (between the right atrium and compact node), and the penetrating bundle (*ie*, His bundle). The penetrating bundle is responsible for conducting the impulse from the AV node to the branching network of Purkinjë fibers, which deliver activating current to the ventricles in a specific spatial and temporal pattern that leads to effective pumping. The penetrating bundle leaves the AV node region and projects through the central fibrous body along the posterior edge of the membranous portion of the atrioventricular septum (*panel A*). At the crest of the interventricular septum, the common bundle divides into the right and left branches. The right bundle branch (RBB) continues as an extension of the main bundle sometimes running deep into the endomyocardium (*panel A*). (*continued on next page*)

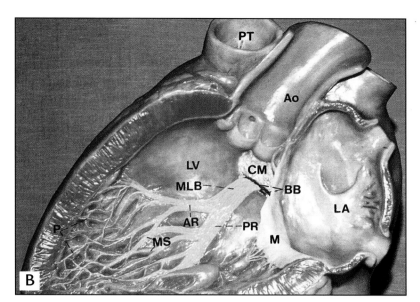

Figure 16-1. (*continued*)
The left bundle branch divides into an extensive array of fascicles along the left side of the interventricular septum (*panel B*). Peripherally, both branches subdivide forming the Purkinjë network, which runs in fine trabeculae within the subendocardium of both ventricles. Ao—aorta; AR—anterior radiation of the left bundle branch; BB—bundle of His, branching portion; C—coronary sinus; CFB—central fibrous body; CM—central fibrous body and membranous portion of the interventricular system; IVC—inferior vena cava; L—limbus of the fossa ovalis; LA—left atrium; LV—left ventricle; M—medial (septal) leaflet of the tricuspid valve; MLB—main left bundle branch; MS—midseptal fibers of the left bundle branch; MV—mitral valve; P—peripheral Purkinjë fibers; PA—pulmonary artery; PB—bundle of His, penetrating portion; PR—posterior radiation of the left bundle branch; PT—pulmonary trunk; PV—pulmonary valve; RA—right atrium; RV—right ventricle; S—septal band of the crista supraventricularis; SVC—superior vena cava. (*From* Bharati and Lev [1]; with permission.)

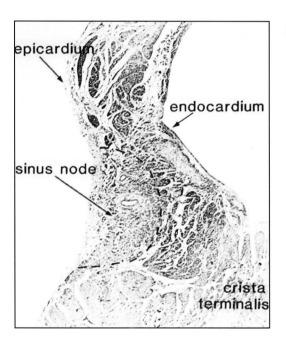

Figure 16-2.
Histology of the sinus node. The sinus node consists of whorled, interwoven muscle fascicles and connective tissue elements surrounded by a fibrous matrix. Sinus node myocytes are small and spindly. They can be differentiated into pacemaker cells and transitional cells by electron microscopy and are easily distinguished from working atrial muscle cells. Note the central location of the sinus node artery (usually the first branch of the right coronary artery) and the subepicardial position of the node in relation to the crista terminalis, a major bundle of atrial muscle that becomes activated by the sinoatrial node and conducts the impulse to the atrioventricular node. (*From* Anderson and Ho [2]; with permission.)

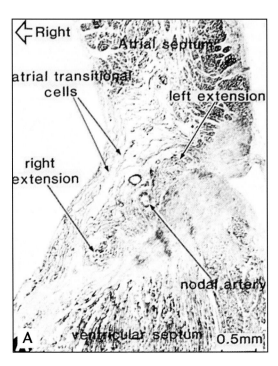

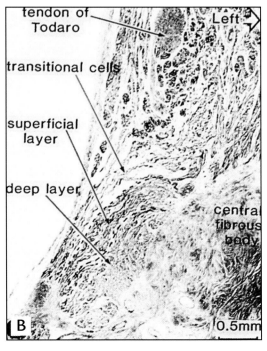

Figure 16-3.
Histology of the atrioventricular (AV) node. The compact AV node consists of interconnecting groups of small cells surrounded by a extensive transitional cell zone (*panel A*). Two posterior extensions of the compact node are shown that bifurcate toward the right and left AV valves. The transitional zone is differentiated into three approaches to the compact node: "superficial" cells run anterior and inferior to the node, "posterior" cells run from the coronary sinus area, and "deep" cells link the left atrium to the node (*panel B*). The node often has a stratified appearance with deep and superficial layers set against the central fibrous body. (*From* Anderson and Ho [2]; with permission.)

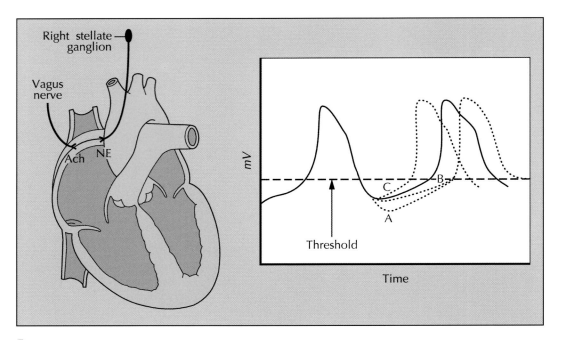

Figure 16-4.

Autonomic nervous system inputs to the sinus node. Automaticity is the property of an electrically excitable cell that enables it to initiate an impulse spontaneously without prior stimulation. Normal automaticity in the sinoatrial node establishes the heart beat. Sinus node myocytes exhibit automaticity caused by inward current during the resting phase of the cardiac cycle (phase 4 or the diastolic phase of the action potential), which depolarizes the cell progressively until it reaches threshold potential and initiates an action potential (*tracing B* in the *inset*). Heart rate is regulated by autonomic neural inputs that change the inherent automaticity of pacemaker cells. For example, parasympathetic stimulation via the vagus nerve releases acetylcholine (Ach), which hyperpolarizes pacemaker cells and decreases the rate of spontaneous depolarization to threshold (*tracing A*). This produces a negative chronotropic response. Sympathetic stimulation via the right stellate ganglion releases norepinephrine (NE), which depolarizes the pacemaker cells, enhances automaticity (*tracing C*), and produces a positive chronotropic response. Abnormal automaticity can occur in virtually all cardiac tissues and may initiate arrhythmias. For example, abnormal automaticity in atrial or ventricular muscle can cause premature beats that activate atrial or ventricular myocardium at ectopic sites and abnormal times during the cardiac cycle. These ectopic beats may serve as triggers of arrhythmias. (*Adapted from* Talano and coworkers [3]; with permission.)

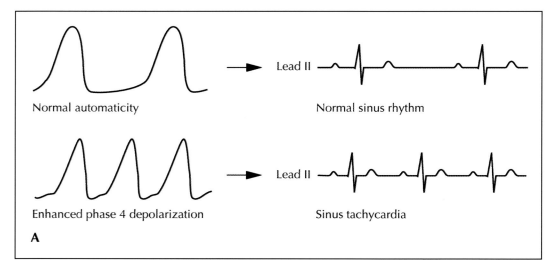

Figure 16-5.

A, The resting sinus heart rate (shown in the lead II electrocardiogram) is determined mainly by basal parasympathetic tone. Normal responses to exercise or psychological stress increase sympathetic tone, which enhances normal automaticity and causes sinus tachycardia. Abnormally enhanced sympathetic tone may result in arrhythmias such as inappropriate sinus tachycardia. (*continued on next page*)

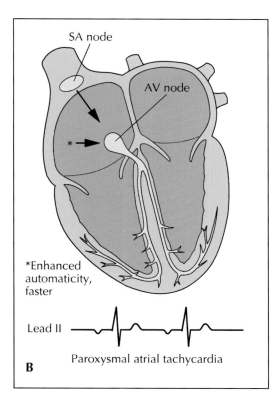

*Enhanced
automaticity,
faster

Lead II

B   Paroxysmal atrial tachycardia

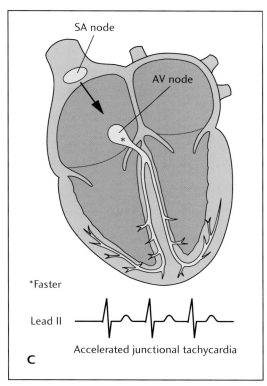

*Faster

Lead II

C   Accelerated junctional tachycardia

Figure 16-5. (*continued*)
B, Certain types of atrial tachycardias can arise because of abnormally enhanced automaticity within cells other than the sinus node. Atrial cells with abnormal automaticity compete with the sinus node, producing paroxysmal atrial tachycardia. Atrial tachycardias originating away from the sinus node region produce an abnormal P wave axis (illustrated as a negative P wave in lead II). **C,** Some types of accelerated junctional tachycardias arise from abnormal enhanced automaticity (in this case, in the atrioventricular node). No specific histopathologic features are typically associated with abnormal automaticity.

CONDITIONS ASSOCIATED WITH SINUS NODE DYSFUNCTION

Intrinsic	Extrinsic
Aging	Hypothermia
Hypertension	Electrolyte abnormalities
Coronary artery disease	Hypothyroidism
Rheumatic heart disease	Abnormalities of autonomic nervous system
Cardiomyopathies	(carotid hypersensitivity)
Pericarditis	Hyperbilirubinemia
Congenital heart abnormalities	Drugs
Collagen vascular disease	Cardiac glycosides
Amyloidosis	β-Adrenergic receptor blockers
Trauma	Calcium-channel blockers
Surgical	Methyldopa
Closure of ASD (sinus venosus type)	Reserpine
Mustard procedure	Lithium carbonate
Placement of caval cannula	Cimetidine
Tumor	Amitriptyline
Irradiation	Phenothiazines

Figure 16-6.
Conditions associated with sinus node dysfunction. Intrinsic sinus node dysfunction may be caused by pathologic processes (*eg*, ischemia, inflammation or fibrosis, infiltration by tumor or amyloid, or iatrogenic causes such as surgical trauma or irradiation) that directly involve the sinus node [4,5]. Extrinsic sinus node dysfunction may be related to systemic metabolic or neural diseases or the use of drugs that have secondary effects on the sinus node. ASD—atrial septal defect.

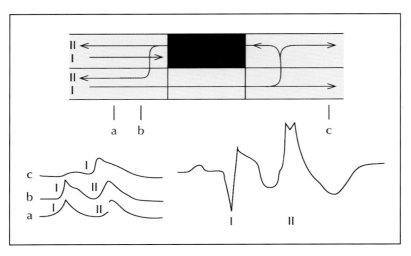

Figure 16-7.

Reentry caused by reflection. Reentry is a major arrhythmia mechanism that probably underlies many tachyarrhythmias, including supraventricular tachycardias, atrial flutter and fibrillation, and ventricular tachycardia and fibrillation. Regardless of its site of origin, reentry has one basic mechanism. During the normal cardiac cycle, electrical activity generated in the sinoatrial (SA) node is conducted throughout the myocardium until the entire heart has been activated. During the absolute refractory period, the impulse has no place to go and dies out. Myocytes recover excitability but normally remain quiescent until the next impulse begins in the SA node. If, however, a group of abnormal myocytes does not become activated

during an initial wave of depolarization because conduction through it is blocked in one direction or because it had not recovered excitability when the impulse first arrived, the wavefront may travel around this region, during which time the abnormal fibers may recover excitability or the impulse may activate the region from another direction or through another conduction pathway. This late-activating region may then serve as an electrical link to reexcite areas that were just discharged and had recovered excitability from the initial depolarization. This process, referred to as reentry, has the primary prerequisite of unidirectional conduction block because of the presence of tissue with altered conduction properties or recovery of excitation (*ie*, refractoriness). Whereas conditions that decrease conduction velocity or decrease refractoriness promote reentry, enhancing conduction and prolonging refractoriness diminish the development of reentry. The *top diagram* demonstrates the way reentry can occur even in a single bundle of muscle or Purkinjë fibers. Conduction through the entire *shaded area* is depressed, but depression in the *darkest area* of the upper fiber is so severe that unidirectional conduction block occurs. *Arrows* indicate the sequence of activation within the fiber bundle. *Arrows* labeled *I* show the impulse entering the bundle, and *arrows* labeled *II* show the reentry impulse returning to its origin. The *lower diagram* shows action potentials measured at sites a, b, and c along with an example of how a surface electrocardiogram may appear. In each of these tracings, deflections labeled *I* are from the normal conducted beat, and deflections labeled *I* are caused by the ventricular extrasystole. (*Adapted from* Wit and Bigger [6]; with permission.)

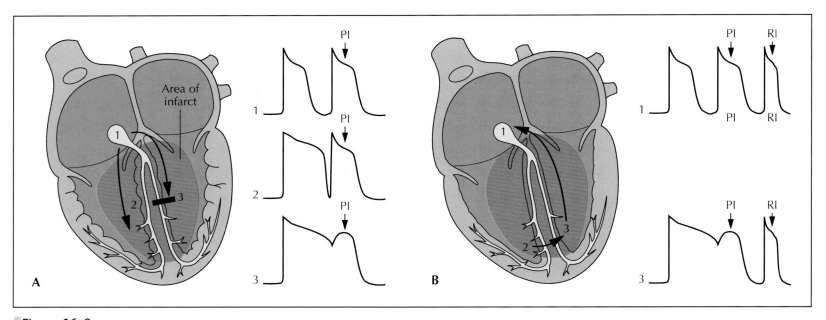

Figure 16-8.

Reentry resulting from dispersion of refractoriness in the subendocardial Purkinjë fiber network over an area of extensive myocardial infarction. Shown is the endocardial surface of a left ventricular papillary muscle. The *colored areas* represent scarred myocardium that is covered by bundles of surviving Purkinje fibers. Purkinje fibers in different regions exhibit markedly different action potentials, reflecting variations in duration and refractory periods. Action potentials are recorded from normal fibers in the proximal His bundle (*site 1*) and from subendocardial Purkinjë fibers surviving in the infarct (at *sites 2* and *3*) and exhibiting prolonged repolarization phases (prolonged action potential durations). **A,** A spontaneous

premature impulse (PI) occurs at the infarct border and conducts into the infarcted regions, as indicated by the *large arrows*. Because the action potential at *site 3* is longer than at *site 2* in the infarcted area, the premature impulse can excite cells at *site 2* but conduction is blocked at *site 3*, which had not recovered excitability when the impulse arrived. **B,** The continuation of these events after the premature impulse conducts through *site 2* and returns from a different direction to activate cells at *site 3* (which had become postrefractory by then). As a reentering impulse (RI), it then proceeds to its site of origin (*site 1*), which also re-excites as a reentry impulse (RI). (*Adapted from* Wit and coworkers [7]; with permission.)

COMPLETE HEART BLOCK

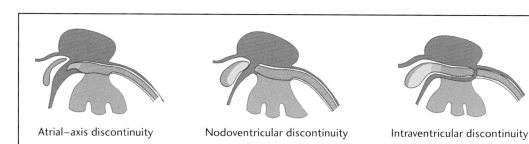

Atrial–axis discontinuity | Nodoventricular discontinuity | Intraventricular discontinuity

Figure 16-9.

Anatomic forms of congenitally complete heart block. Complete heart block is the total failure of electrical impulse propagation from the atria to the ventricles. Complete heart block may be congenital or acquired. It is often associated with anatomically identifiable discontinuities or disruptions in the conduction system in the vicinity of the atrioventricular (AV) junction. Congenital heart block may exist in an otherwise normal heart or in hearts with grossly apparent malformations such as ventricular inversion or atrioventricular canal defects [8]. Lev [8] and Husson *et al.* [9] described three pathologic patterns of congenitally complete heart block involving the AV node and proximal His-Purkinje system. Congenital heart block in the absence of structural heart disease has also been associated with maternal connective tissue disease, especially systemic lupus erythematosus [10,11]. Recent studies have shown that in the presence of placentally transmitted maternal SS-A/Ro or SS-B/La autoantibodies, the incidence of congenitally complete heart

block approaches 100% [12,13]. The most common causes of acquired heart block involve direct injury to the AV junction region as a result of infarction, inflammatory or infiltrative diseases, cardiac surgery, or catheterization.

Three pathologic patterns of congenitally complete heart block have been elucidated. The first (*left*) is lack of communication between the atria and the AV node (*ie*, atrial–axis discontinuity). In this form, the AV node may be totally absent. The second (*middle*) is interruption of the AV bundle (*ie*, nodoventricular discontinuity), in which the penetrating part of the bundle is disrupted but the distal bundle branches are intact. The third form (*right*) is less common and consists of disruption of the interventricular bundle branches (*ie*, intraventricular discontinuity). This latter form is more commonly seen with ventricular inversion. (*Adapted from* Gillette and Garson [14].)

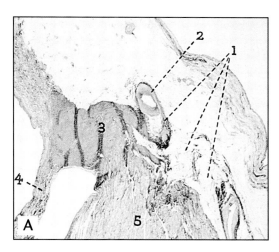

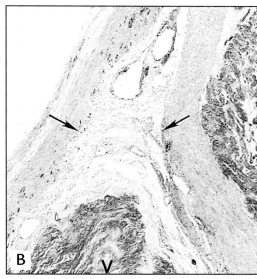

Figure 16-10.

Histopathology of congenitally complete heart block. **A,** Atrial-axis discontinuity. In this example, there is anatomic disruption between the atria and the region normally occupied by the atrioventricular (AV) node (these areas are indicated by *1*). **B,** Nodoventricular discontinuity. In this example, the connection between the penetrating portion of the bundle of His and the more distal bundle branches is disrupted. The area normally occupied by the penetrating portion of the bundle (*arrows*) is replaced by loose connective tissue. 2—AV node artery; 3—central fibrous body; 4—mitral valve; 5—ventricular muscle; V—ventricular muscle. (*Adapted from* Lev [8].)

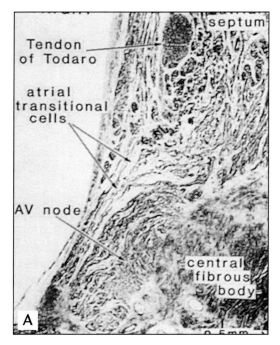 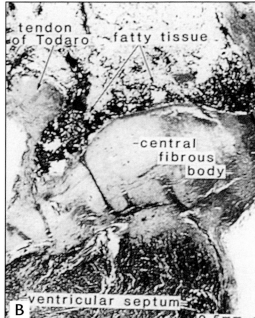 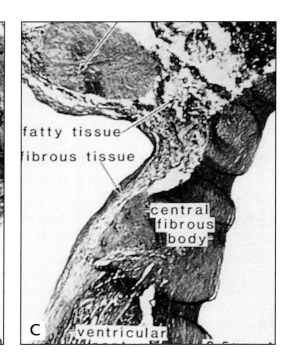

Figure 16-11.

Congenitally complete heart block associated with maternal systemic lupus erythematosus. Three histologic sections through the posterior atrioventricular (AV) junctional area have been taken at similar levels showing the AV node situated between the tendon of Todaro and the central fibrous body. **A,** Section from a normal heart. **B** and **C,** Sections from subjects with congenital heart block related to the presence of maternal serum anti-Ro antibodies. Fibrofatty tissue replaces areas of the AV node in these sections, resulting in discontinuity of the atria and distal conduction system. (*From* Ho and coworkers [15]; with permission.)

BUNDLE BRANCH BLOCK

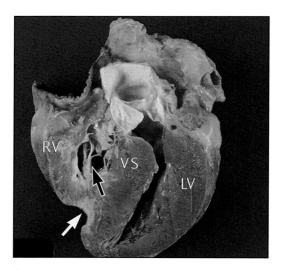

Figure 16-12.

Gross photograph showing the heart of a 55-year-old woman with metastatic carcinoma of the cervix who presented with dyspnea, tachypnea, and distended neck

veins. Occasionally, a bundle branch block (BBB) pattern on the electrocardiogram can be attributed to a specific pathologic finding in the heart. Two-dimensional echocardiogram revealed an echogenic mass in the right ventricle (RV) deforming the RV cavity. The electrocardiogram showed normal sinus rhythm with right BBB (RBBB) that had developed since a study 10 months earlier. The patient died as a result of pulmonary thromboemboli. At autopsy, the heart showed a localized deformity of the RV free wall (*white arrow*). The moderator band, anterior papillary muscle of the tricuspid valve (*black arrow*), and a circumscribed transmural region of the RV free wall were extensively replaced by nests of carcinoma cells in a dense, desmoplastic stroma. In most individuals, the moderator band, a discrete band of muscle that connects the ventricular septum (VS) to the RV free wall, originates at the apical limit of the septal band of the crista terminalis and inserts on the free wall at the base of the anterior papillary muscle. The moderator band usually contains a branch of the right coronary artery that supplies the anterior papillary muscle and the RV free wall in the same distribution observed to be replaced by tumor in this case. Thus, the pattern of metastatic tumor involvement of the RV strongly suggests hematogenous metastasis via the moderator band artery. The moderator band also carries a major branch of the right bundle of the cardiac conduction system that is responsible for conducting depolarizing current from the basal portion of the VS to the RV free wall. Destruction of the moderator band by tumor clearly accounted for the development of RBBB in this patient. LV—left ventricle.(*From* Jaffe and coworkers [16]; with permission.)

SUPRAVENTRICULAR TACHYCARDIA

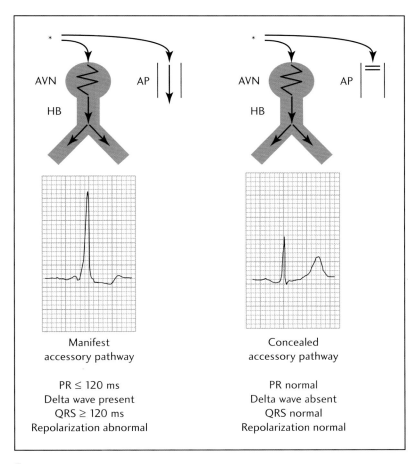

Manifest
accessory pathway

PR ≤ 120 ms
Delta wave present
QRS ≥ 120 ms
Repolarization abnormal

Concealed
accessory pathway

PR normal
Delta wave absent
QRS normal
Repolarization normal

Figure 16-13.

Manifest and concealed accessory pathways. Supraventricular tachycardia (SVT) is defined as any rapid rhythm arising from the atrium, atrioventricular (AV) junction, or an accessory pathway (an abnormal electrical connection between the atria and ventricle). One mechanism of SVT is abnormal automaticity. This occurs when a group of cells distinct from the sinus node exhibits enhanced spontaneous depolarization, resulting in an accelerated rhythm with features similar to sinus tachycardia. Ectopic atrial tachycardia occurs when the abnormal automatic focus is located within the atrium, usually near the orifices of the pulmonary veins or along the crista terminalis. Junctional tachycardia occurs when the automatic focus arises in the AV node or His bundle. Typically, there are no histopathologic correlates in ectopic atrial or junctional tachycardias.

Reentry is the most common mechanism of SVT and usually involves the AV node as a critical component of the tachycardia circuit (AV node dependent). Accessory connection–mediated tachycardia occurs when a second discrete conduction pathway exists separate from the AV node. Typical accessory connections may arise from the atria anywhere along the right or left AV groove and connect with the ventricle to give rise to the Wolff-Parkinson-White syndrome. Mahaim fibers are an uncommon type of accessory pathway that was originally thought to arise from the AV node or His bundle and insert into the right ventricle. More recent studies [17] have demonstrated that the majority of Mahaim fibers are atriofascicular pathways that generally arise from atrial tissue on the lateral aspect of the tricuspid annulus and insert into the distal right bundle branch.

Atrioventricular node reentry tachycardia involves conduction along dual pathways within the AV junction region. Disparate conduction and refractory properties of the two pathways underlie the mechanism for reentry. Although the dual pathway concept is well documented electrophysiologically, the anatomic correlates have not been well defined and remain a subject of current debate.

In patients with accessory connections, conduction from the atria to the ventricles during sinus rhythm may occur in the anterograde direction through both the AV node (AVN) and the accessory pathway (AP) (ie, manifest accessory pathway) (left). Conduction via the accessory pathway is generally faster than conduction through the AV node, "preexciting" some portion of the ventricle and resulting in a short PR interval, a slurred initial portion of the surface QRS (delta wave), and a prolonged QRS interval. In the case of a concealed accessory pathway (right), anterograde conduction does not occur through the accessory pathway during sinus rhythm resulting in a normal-appearing electrocardiogram. HB—His bundle.

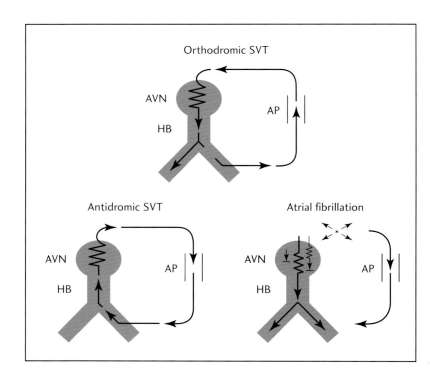

Orthodromic SVT

AVN

HB

AP

Antidromic SVT

AVN

HB

AP

Atrial fibrillation

AVN

HB

AP

Figure 16-14.

Wolff-Parkinson-White (WPW) syndrome and supraventricular tachycardia (SVT). The most common type of arrhythmia observed in WPW syndrome is orthodromic reciprocating SVT (*top*). This consists of anterograde conduction from atrium to ventricle through the atrioventricular node (AVN) and His bundle (HB) and retrograde conduction from ventricle to atrium through the accessory pathway (AP). This arrhythmia produces a normal, narrow QRS during tachycardia because the ventricles are being activated via the His-Purkinjë system. The reverse of this circuit (antidromic reciprocating SVT [*bottom left*]) is less common and results in a wide complex QRS during tachycardia. The wide QRS reflects ectopic activation of the ventricles. Sudden death associated with WPW is rare and is related to the development of ventricular fibrillation in response to rapid anterograde conduction through the accessory connection during any rapid atrial tachycardia (usually atrial fibrillation [*bottom right*] or flutter). (*Adapted from* Lindsay [18]; with permission.)

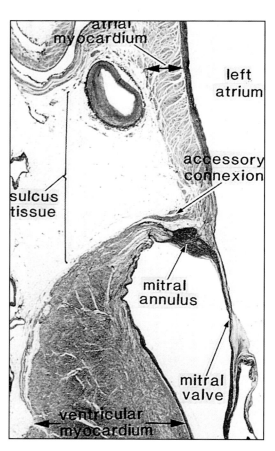

atrial myocardium

left atrium

accessory connexion

sulcus tissue

mitral annulus

mitral valve

ventricular myocardium

Figure 16-15.

Histologic demonstration of a left-sided accessory connection associated with the Wolff-Parkinson-White syndrome. An accessory strand of cardiac muscle arising in the left atrium is shown on the epicardial aspect of the mitral annulus coursing through the adipose tissue of the atrioventricular sulcus and connecting to ventricular myocardium. (*From* Anderson and Ho [2]; with permission.)

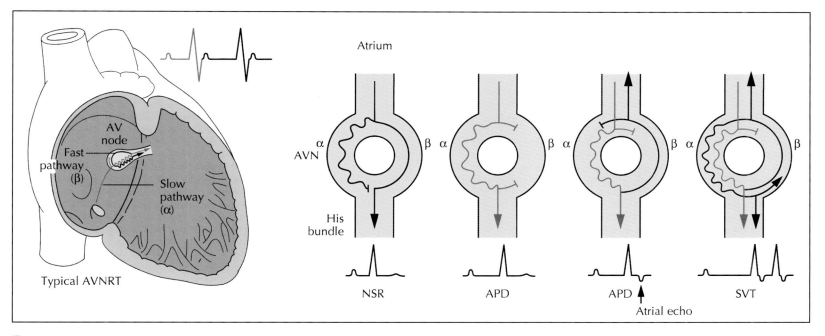

Figure 16-16.

Arrhythmia circuits in typical atrioventricular (AV) node reentry tachycardia (AVNRT). In this arrhythmia, dual pathways with different conduction properties have been demonstrated by electrophysiologic testing, but the exact anatomic basis has been debated. The actual circuit is not confined to the compact AV node. One pathway (α) typically exhibits slow conduction velocity with a short refractory period. Slow anterograde conduction in this pathway (*wavy line*) occurs along the septal aspect of the tricuspid annulus. The other pathway (β) conducts more rapidly but has a longer refractory period. During normal sinus rhythm (NSR), an impulse from the atrium travels down both the slow and fast pathways. It travels more rapidly down the fast pathway, activating the ventricle with a relatively short PR interval. The impulse also travels down the slow pathway but blocks at the terminal portion

of the AV node because the tissue at this site is still refractory. A spontaneously occurring atrial premature depolarization (APD) is blocked in the fast pathway because of its longer refractory period but conducts through the slow pathway, resulting in ventricular depolarization with a long PR interval. If the tissue of the fast pathway regains excitability, the impulse traveling down the slow pathway can return and travel retrogradely up the fast pathway and activate the atria, resulting in an atrial echo beat. This reentry circuit leads to a narrow complex supraventricular tachycardia (SVT) with a short RP interval (rapid retrograde activation through the fast pathway). Atypical AV node reentry tachycardia occurs when the circuit is reversed: anterograde conduction through the fast pathway and retrograde conduction through the slow pathway. This results in a narrow complex SVT with a long RP interval.

Figure 16-17.

Ablation of atrioventricular node reentry tachycardia with radiofrequency (RF) current. Shown is the explanted heart of a patient with refractory AV node reentry who eventually underwent cardiac transplantation. The patient was treated with RF current through a percutaneous catheter to ablate his slow pathway and terminate his supraventricular tachycardia (SVT). The oblong lesion induced by RF current is located along the tricuspid annulus (TA) midway between the os of the coronary sinus (CS) and the anterior aspect of the atrial septum (AS). (*From* Gamache and coworkers [19]; with permission.)

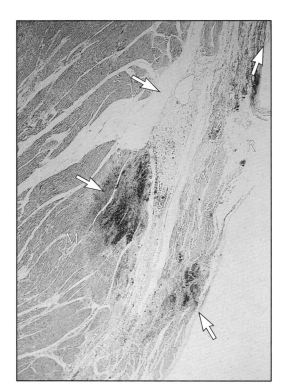

Figure 16-18.

Figure 16-18.
Photomicrograph of the lesion shown in Figure 16-22. A region of myocardial injury (bounded by *arrows*) induced by radiofrequency current extends from the approaches to the atrioventricular node (A) in the right atrial myocardium into the right ventricular septal myocardium (M). The right atrial endocardium has been disrupted by the radiofrequency current (R). The lesion (5 × 5 × 4 mm) exhibits myocyte necrosis with hemorrhage, edema, and chronic inflammatory cells. These observations support the hypothesis that the slow pathway of atrioventricular (AV) nodal reentry is anatomically distinct from the AV node and is composed of atrial tissue located posteriorly in the septum close to the posterior end of the AV node. (*From* Gamache and coworkers [19]; with permission.)

ATRIAL FLUTTER

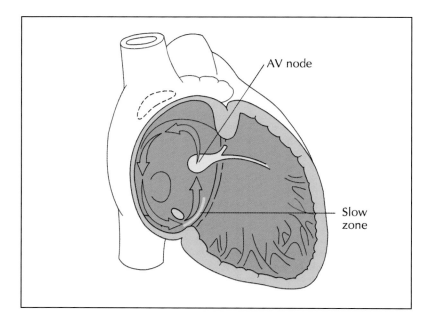

Figure 16-19.
Macroreentrant circuit of typical atrial flutter characterized by counterclockwise rotation in the right atrium. Ablation of tissue between the tricuspid valve and the inferior vena cava (slow zone) interrupts conduction through this isthmus of tissue and prevents atrial flutter.

Atrial flutter is a rapid macroreentrant atrial arrhythmia (atrial rate of 250 to 300 bpm). The most common type of atrial flutter circuit involves the right atrium, in which the wavefront of activation circulates down the lateral wall of the right atrium, across the isthmus of tissue between the inferior vena cava and the tricuspid valve, up the septum, and back across the roof of the right atrium [20–22]. Less common forms of atrial flutter circulate around surgical scars or other functional or fixed anatomic barriers [23]. Catheter-guided applications of radiofrequency energy are commonly used to ablate tissue between the inferior vena cava and tricuspid valve to block the conduction of electrical impulses through this isthmus and thereby prevent the common form of atrial flutter. Patients who have undergone ablation of common atrial flutter typically exhibit a line of fibrotic lesions 1 to 2 cm thick between the tricuspid valve and inferior vena cava.

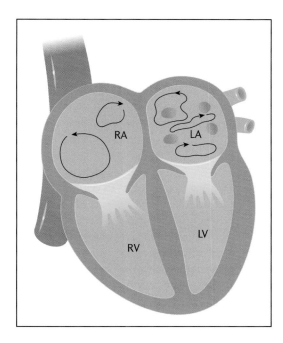

Figure 16-20.

Mechanism of atrial fibrillation. Atrial fibrillation is generally thought to be caused by multiple wavelets of reentry that migrate throughout the atria with rapidly changing activation patterns. A focal source of high-frequency discharges generally emanating from one of the pulmonary veins is a less common cause of atrial fibrillation.

In 1962, Moe [24] proposed the multiple wavelet hypothesis to explain the characteristics of atrial fibrillation. In this model, persistent reentrant activity is sustained by five or six wavelets that migrate over the surface of the atria, coalescing and fractionating in constantly changing patterns. This concept is supported by independent investigations by Cox *et al.* [25] and Konings *et al.* [26], who performed intraoperative mapping of atrial fibrillation using epicardial electrode arrays. A surgical procedure called the maze operation was designed to test Moe's multiple wavelet hypothesis and has proven effective in preventing both chronic and paroxysmal atrial fibrillation. This operation uses several strategically placed atrial incisions that prevent multiple wavelets of atrial reentry from developing. Both atrial appendages are amputated. The incisions are positioned to allow sinus impulses to activate the entire right atrium (RA) and left atrium (LA) except for a region within an incision that encircles the pulmonary veins. Subsequent studies [27] have confirmed that focal mechanisms of atrial fibrillation also exist and can be ablated by catheter-guided applications of radiofrequency energy.

Patients with chronic atrial fibrillation usually have structurally abnormal atria, but the pathologic anatomy of atrial fibrillation is nonspecific. Most commonly, the atria are dilated and show interstitial fibrosis. These changes probably affect atrial conduction pathways and, in a general sense, increase the risk of developing a localized reentrant circuit. LV—left ventricle; RV—right ventricle.

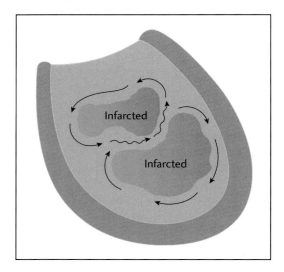

Figure 16-21.

View of a reentrant circuit in ventricular tachycardia. In this depiction, a reentrant wavefront of electrical activation propagates slowly (*wavy lines*) through surviving strands of myocardial tissue between two regions of infarcted tissue and circles back around the infarcted myocardium before reentering the zone of slow conduction. The slow conduction of electrical impulses through viable but structurally altered tissue between the zones of infarct scar allows the remaining myocardium to recover from the preceding wavefront and propagate the next wave of activation. This cycle of reentry is a common cause of ventricular tachycardia in patients with healed infarcts.

Sustained ventricular arrhythmias are the most common cause of sudden death. They often occur in patients with coronary artery disease but are not necessarily associated with acute infarction. Sustained ventricular tachycardia may occur as a spontaneous event independent of acute myocardial infarction (MI). These arrhythmias are especially common in patients who have had a previous MI. Once initiated, the ventricular tachycardia may terminate spontaneously or degenerate into ventricular fibrillation and cause sudden death. Several studies have shown that reentry is the predominant mechanism of ventricular tachycardia. In patients with healed infarcts, regions of slow conduction and unidirectional conduction block typically map to areas of viable but structurally altered muscle at the edges of healed infarcts or ventricular aneurysms [28,29]. Remodeling of intercellular connections at gap junctions is thought to play an important role in altering conduction in these areas and contributing to reentry. These regions typically contain strands of surviving myocardium within a background of extensive interstitial and replacement fibrosis. Although this histopathologic appearance is commonly seen in areas of slow conduction and block critical to the reentrant circuit, similar structural alterations are present in the hearts of most patients with healed infarcts, including those with no history of ventricular arrhythmias. Thus, it seems likely that an appropriate anatomic substrate is only one of multiple determinants of ventricular tachycardia. Other factors, including the location, frequency, and timing of ventricular premature beats; the onset of acute conduction derangements triggered by acute ischemia; and complex interactions between areas of anatomically fixed conduction block (scar tissue) and functional block (related to alterations in refractoriness) combine to make the development of ventricular tachycardia a stochastic process.

Nonischemic cardiomyopathies, myocardial tumors, and infiltrative diseases such as amyloidosis or sarcoidosis are among the other potential causes of ventricular arrhythmias. Each of these diseases may result in surviving muscle fibers interspersed through regions of fibrosis that could provide the substrate for reentry. However, the mechanisms of ventricular tachycardia in these conditions have not been completely determined nor have the anatomic substrates been as well characterized as in ischemic heart disease. In most patients with reentrant ventricular tachycardia in the setting of healed MI, the arrhythmia circuit involves the ventricular myocardium per se with little or no involvement by the conduction system. However, in some patients, including those with nonischemic cardiomyopathies and conduction system disease, the bundle branches may participate in the reentry circuit.

Arrhythmogenic right ventricular cardiomyopathy, hypertrophic cardiomyopathy, and long QT syndrome are three genetically transmitted disorders that cause ventricular arrhythmias associated with syncope or sudden death in children and young adults. Ventricular arrhythmias are especially likely to occur with physical exertion in each of these conditions.

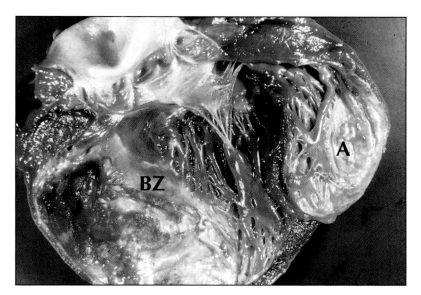

Figure 16-22.
Typical gross appearance of a left ventricular aneurysm. The left ventricle is half opened. The border zone (BZ) covered by the whitish endocardial fibrosis circumscribes the central fibrotic segment of the aneurysm (A). Reentrant ventricular tachycardia is especially common in patients with left ventricular aneurysms.

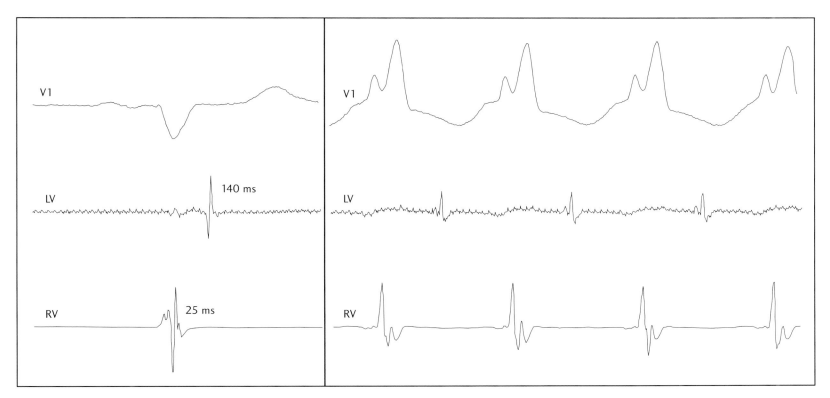

Figure 16-23.
Slow conduction at the margin of a ventricular aneurysm. Sinus rhythm is illustrated on the *left*. Surface lead V1, and intracardiac electrograms from the left ventricle (LV) and apex of the right ventricle (RV) are displayed. A catheter was positioned in the LV at the margin of a large aneurysm. Ventricular activation at this site during sinus rhythm was delayed, occurring 140 ms after the onset of the surface QRS and well after the end of the QRS complex, which was only 110 ms in duration. In contrast, activation of the RV apex occurred 25 ms after the onset of the surface QRS.

Ventricular tachycardia is illustrated on the *right*. During ventricular tachycardia, activation at the same LV site occurred in diastole 190 ms after the onset of the surface QRS and 140 ms before the next complex. This region corresponded to a zone of slow conduction within the reentrant circuit.

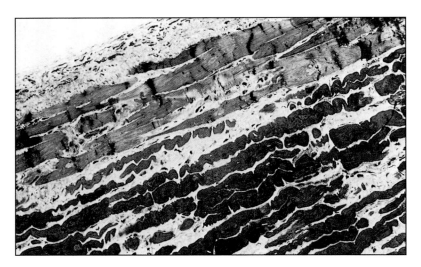

Figure 16-24.

The typical histologic substrate of sustained ventricular tachycardia (VT) in the setting of healed myocardial infarction. This section is from a patient who underwent surgery to remove a portion of the endomyocardium in which slow conduction and conduction block were responsible for his VT. These areas were characterized by interdigitation of scar and relatively normal surviving muscle bundles. Microelectrode experiments indicate that the surviving muscle cells at the edges of healed infarcts usually have relatively normal action potential characteristics, with normal resting membrane potential and action potential upstroke. Therefore, VT does not result from any abnormality of the cellular electrophysiologic properties themselves; rather, patchy scarring disrupts the normal cell-to-cell pathway for current spread, resulting in serpiginous, slow conduction. This nonuniformly anisotropic substrate has the characteristics required for sustained reentrant tachycardia. (*From* Wit and Josephson [30]; with permission.)

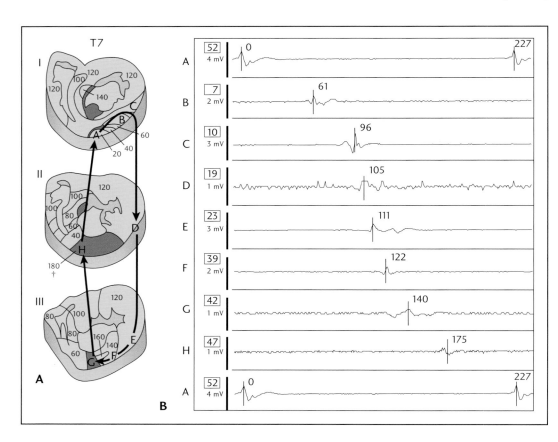

Figure 16-25.

Detailed three-dimensional isochronal map of a reentrant pathway during ventricular tachycardia in a patient with a healed anterior infarct. This isochronal map depicts the sequential spread of electrical activation in increments of 20 ms. The heart has been sliced transversely (in the short axis) with the base on top and the apex on bottom. The anterior wall of the left ventricle is at the lower edge and the right ventricle at the left edge of each slice. Zones or lines of conduction block are denoted by *blackened areas* or *thickened lines*. **A**, Activation sequences in slices I, II, and III during the seventh beat (T7) of ventricular tachycardia. *A* to *H* denote recording sites along the reentrant pathway. The *arrows* denote the reentrant pathway leading to the initiation of the next beat, T8, at site A. **B**, Continuous activation along the reentrant pathway.

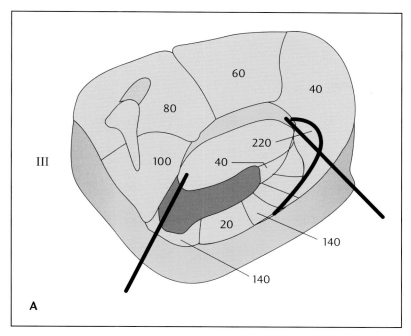

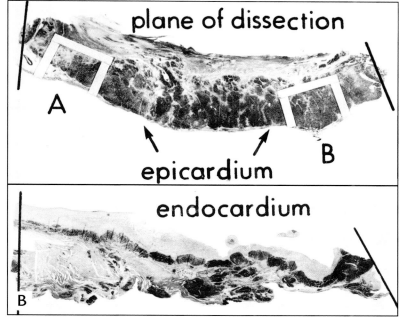

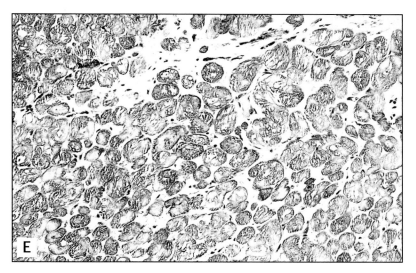

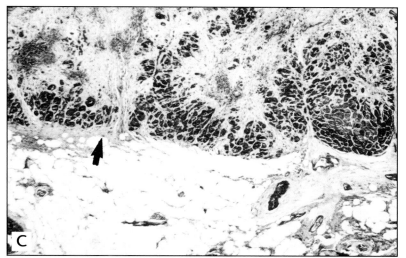

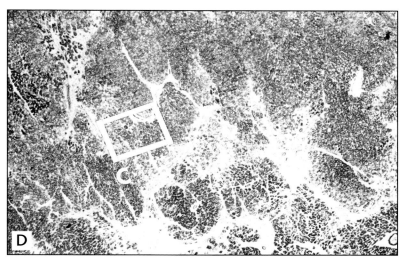

Figure 16-26.

Spatial correlation between histopathology and reentry in ventricular tachycardia in a patient who underwent a surgical procedure to map ventricular tachycardia and resect tissues responsible for conduction block. **A,** Isochronal map of ventricular activation during a beat of ventricular tachycardia. Mapping at this level demonstrated areas of both fixed and functional conduction block (*solid black*

area and *heavy curved line*) as well as delayed activation and a reentry circuit. **B,** Histologic sections of tissue removed at the time of surgery and cut in a plane perpendicular to the apex-base axis. Endocardial and epicardial portions of the resection are labeled; the *straight lines* indicate the position of the resected tissues with respect to the ventricular activation map. Note that areas of fixed conduction block (*solid black*) correspond to areas of infarct scar that extend nearly transmurally in the anteroseptal wall of the left ventricle (*arrows*). **C,** Magnification of "A" in *panel B.* The remainder of the epicardial histologic preparations demonstrated an epicardial mantle of surviving muscle of varying thickness with significant interstitial fibrosis. This area was the site of delayed activation and reentry. **D,** Magnification of "B" in *panel B.* The region of functional conduction block and delayed activation shown in greater detail is demonstrating surviving muscle bundles with highly variable and extensive degrees of interstitial fibrosis. **E,** Higher-magnification view of *boxed area* in *panel D.* Myocyte profiles are cut in cross section indicating the transverse orientation of myocyte fibers with respect to the direction of the reentrant wavefront. These findings demonstrate that surviving muscle fibers conducted electrical impulses slowly through peri-infarct regions and created the substrate required for reentry. Slowing of conduction occurred in a direction transverse to fiber orientation.

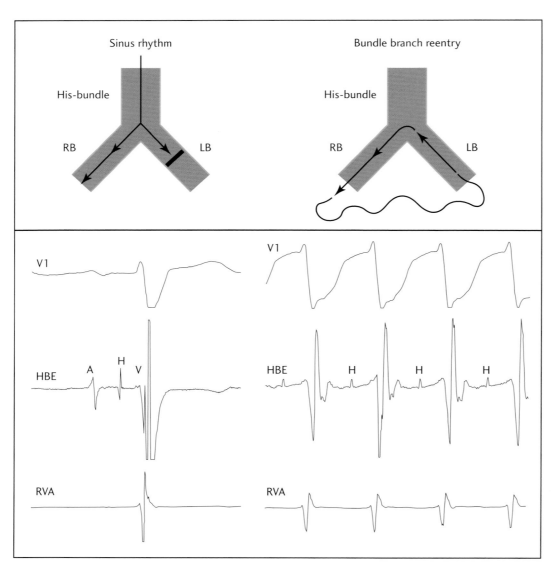

Figure 16-27.

View of bundle branch reentry in a patient with a nonischemic cardiomyopathy. Bundle branch reentry may account for ventricular tachycardia in as many as 6% of patients with nonischemic cardiomyopathies and conduction system disease [31]. In the example shown on the *top*, left bundle branch block was present during sinus rhythm because the left bundle (LB) did not conduct anterogradely. However, it was capable of retrograde conduction. During bundle branch reentry, the electrical impulse proceeded down the right bundle (RB) to activate the myocardium and then conducted retrogradely up the left bundle. Surface lead V1 and intracardiac recordings from the His-bundle electrogram (HBE) and right ventricular apex (RVA), are shown on the *bottom*. The His-bundle electrogram, which is recorded near the atrioventricular junction, reveals atrial activation (A), conduction through the His-bundle (H), and local ventricular activation (V). During ventricular tachycardia, the His-potential (H) is observed 70 ms before the onset of ventricular activation because it must pass through the His-bundle with each revolution of the reentrant circuit.

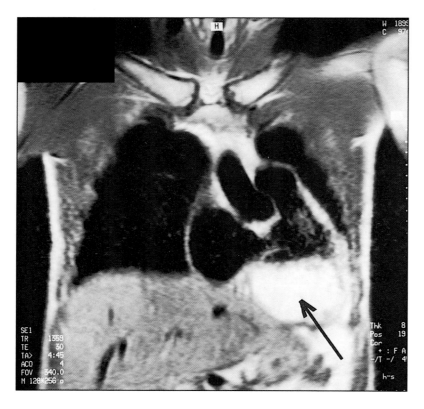

Figure 16-28.

Magnetic resonance image of a patient with a large hemangioma (*arrow*) involving the right ventricle, which was associated with recurrent episodes of ventricular fibrillation. Although the mechanism leading to arrhythmias has not been established in patients with tumors or other infiltrative diseases, potential explanations include damage to cell membranes, which may destabilize the electrical properties of cells, or separate myofibers, which may slow conduction and provide an anatomic substrate for reentry.

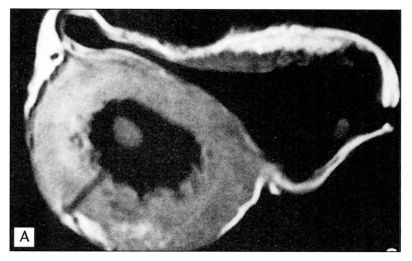

Figure 16-29.

An in vitro magnetic resonance image (*panel A*) and a gross photograph (*panel B*) of a transverse slice of the heart of a 17-year-old boy who died suddenly in a soccer game as the result of arrhythmogenic right ventricular dysplasia. This fascinating condition is probably more appropriately referred to as arrhythmogenic right ventricular cardiomyopathy because the basic pathologic process does not appear to be truly dysplastic in nature. This heart muscle disease is characterized by severe, often lethal, ventricular arrhythmias (ventricular tachycardia and ventricular fibrillation) and fibrofatty replacement of the right ventricular myocardium [32]. The extent and distribution of the pathologic alterations and the associated clinical manifestations vary, but the heart typically shows extensive loss of muscle of the right ventricular free wall with apparent replacement by mature adipose tissue. The cause of this disease is unknown, but a familial occurrence with autosomal dominant inheritance, variable penetrance, and highly variable phenotypic expression is well documented [33]. Three loci linked to this clinical disease have been mapped to two different chromosomes [34–36]. (*From* Basso and coworkers [32]; with permission.)

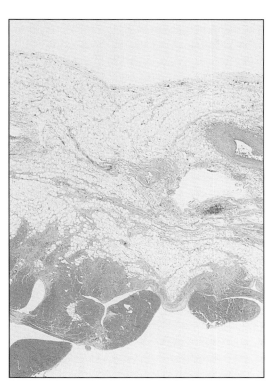

Figure 16-30.

Section of the right ventricular free wall of a 20-year-old woman who underwent cardiac transplantation after failing medical therapy for recurrent ventricular fibrillation and in whom more than 400 episodes of fibrillation were documented and terminated by an implanted cardioverter/defibrillator. Much of the right ventricular myocardium has been replaced by fibrofatty tissue; only the subendocardial trabeculae have been spared. Although this pathologic picture was most dramatic in the right ventricle, other areas of this patient's heart, including the left ventricle and the atria, showed focal accumulation of adipose tissue.

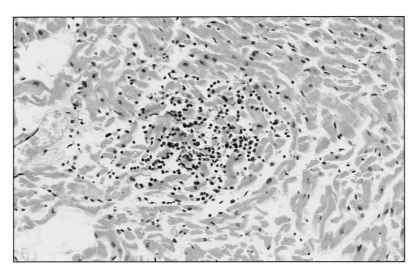

Figure 16-31.

A section of the right ventricle from the father of the patient whose heart is shown in Figure 16-30. The father was a 46-year-old man in apparent good health who died suddenly. His heart showed multiple foci of nongranulomatous, lymphocytic myocarditis in both ventricles but only modest, focal accumulation of mature adipose tissue seen primarily in the right ventricle. Cellular inflammation is a well-documented histopathologic feature of arrhythmogenic cardiomyopathy [32] and is often observed to a variable extent in patients with massive fibrofatty replacement of the right ventricle. In the material shown here, however, myocarditis was the dominant feature and fibrofatty replacement was quite limited. An association between myocarditis and arrhythmogenic cardiomyopathy in first-degree relatives has been reported [36].

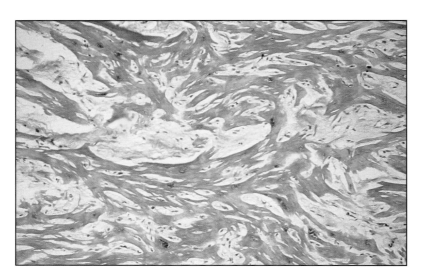

Figure 16-32.

Typical histologic appearance in hypertrophic cardiomyopathy. Hypertrophic cardiomyopathy is a heterogeneous disease affecting patients of all ages. It is characterized by diverse morphologic, functional, and clinical features. Familial hypertrophic cardiomyopathy is a common genetic disease that has a prevalence of approximately one in 500 and is caused by mutations in genes encoding sarcomeric proteins, including beta-myosin heavy chain, cardiac troponin-T, α-tropomyosin, and myosin-binding protein C. The annual mortality from hypertrophic cardiomyopathy is 1% to 4% for adults and 6% for children [37]. Ventricular arrhythmias, which are the primary cause of sudden death, may occur as a primary event or may develop secondary to ischemia, hypotension, or supraventricular arrhythmias that result in hemodynamic compromise. Hypertrophic cardiomyopathy is an especially important cause of sudden death among young athletes. Mechanisms of arrhythmias in patients with hypertrophic cardiomyopathy are poorly understood. Histologically, the left ventricle in hypertrophic cardiomyopathy exhibits disarray of myofibers and often extensive interstitial fibrosis. The contributions of altered structure to electrophysiological derangements and arrhythmia mechanisms in hypertrophic cardiomyopathy have not been elucidated.

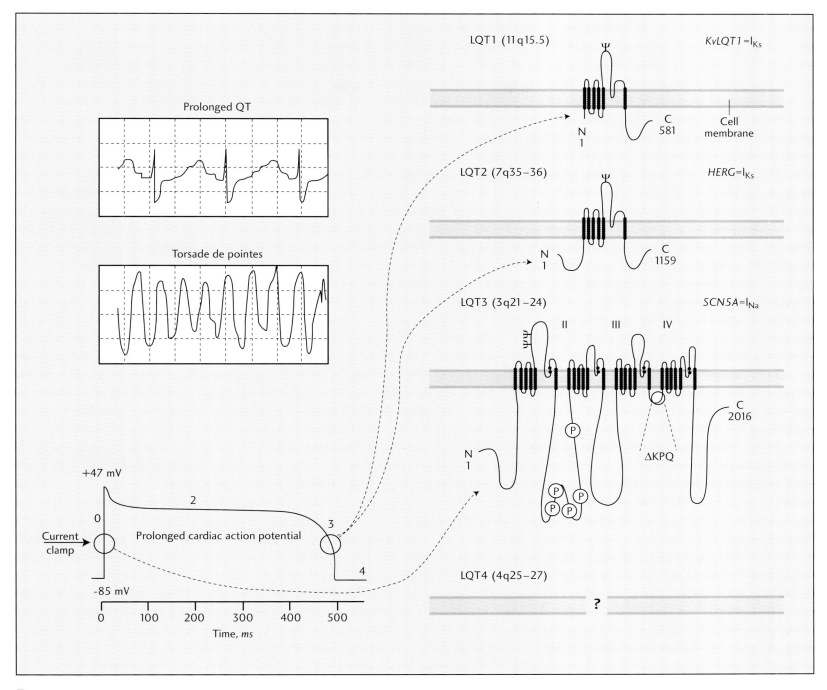

Figure 16-33.

The long QT syndrome. A prolonged corrected QT interval (QTc) on the surface electrocardiogram reflects an abnormality of ventricular repolarization that may arise as a congenital disorder or as a result of certain drugs, toxins, or metabolic abnormalities. Syncope and/or sudden death associated with long QT syndrome often occur during times of physical or emotional stress and are typically the result of a recurrent polymorphic ventricular tachycardia referred to as "torsades de pointes." Congenital long QT syndrome is usually a familial disorder with both autosomal dominant and autosomal recessive patterns of inheritance. The autosomal recessive disorder is associated with deafness and may be a homozygous form of the disease [38]. In 1991, Keating *et al.* [39] first demonstrated linkage of the disorder

to a gene on chromosome 11. It was later found that this gene encoded a cardiac potassium channel protein, KvLQT1, which is responsible for the slow inward rectifying current during repolarization of the action potential [40]. Mutations in this gene disrupt normal repolarization and result in a long QT interval on the surface electrocardiogram. Multiple mutations have since been described in genes encoding for HERG (a cardiac potassium channel) on chromosome 7, SCN5A (a cardiac sodium channel) on chromosome 3, and a gene (LQT4) linked to chromosome 4 [41,42]. There are no consistent gross or microscopic pathologic correlates in the long QT syndrome. (*Adapted from* Ackerman and Clapham [43].)

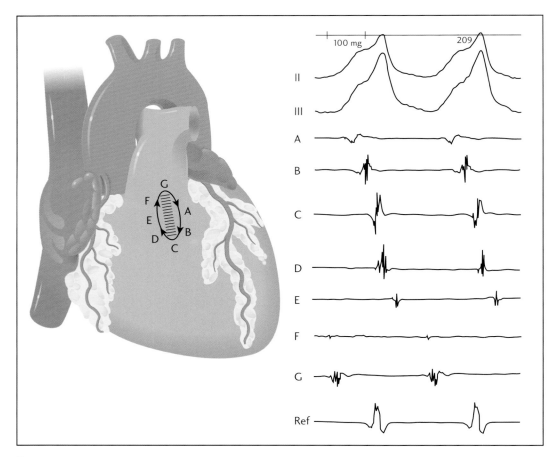

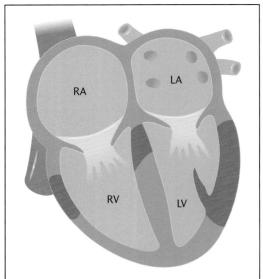

Figure 16-34.

Ventricular tachycardia in congenital heart disease. Shown is ventricular tachycardia resulting from reentry around a surgical scar after a right ventriculotomy. Surface electrogram leads II and III are shown with intraoperative epicardial electrograms from different sites within the tachycardia circuit. The timing of the electrograms seen at sites *A* through *G* with respect to the onset of the surface QRS demonstrates a clockwise rotation of the tachycardia circuit around the surgical scar.

Figure 16-35.

Ventricular arrhythmias in sarcoidosis. Cardiac sarcoidosis is a highly destructive, granulomatous disease of the myocardium that is often associated with serious arrhythmias. The *dark areas* show the distribution of regions most frequently affected by sarcoidosis in 34 autopsy patients. The marked predilection of sarcoidosis for the basal portions of the ventricular septum explains its frequent association with heart block, bundle branch block, ventricular tachycardia, and sudden death. LA—left atrium; LV—left ventricle; RA—right atrium; RV—right ventricle.

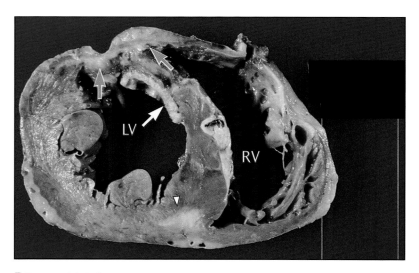

Figure 16-36.

Gross photograph of the heart of a 43-year-old man who died as a result of complications of cardiac sarcoidosis associated with refractory ventricular arrhythmias. He first noted episodes of palpitations 3 years earlier. A routine electrocardiogram 8 months before he died revealed right bundle branch block. Three months before death, the patient experienced abrupt onset of palpitations, diaphoresis, light headedness, and dyspnea demonstrated to be caused by wide complex ventricular tachycardia at 260 bpm. Subsequently, he underwent several electrophysiologic studies in which ventricular tachycardia originating from the right ventricular outflow tract (RVOT) was readily induced but not prevented by multiple antiarrhythmic drugs. Attempts to ablate the arrhythmia focus in the RVOT were unsuccessful. He then underwent attempted surgical resection of the ventricular tachycardia focus. The anterobasal portion of the ventricular septum was found at surgery to be replaced by dense, gray-white scar tissue. Attempts to resect this area resulted in a septal defect that required patch closure. After surgery, ventricular tachycardia recurred and complete heart block subsequently developed. The patient eventually died of progressive hemodynamic deterioration. At autopsy, extensive fibrosis was observed in the anterior left and right ventricular free walls (*gray arrows*) abutting regions previously resected and replaced surgically by a patch (*white arrow*). Additional fibrous areas were apparent in the posterior left and right ventricular free walls near their junction with the posterobasal ventricular septum (*arrowhead*). (*From* Geltman and coworkers [44]; with permission.)

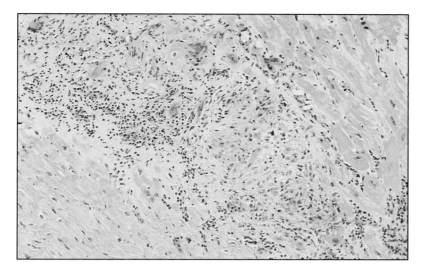

Figure 16-37.
Active sarcoid granulomas containing numerous giant cells present at the junction of the fibrous tissue and viable myocardium.

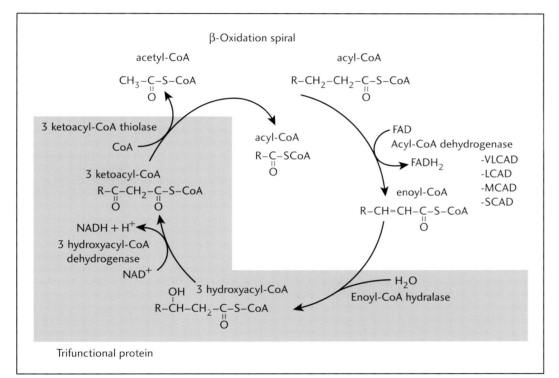

β-Oxidation spiral

acetyl-CoA

$CH_3-C-S-CoA$
$\quad\quad\overset{\|}{O}$

3 ketoacyl-CoA thiolase

CoA

3 ketoacyl-CoA

$R-C-CH_2-C-S-CoA$
$\quad\overset{\|}{O}\quad\quad\overset{\|}{O}$

NADH + H$^+$

3 hydroxyacyl-CoA
dehydrogenase

NAD$^+$

$\quad\quad\quad$ OH $\quad$ 3 hydroxyacyl-CoA

$R-CH-CH_2-C-S-CoA$
$\quad\quad\quad\quad\overset{\|}{O}$

Trifunctional protein

acyl-CoA

$R-CH_2-CH_2-C-S-CoA$
$\quad\quad\quad\quad\overset{\|}{O}$

acyl-CoA

$R-C-SCoA$
$\quad\overset{\|}{O}$

FAD
Acyl-CoA dehydrogenase

FADH$_2$

enoyl-CoA

$R-CH=CH-C-S-CoA$
$\quad\quad\quad\quad\overset{\|}{O}$

H$_2$O
Enoyl-CoA hydralase

-VLCAD
-LCAD
-MCAD
-SCAD

Figure 16-38.
The genetic basis of cardiovascular disease caused by defects in fatty acid β-oxidation [35,36]. The normal heart oxidizes fatty acids through a cyclical enzymatic pathway to produce adenosine triphosphate (ATP). Critical enzymes include a group of acyl-CoA dehydrogenases that act on fatty acids of different chain lengths and a trifunctional protein that consists of a complex of three separate enzymes. Mutations in genes encoding each of these enzymes impair normal fatty acid oxidation. Individuals with these inborn errors of metabolism are more dependent on cardiac energy production from glucose than normal individuals. At times of fasting (when glycogen stores are depleted) or metabolic stress (when energy requirements are increased), these individuals may experience cardiac dysfunction and sudden death, presumably caused by lethal ventricular arrhythmias. LCAD—long chain acyl-CoA dehydrogenase; MCAD—medium chain acyl-CoA dehydrogenase; SCAD—short chain acyl-CoA dehydrogenase; VLCAD—very long chain acyl-CoA dehydrogenase. (*Courtesy of* Arnold W. Strauss, Washington University.)

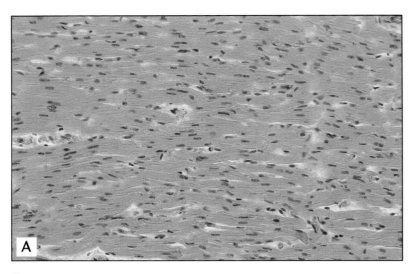 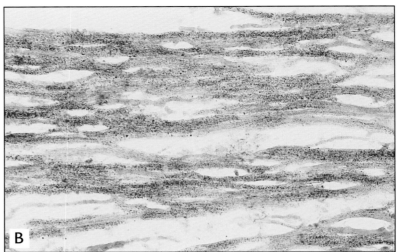

Figure 16-39.

Sections of the heart of a previously healthy 2-year-old girl who developed a viral upper respiratory tract infection and then had a fatal cardiac arrest. Routine hematoxylin and eosin–stained sections of the ventricles (*panel A*) were unremarkable, but an oil-red-O stain of a frozen section (*panel B*) revealed marked accumulation of lipid droplets in myocytes. This finding is typical in children with fatty acid oxidation defects.

REFERENCES

1. Bharati S, Lev M: *The Cardiac Conduction System in Unexplained Sudden Death.* New York: Futura Publishing Company; 1990.

2. Anderson RH, Ho SY: Cardiac conduction system in normal and abnormal hearts. In *Cardiac Arrythmias in the Neonate, Infant and Child.* Edited by Roberts NK, Gelband H. Connecticut: Appleton-Century-Crofts; 1983.

3. Talano, JR. Euler D, Randall WC, *et al.*: Sinus mode dysfunction: an overview with emphasis on autonomic and pharmacologic considerations. *Am J Med* 1978, 64:773–781.

4. Evans R, Shaw BD: Pathological studies in sinoatrial disorder (sick sinus syndrome). *Br Heart J* 1997, 39:778–786.

5. Demoulin J-C, Kulbertus HE: Histopathological correlates of sinoatrial disease. *Br Heart J* 1978, 40:1384–1389.

6. Wit AL, Bigger JT: Possible electrophysiologic mechanisms for lethal arryhthmias accompanying myocardial ischemia and infarction. *Circulation* 1975, 3 (suppl 51,52):96.

7. Wit AL, Rosen MR, Hoffman BF: Electrophysiology and pharmacology of cardiac arrhythmias. II:Relationship of normal and abnormal electrical activity of cardiac fibers to the genesis of arrhythmias. B: Reentry. *Am Heart J* 1974, 88:799.

8. Lev M: Pathogenesis of congenital atrioventricular block. *Prog Cardiovasc Dis* 1972, 15:145–157.

9. Husson GS, Blackman MS, Rogers MC, *et al.*: Familial congenital bundle branch system disease. *Am J Cardiol* 1973, 32:365–369.

10. Chameides L, Truex RC, Vetter V, *et al.*: Association of maternal systemic lupus erythematosus with congenital complete heart block. *N Engl J Med* 1977, 2907:1204–1207.

11. McCue CM, Mantakas ME, Tinglestad JB, Ruddy S: Congenital heart block in mothers with connective tissue disease. *Circulation* 1977, 56:82–92.

12. Taylor PV, Taylor KF, Norman A, *et al.*: Prevalence of maternal Ro (SS-A) and La (SS-B) autoantibodies in relation to congenital AV block. *Br J Rheumatol* 1988, 27:128–132.

13. Provost TT, Watson R, Gammon WR, *et al.*: The neonatal lupus syndrome associated with U1RNP (nRNP) antibodies. *N Engl J Med* 1987, 316:1135–1138.

14. Gillette PC, Garson A, Jr (eds): *Pediatric Arrythmia: Electophysiology and Pacing.* Philadelphia: WB Saunders Co.; 1990.

15. Ho SY, Esscher E, Anderson RH, Michaelsson M: Anatomy of congenital complete heart block and relation to maternal anti-Ro antibodies. *Am J Cardiol* 1986, 58:291–294.

16. Jaffe A, Safdar S, Barzilai B, *et al.*: Clinicopathologic Conference: cardiovascular collapse and death in a 55 year old woman with cervical cancer. *Am J Med* 1988, 84:463–474.

17. McClelland JH, Wang X, Beckman KJ, *et al.*: Radiofrequency catheter ablation of right atriofascicular (Mahaim) accessory pathways guided by accessory pathway activation potentials. *Circulation* 1994, 89:2655–2666.

18. Lindsay BD: Accessory pathway mediated tachycardias. In *Medical Management of Heart Disease.* Edited by Sobel BE. New York: Marcel Dekker; 1996.

19. Gamache MC, Bharati S, Lev M, Lindsay BD: Histopathologic study following catheter guided radiofrequency current ablation of the slow pathway in a patient with atrioventricular nodal reentrant tachycardia. *PACE* 1994, 17:247–251.

20. Disertori M, Inama G, Vergara G, *et al.*: Evidence of a reentry circuit in the common type of atrial flutter in man. *Circulation* 1983, 67:434–440.

21. Klein GJ, Guiradon GM, Sharma AD, Milstein S: Demonstration of macroreentry and feasibility of operative therapy in the common type of atrial flutter. *Am J Cardiol* 1986, 57:587–591.

22. Feld GK, Fleck RP, Chen PS, *et al.*: Radiofrequency catheter ablation for the treatment of human type 1 atrial flutter: identification of a critical zone in the reentrant circuit by endocardial mapping techniques. *Circulation* 1992, 86:1233–1240.

23. Baker B, Lindsay BD, Bromberg BI, *et al.*: Catheter ablation of clinical intra-atrial reentrant tachycardias resulting from prior atrial surgery: localizing and transecting the critical isthmus. *J Am Coll Cardiol* 1996, 28:411–417.

24. Moe GK: On the multiple wavelet hypothesis of atrial fibrillation. *Arch Int Pharmacodyn Ther* 1962, 140:183.

25. Cox JL, Canavan TE, Schuessler RB, *et al.*: The surgical treatment of atrial fibrillation: II. Intraoperative electrophysiologic basis of atrial flutter and atrial fibrillation. *J Thorac Cardiovasc Surg* 1991, 101:406.

26. Konings KTS, Kirchhof CJHJ, Smeets JRLM, *et al.*: High-density mapping of electrically induced atrial fibrillation in humans. *Circulation* 1994, 89:1665.

27. Jais P, Haissaguerre M, Shah DC, *et al.*: A focal source of atrial fibrillation treated by discrete radiofrequency ablation. *Circulation* 1997, 95:572–576.

28. de Bakker JMT, van Capelle FJ, Janse MJ, *et al.*: Reentry as a cause of ventricular tachycardia in patients with chronic ischemic heart disease: electrophysiologic and anatomic correlation. *Circulation* 1988, 77:589–606.

29. Pogwizd SM, Hoyt RH, Saffitz JE, *et al.*: Reentrant and focal mechanisms underlying ventricular tachycardia in the human heart. *Circulation* 1992, 86:1872–1887.

30. Wit AW, Josephson ME: Fractionated electrograms and continuous electrical activity: fact or artefact. In *Cardiac Electrophysiology and Arrhythmias.* Edited by Zipes DP, Jalife J. New York: Grune and Stratton; 1985:350–361.

31. Caceres J, Jazayeri M, McKinnie J, *et al.*: Sustained bundle branch reentry as a mechanism of clinical tachycardia. *Circulation* 1989, 79:256–270.

32. Basso C, Thiene G, Corrado D, *et al.*: Arrhythmogenic right ventricular cardiomyopathy: dysplasia, dystrophy, or myocarditis? *Circulation* 1996, 94:983–991.

33. Nava A, Thiene G, Canciani B, *et al.*: Familial occurrence of right ventricular dysplasia: a study involving nine families. *J Am Coll Cardiol* 1988, 12:1222–1228.

34. Rampazzo A, Nava A, Danieli GA, *et al.*: The gene for arrhythmogenic right ventricular cardiomyopathy maps to chromosome 14q23-q24. *Hum Molec Genet* 1994, 3:959–962.

35. Severini GM, Krajinovic M, Pinamonti B *et al.*: A new locus for arrhythmogenic right ventricular dysplasia on the long arm of chromosome 14. *Genomics* 1996, 31:193–200.

36. d'Amati G, Fiore F, Giordano C, *et al.*: Pathologic evidence of arrhythmogenic cardiomyopathy and myocarditis in two siblings. *Cardiovasc Pathol* 1998, 7:39–46.

37. Spirito P, Seidman C, McKenna WJ, Maron BJ. The management of hypertrophic cardiomyopathy. *N Engl J Med* 1997, 336:775–785.

38. Neyroud N, Tesson F, Denjoy I, *et al.*: A novel mutation in the potassium channel gene KvLQT1 causes the Jervell and Lange-Nielsen cardioauditory syndrome. *Nat Genet* 1997, 15:186–189.

39. Keating M, Atkinson D, Dunn C, *et al.*: Linkage of a cardiac arrhythmia, the long QT syndrome, and the Harvey ras-1 gene. *Science* 1991, 252:704–706.

40. Wang Q, Curran ME, Splawski I, *et al.*: Positional cloning of a novel potassium channel gene: LvLQT1 mutations cause cardiac arrhythmias. *Nat Genet* 1996, 12:17–23.

41. Curran ME, Splawski I, Timothy KW, *et al.*: A molecular basis for cardiac arrhythmias: HERG mutations cause long QT syndrome. *Cell* 1995, 80:795–803.

42. Wang Q, Shen J, Splawski I, *et al.*: SCN5A mutations associated with an inherited cardiac arrhythmia, long QT syndrome. *Cell* 1995, 80:805–811.

43. Ackerman MJ, Clapham DE: Ion channels: basic science and clinical disease. *N Engl J Med* 1997, 336:1557–1586.

44. Geltman EM, Levitt RR, Barzilai B, *et al.*: Refractory ventricular arrhythmias and death in a 43 year old man (CPC). *Am J Med* 1990, 89:496–506.

Diseases of the Aorta

Stanley J. Radio
Maurice Godfrey
Timothy Baxter

The aorta is the largest of the elastic arteries, and it performs two important functions: 1) it acts as a large conduit of oxygenated blood from the heart to the rest of the body, and 2) it reduces cardiac workload by absorbing energy as blood is ejected from the heart. The aorta is divided into several anatomic segments: ascending, arch, descending (thoracic), and abdominal. The normal aorta consists of collagen fibers, especially types I and III; elastin fibers; smooth muscle cells; and acid mucopolysaccharide ground substance [1]. Collagens mainly impart tensile strength to the aorta but also contribute to the extensile properties; the elastin fibers are responsible primarily for the viscoelastic properties. The elastin fibers fragment with advancing age, at which time the smooth muscle cells also decrease in number while the collagen fibers and the amount of acid mucopolysaccharide ground substance increases. These changes result in a generalized dilatation process referred to as *ectasia*. The aorta is subject to several acquired and congenital diseases, the most important of which is atherosclerosis and its complications of aneurysm formation, occlusive disease, and embolic pheneomon. Aortic dissection, acute and chronic aortitis, medial degeneration with and without Marfan syndrome, and trauma are other important processes.

Atherosclerosis is more commonly located in the abdominal aorta below the renal arteries, and it is a diffuse process in this region. When present in the thoracic aorta, atherosclerosis tends to be more patchy in distribution. Significant plaque development is uncommon in the ascending aorta unless the patient has diabetes mellitus, type II familial hyperlipidemia, or previous aortitis. The cause of aneurysms can be related to their location. In the abdominal aorta, the classic fusiform aneurysm is of atherosclerotic origin and is by far the most common type of aneurysms in all locations. Isolated atherosclerotic aneurysm of the thoracic aorta is rare; more commonly they are associated with abdominal aortic involvement. Aneurysms of the aortic sinus region are usually congenital or infectious in origin [1–3].

Abdominal aortic aneurysm (AAA), is the tenth leading cause of death in men older than 55, affecting 1.6% to 3.3% [4]. More than 40,000 patients per year require treatment in the United States, where there are more than 15,000 deaths per year associated with aneurysm rupture [5]. Currently, no medical therapy exists that can inhibit the growth of small aneurysms and, thus, it is not generally considered cost effective to screen for aneurysms. Aneurysmal disease appears to be a complex remodeling process associated with increased activity of a family of metallopeptidases, the matrix metalloproteinases [6]. These enzymes are thought to be responsible for the matrix degradation that occurs with aneurysm growth. During the initial stages of AAA growth, synthesis of collagen reinforces the vessel wall, making rupture of small aneurysms (< 5 cm) rare. This compensatory process eventually fails, and both growth rate and rupture risk increase exponentially [7]. Lesser invasive endovascular procedures are now being explored in an effort to lessen morbidity associated with aneurysmal repair. The mid- and long-term results of these new approaches are unknown, and the only proven treatment to prevent rupture is surgical repair. There are two goals for future therapy: 1) to develop a pharmacologic means of inhibiting the growth of small aneurysms, and 2) to identify aneurysm-associated genes.

Aortitis may be caused by mechanical , toxic , infectious, or idiopathic factors. As is true with other blood vessels, when the aorta has been injured, it has a limited number of morphologic patterns of response regardless of the nature of the inciting injury. Thus, a similar morphology may be seen in several aortitides during either the acute or healing phase. The inflammatory response in most types of aortitis is limited to the media and adventitia with relative sparing of the intima. A notable exception is aortitis in the setting of rheumatic fever in which there is fibrinoid necrosis and inflammatory reaction in the intima or the media and adventitia. In the healing or chronic phase of aortitis, as the infiltrates subside, the damaged tissue is replaced with collagen. Retraction of the collagen that accompanies maturation results in wrinkling and a "tree-bark" texture. This appearance of the internal surface of the aorta is characteristic for most forms of aortitis, regardless of the cause. In advanced aortitis, the characteristic appearance of the aortic intima is frequently altered by secondary dystrophic calcification and atherosclerosis. Thus, although there are important gross and microscopic feature characteristics that are usually not pathognomonic of some types of aortitis, a great deal of overlap exists between entities. The pathologist, therefore, must have a detailed clinical history, findings of the physical examination, laboratory results, and the results of any specific investigation (*eg*, aortogram, CT scan, echocardiographic findings) to formulate a meaningful pathology consultation [8].

It has long been recognized that congenital malformations and inherited disorders manifest as abnormalities of the aorta. These are in addition to disease caused by numerous predisposing factors, including genetic ones. Structural abnormalities comprise a large set of aortic disease, and those caused by defects in components of the extracellular matrix are referred to as heritable disorders of connective tissue (HDCT). Perhaps the prototypical HDCT is Marfan syndrome. Marfan syndrome is an autosomal dominant disorder manifested by abnormalities in the ocular, skeletal, and cardiovascular systems. The cardiovascular manifestations include mitral valve prolapse and regurgitation, dilatation of the aortic root, and aortic regurgitation. The major causes of morbidity and mortality in Marfan syndrome are aortic aneurysm and dissection. Echocardiographic monitoring is essential because approximately one third of individuals with aortic root dilatation, mitral valve prolapse, or both, have normal auscultatory findings on cardiac examination. CT and magnetic resonance imaging are additional tools with a role in evaluation of the aorta in Marfan syndrome. Management revolves around prevention of complications and their correction when they occur. Careful follow-up of patients with Marfan syndrome has permitted preemergent composite graft repair, the results of which have significantly increased life expectancy.

Numerous genetic disorders present with aortic and other cardiovascular complications. Careful and deliberate examination by multiple subspecialists is often required to provide an accurate diagnosis. People with pleiotropic and variable disorders, such as Marfan syndrome, are best followed in a multidisciplinary clinic. Current progress toward understanding the basic defects in relatively rare disorders will provide the essential framework to understanding the pathophysiology in common cardiovascular disease.

Congenital malformations of the aorta include supravalvular aortic stenosis, coarctation, fibromuscular subvalvular aortic stenosis, arch interruption, sinus of Valsalva aneurysm, and aortic rings.

The diagnosis of coarctation is usually made on physical examination, which reveals unequal pulses and blood pressure between the upper and lower extremities. The major physiologic effects of coarctation are systolic hypertension in arteries arising proximal to the coarctation, systolic hypotension in those arising distal, and left ventricular hypertrophy. Pure isolated coarctation discovered after infancy is usually asymptomatic. The coarctation syndrome in infants is usually caused by associated cardiac abnormalities, most commonly a ventricular septal defect and a patent ductus arteriosus.

Fibromuscular subvalvular aortic stenosis is the second most common fixed cause of aortic stenosis. Associated cardiovascular anomalies are present in 50% to 65% of patients and include ventricular septal defect, coarctation, patent ductus arteriosus, left superior vena cava, and aortic valvular stenosis. Subvalvular aortic stenosis can be caused by a thin discrete membrane, a thicker diaphragm with a muscular base, or a diffuse tunnel-like narrowing. Most patients have a thin membrane. The physiology of subvalvular aortic stenosis is identical to valvular stenosis with resultant left ventricular hypertrophy. In many patients, associated thickening of the aortic valve and abnormal flow producing aortic insufficiency are present. Most patients with subvalvular aortic stenosis are identified because of associated cardiac malformations. Subvalvular aortic stenosis is a progressive lesion in most patients with up to 75% demonstrating a gradient of 25 mm Hg or more over a 5-year period.

Supravalvular stenosis is the least common form of aortic stenosis and can be further divided into "hourglass" deformity (in 50% to 75% of patients) with a constricting ridge above the sinus of Valsalva or diffuse types. Approximately 30% to 50% of patients with supravalvular aortic stenosis have Williams syndrome, which includes moderate to severe mental retardation, "elfin" facial features, a stellate iris pattern, and a husky voice.

Aortic dissection is a disruption of the media by a column of blood parallel to the longitudinal axis of the aorta. Aortic dissection typically begins within a few centimeters of the aorta valve annulus with a transverse interomedial tear involving one third to one half of the circumference. The most common location is above the aortic valve or in the descending thoracic aorta. The dissection may then extend distally or away from the heart as far distal as the abdominal aorta and into its branches, including the mesenteric vessels or the iliac arteries, with resultant regional ischemia. The mean age of patients with aortic dissection is 60 years, and it occurs two to three times more frequently in men than in women. At least 70% of patients with aortic dissection have essential hypertension. The predominant pathologic finding in aortic dissection is a multifocal disruption and loss of elastic lamellae and smooth muscle cells that are filled in by pools of acid mucopolysaccharides. In older patients, the histologic picture is predominated by smooth muscle cell loss; in younger patients with Marfan syndrome, Ehlers-Danlos, osteogenesis imperfecta, or cutis laxa, elastin loss is more prominent [1–2].

The exact pathophysiology of aortic dissection is still unknown. Although many believe medial destruction is the cause of aortic dissection, there is some evidence to the contrary. Schlatmann and Becker [9] and others in a study of 100 aortas at autopsy found that cystic medial destruction is present to varying degrees with advancing age and therefore may be a consequence of hemodynamic damage and not necessarily a predisposing condition for dissection.

ATHEROSCLEROSIS

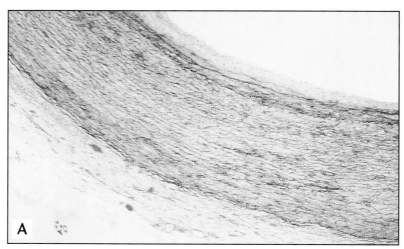

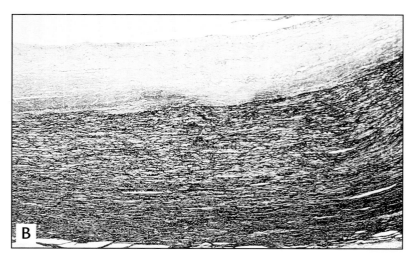

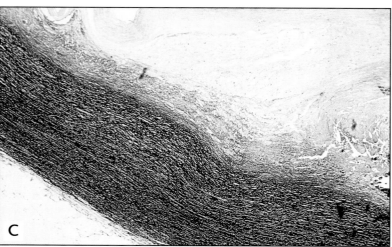

Figure 17-1.

Ascending aorta and abdominal aorta. **A,** Segment of abdominal aorta. The wall thickness and number of elastic lamellae change along the course of the aorta with a progressive decrease from proximal to distal aorta. The adventitia has increased collagen (Movat's pentachrome stain × 40). **B,** Section of abdominal aorta where atherosclerosis is typically first affected with lesser involvement of the more proximal aorta. Histologically, this fibrofatty plaque contains a thickened intima toward the *top* of the photograph. This plaque formation results in medial attenuation and loss of the distinct lamellar architecture (Movat's pentachrome stain × 40). **C,** Section of abdominal aorta with advanced atherosclerotic plaque including fibrous cap, deeper necrotic core with extracellular lipids, and calcification. Medial atrophy is also present (Movat's pentachrome stain × 40).

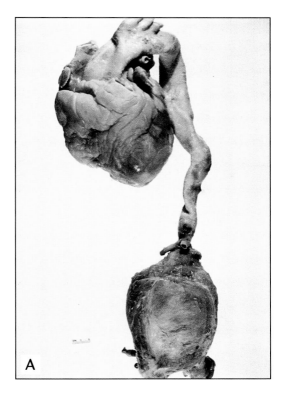

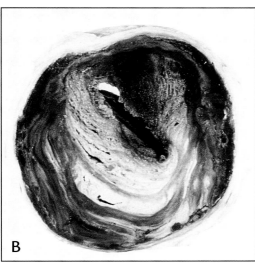

Figure 17-2.

Fusiform aneurysm. **A,** Autopsy specimen from a 74-year-old man with severe athero-sclerosis of the aorta, including diffuse ectasia of thoracic aorta as well as a massive fusiform abdominal aortic aneurysm. The infrarenal aorta is the most common site of atherosclerotic aneurysm formation. This occurs in the presence of significant athero-sclerotic plaque and degradation of the medial elastic lamellae. It is typically accompanied by significant atherosclerosis in the more proximal aorta. **B,** Transverse sections of abdominal aortic aneurysm from the same 74-year-old man demon-strating concentric dilatation of the entire circumference of the aorta. Laminated layers of tan and red-brown mural throm-bus (lines of Zahn) occupy most of the intra-aneurysmal space. A residual central lumen remains to provide a blood conduit.

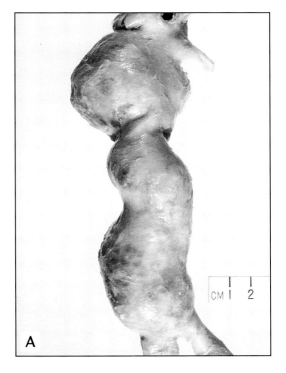

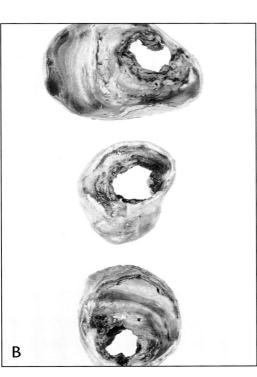

Figure 17-3.

Saccular aneurysm. **A,** Close-up view of abdominal aortic aneurysms. **B,** Transverse sections of abdominal aortic aneurysms in *panel A.* The uppermost of the three sec-tions corresponds to the aneurysm with the more saccular shape and less than total cir-cumference involvement by the aneurysm.

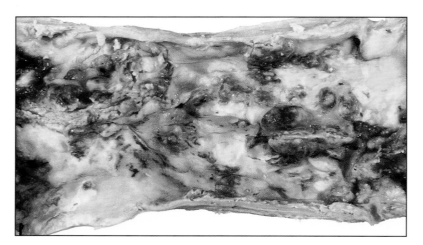

Figure 17-4.

Intimal surface. Autopsy specimen of fusiform abdominal aortic aneurysm open longitudinally demonstrating diffuse involvement with complicated atherosclerotic plaque. Areas of plaque calcification are present, and the large plaques are soft in many areas with a friable surface predisposed for embolization.

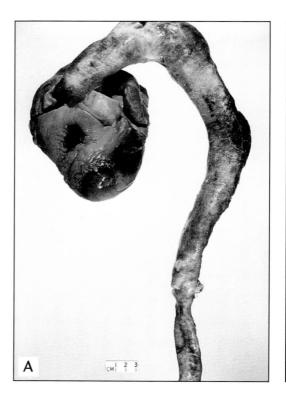

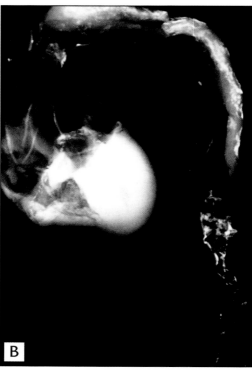

Figure 17-5.

Aortic ectasia and saccular aneurysm. **A,** Autopsy specimen from 82-year-old man with history of hypertension and atherosclerosis with diffuse dilatation of the thoracic aorta (ectasia) with a saccular aneurysm just distal to the left subclavian artery. **B,** Specimen radiograph demonstrating calcification of atherosclerotic plaques in coronary arteries as well as in the atherosclerotic plaques and aneurysm of the thoracic aorta.

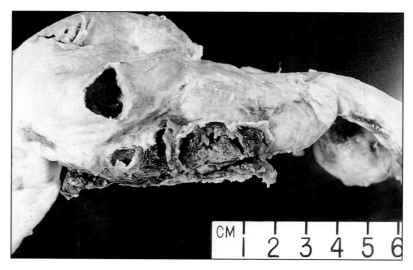

Figure 17-6.

Aneurysm rupture. Autopsy specimen of fusiform aortic abdominal aneurysm from a 65-year-old man with a history of essential hypertension and atherosclerosis who died from massive retroperitoneal hemorrhage. Rupture site of the large aneurysm is evident with a defect in the lateral aspect. The site of aneurysm rupture depends on the location of the aneurysm. Abdominal aneurysms usually rupture into the retroperitoneal space or less commonly into the duodenum. Descending aortic aneurysms commonly rupture into the left pleural space or the esophagus, and ruptures of the aortic arch may involve the mediastinum structures [2].

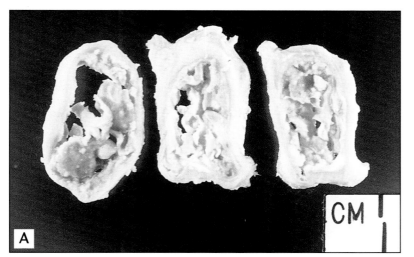

A

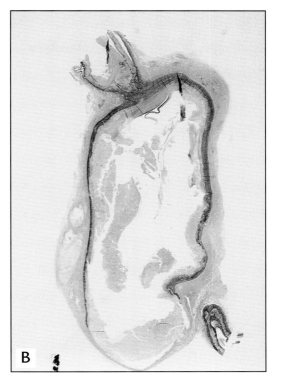

B

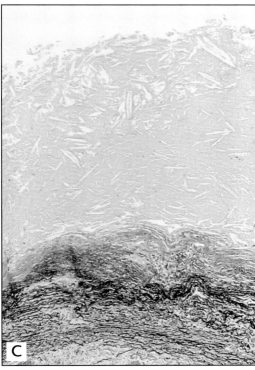

C

Figure 17-7.

Embolic complication of aortic atherosclerosis. Autopsy specimen of an aorta from a 65-year-old woman with ischemic bowel necrosis caused by embolic occlusion of preexisting atherosclerotic narrowing of the superior mesenteric artery. As is common in patients with mesenteric artery narrowing, she also had aortic and coronary artery atheroma and diabetes.

A, Transverse sections of a long but only moderately dilated diameter fusiform abdominal aortic aneurysm involving the infrarenal aorta with extensive central soft, friable atheroma. The ascending and thoracic segments are relatively free of atherosclerosis and aneurysm formation.

B, Whole-mount section of aorta from the middle segment of row from Figure 17-7A demonstrating aneurysm formation, especially prominent toward the top of the photograph. Intima thickening caused by atherosclerotic plaque formation is present along with secondary medial atrophy (elastin van Gieson stain, whole mount).

C, Histologic section of abdominal aorta in region of aneurysm with large amount of yellow amorphous plaque with abundant extracellular lipids in the form of cholesterol clefts (crystaline-like clear spaces). Marked medial atrophy is apparent toward the bottom of the photograph (elastin van Gieson stain × 40).

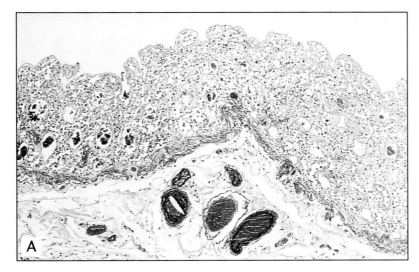

A

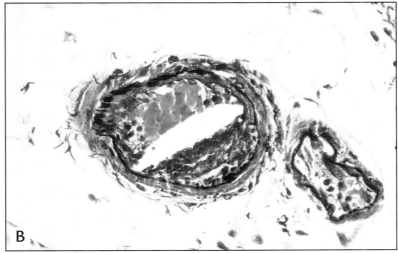

B

Figure 17-8.

Ischemic colitis secondary to emboli. **A,** Histologic section of ascending colon of same patient as Figure 17-7 demonstrating cholesterol emboli and fibrin-platelet rich emboli in submucosal vessels with ischemic necrosis of overlying mucosa (elastin van Gieson stain × 100). **B,** Higher magnification of section shown in *panel A* (elastin van Gieson stain × 400). (*continued on next page*)

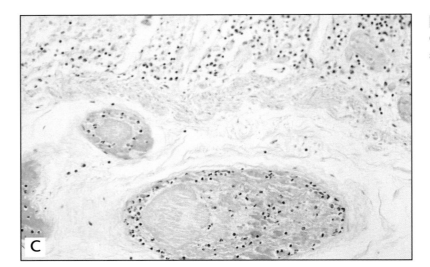

Figure 17-8. (*continued*)
C, Fibrin-platelet rich emboli filling submucosal vessel of
ascending colon (hematoxylin and eosin stain × 200).

AORTITIS

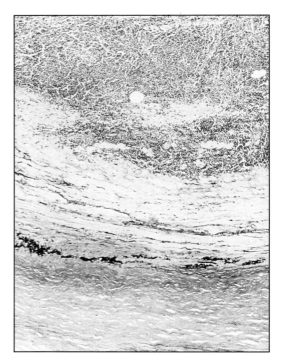

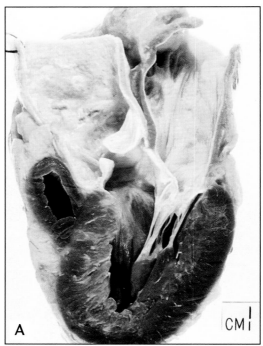

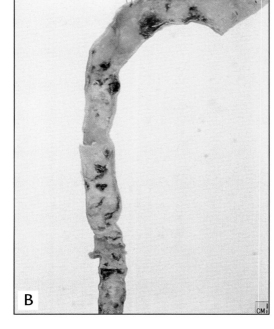

Figure 17-9.
Chronic aortitis. Histologic section of non-specific chronic aortitis. Although there are several possible causes of aortitis, the pattern of injury and repair is somewhat limited. This photomicrograph demonstrates a typical pattern of marked destruction of the medial elastin and fibrosis and prominent inflammatory infiltrate in the outer media and adventitial layers. Secondary fibrous thickening of the intima is present (elastin van Gieson stain × 40).

Figure 17-10.
Chronic syphilitic aortitis. **A,** Autopsy specimen from a 65-year-old man with syphilitic aortitis. The aortic root and ascending aorta are markedly dilated, resulting in aortic valve insufficiency. Secondary superimposed atherosclerosis is present throughout the ascending aorta including the coronary artery ostia. **B,** Longitudinally opened aorta from same patient in *panel A* demonstrating intimal fibrosis and wrinkling ("treebarking") along with superimposed secondary atherosclerosis in both the thoracic and abdominal aorta. (*continued on next page*)

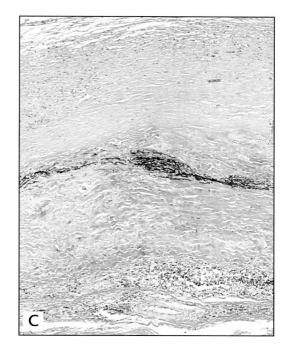

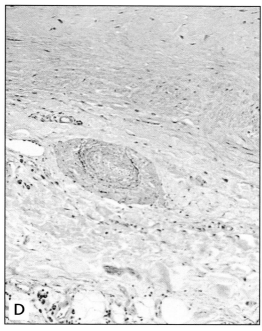

Figure 17-10. (*continued*)
C, Histologic section of aorta from a patient with syphilitic aortitis demonstrating marked destruction of elastin with only focal small amount of medial elastin remaining. Infiltrate of lymphocytes and plasma cells is present in the adventitia toward the *bottom*. In addition, the superimposed atherosclerotic plaque is present at the *top* (elastin van Gieson stain × 40). **D,** Histologic section of adventitia with fibrosis and endarteritis obliterans present in vasa vasora (Movat's pentachrome stain × 200).

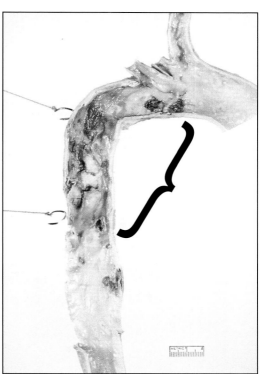

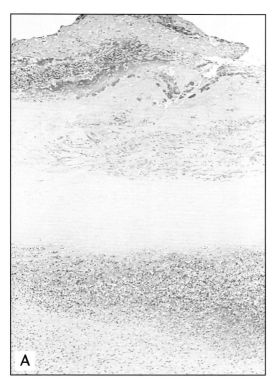

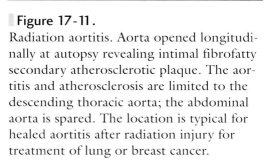

Figure 17-11.
Radiation aortitis. Aorta opened longitudinally at autopsy revealing intimal fibrofatty secondary atherosclerotic plaque. The aortitis and atherosclerosis are limited to the descending thoracic aorta; the abdominal aorta is spared. The location is typical for healed aortitis after radiation injury for treatment of lung or breast cancer.

Figure 17-12.
Infective aortitis. **A,** Aorta removed from a 35-year-old woman with Marfan syndrome who had undergone previous aortic root repair and valve replacement. Bacterial aortitis developed as a complication of infective endocarditis of the left ventricle. Friable fibrinous vegetation is present on the intimal surface toward the *top*. Fibrotic intima and media are present in the *middle*, and dense infiltrate of acute inflammation with associated necrosis and bacterial colonies is present at the *bottom* (hematoxylin and eosin × 40).

B, Marked intimal thickening and fibrosis are present in the aorta damaged by bacterial aortitis. Extensive destruction of medial elastin is demonstrated as well as fibrosis in the adventitia along with adventitial inflammation toward the *bottom* (elastin van Gieson stain × 40). The source of infection in mycotic aneurysms is thought to be 1) embolic from infective endocarditis; 2) bacterial with normal artery, previous atherosclerosis, previous syphilis, or a congenital anomaly; 3) contiguous infection secondary to osteomyelitis, abcesses, cellulitis, or lypmphadenitis; and 4) arterial trauma, including aortectomy or other aortic surgery. *Salmonella* species have emerged as the most common etiologic agent followed by staphylococcal, streptococcal, and pneumococcal infections (elastin van Gieson × 40).

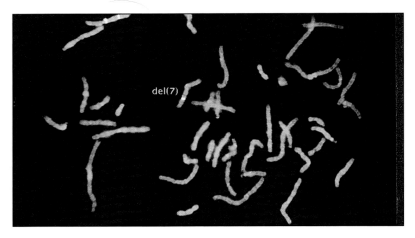

Figure 17-13.

Chromosomal deletion in Williams syndrome. Two-color WSCR (elastin Williams syndrome chromosome region) fluorescence in situ hybridization of a metaphase chromosome preparation from a patient with Williams syndrome. Shown is the hybridization pattern of the WSCR probe (*red*) and chromosome 7 control region (D7S522 to 7q31; *green*). The aortic manifestations of Williams syndrome include supravalvular aortic stenosis, known to be caused by mutations in the gene encoding elastin. The chromosomal deletion (del 7q 11) shown includes the region that encodes elastin. Therefore, the absence of one elastin allele is sufficient to cause aortic disease.

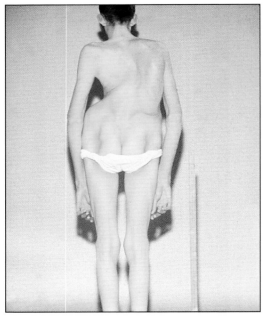

Figure 17-14.

Marfan syndrome body type. Marfan syndrome is an autosomal dominant heritable connective tissue disorder that affects primarily the ocular, skeletal, and cardiovascular systems. Typical skeletal features, such as those shown here, include tall stature, especially when compared with unaffected first-degree relatives; dolichostenomelia; scoliosis; arachnodactyly; and pes planus. It is now known that mutations in the gene encoding fibrillin-1 cause Marfan syndrome.

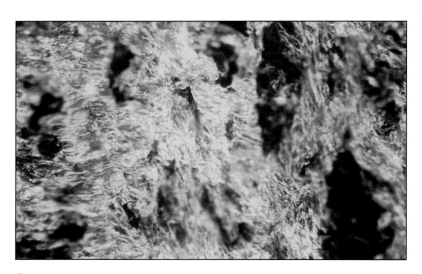

Figure 17-15.

Aortic fibrillin. Immunofluorescence photomicrograph of a section from a normal aorta after limited digestion with elastase and immunostaining with antibodies to fibrillin-1. The microfibrillar structures emerge after enzymatic digestion to show the scaffolding that elastin-associated microfibrils form for deposition of elastin in forming the aorta.

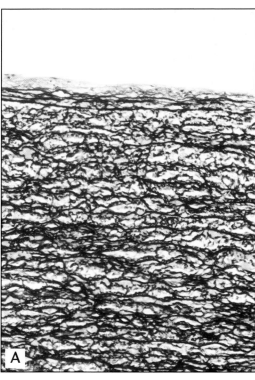

Figure 17-16.
Histologic changes of medial degeneration of the aorta. **A,** Normal aorta. (*continued on next page*)

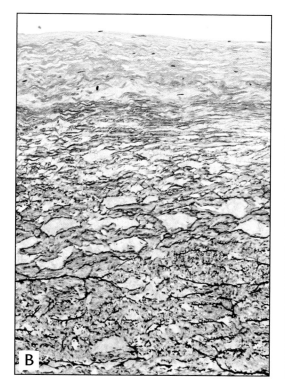

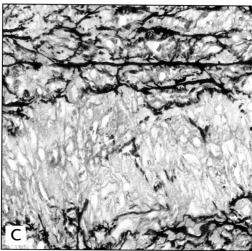

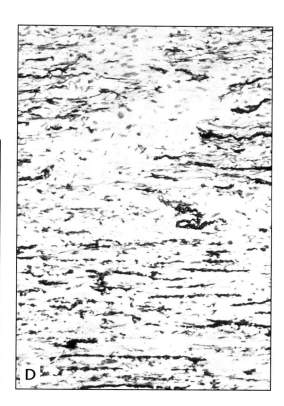

Figure 17-16. (*continued*)

B, Depletion of elastic tissue, focal loss of medial smooth muscle cells, and mucopolysaccharide accumulation, which stains *light green*. **C,** Higher-power photomicrograph of a section of the aortic wall from another patient demonstrating mucopolysaccharide accumulation, which stains *light green*. These accumulations are the so-called "cysts" of cystic medial necrosis. **D,** Advanced medial degeneration with gross deficiency of elastic tissue (Movat's pentachrome stain: *panels A and B × 100, panel C × 400, panel D × 200*).

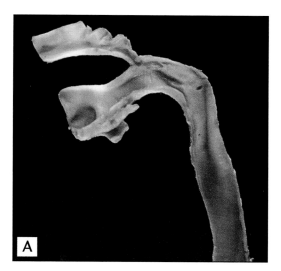

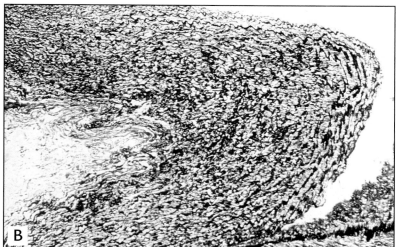

Figure 17-17.

Coarctation of the aorta. **A,** Autopsy specimen from a patient with coarctation of the aorta demonstrating preductal narrowing of the aorta along with marked dilatation of a ductus arteriosus. Coarctation of the aorta is narrowing of the aortic lumen caused by a ridgelike thickening of the media that protrudes from the posterior and lateral wall. Coarctation of the aorta that consists of a short, discrete, abrupt narrowing located just distal to the insertion of the ductus arteriosus has been traditionally designated as the adult or postductal form. Alternatively, if the coarctation is located between the left subclavian artery and the ductus, it is considered the infantile or preductal form. In the infantile form, a long segment of aortic tubular hypoplasia (combination of small diameter and abnormal length) is usually present in addition to the area of more discrete stricture in the isthmus. **B,** Low-power photomicrograph of coarctation of the aorta demonstrating the shelf-like thickening of the aortic wall consisting of multiple laminae of elastin fibers. In some patients with long-standing coarctation, intimal fibrous thickening also contributes to the luminal narrowing (elastin van Gieson stain × 40).

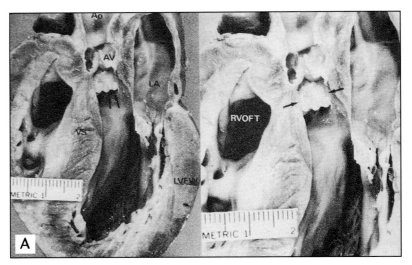

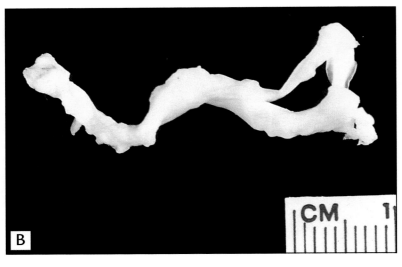

Figure 17-18.

Subaortic discrete membrane. **A,** Four-chamber echocardiographic view of an autopsy heart with subaortic discrete membrane. **B,** Discrete subaortic membrane removed during life showing a white fibrotic surface. **C,** Histologic section of a subaortic discrete membrane with mucopolysaccharide-rich endocardial surface along with deeper layers of black elastin fibers and increased yellow collagen (Movat's pentachrome stain × 100).

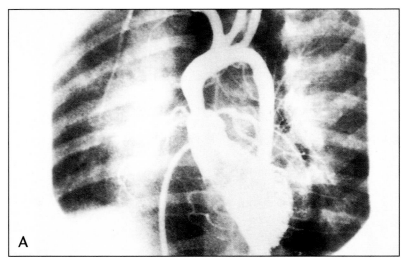

Figure 17-19.

Manifestations of Williams syndrome. **A,** Angiogram of aortic root of child with Williams syndrome demonstrating supravalvular aortic stenosis. (*continued on next page*)

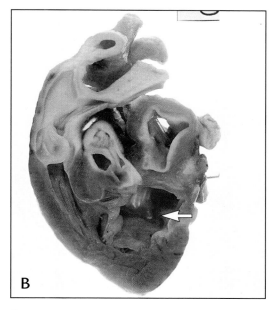

B

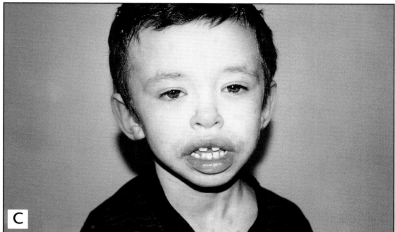

C

Figure 17-19. (*continued*)

B, Gross autopsy heart specimen with features of Williams syndrome. The right ventricular outflow tract has been opened to display the normal tissue of the pulmonic valve with slight narrowing of the immediate suprapulmonic region. *Arrow* indicates the conal musculature. The gelatinous cusps of the aortic valve are seen immediately adjacent to the conus. **C,** Clinical features of a typical patient with Williams syndrome. Patients with Williams syndrome have mild midface hypoplasia, epicanthal folds, strabismus, long philtrum, and anteverted nostrils.

AORTIC DISSECTION

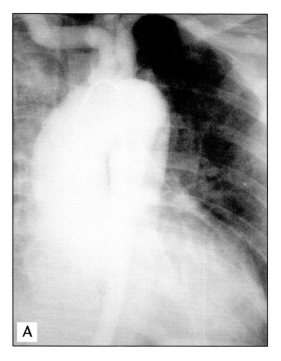

A

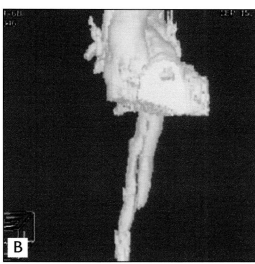

B

Figure 17-20.

Development of aortic dissection. Aortic dissection typically begins in the ascending aorta near the aortic valve annulus or in the descending thoracic aorta. The dissection may then extend toward or away from the heart as far distal as the abdominal aorta and into its branches, including the mesenteric vessels or the iliac arteries. **A,** Both the true and the false lumens are also easily identified on the arteriogram because of the differing amounts of contrast in these two lumens. **B,** The reconstruction of a dynamic contrast scan demonstrates septum and the true and false lumens in the descending thoracic and abdominal aorta.

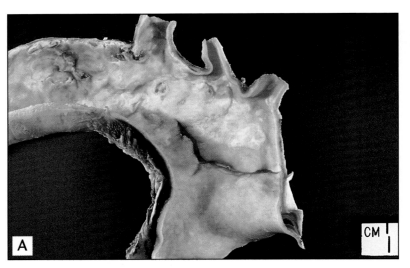

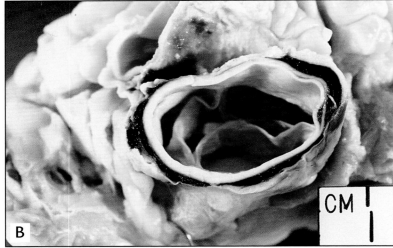

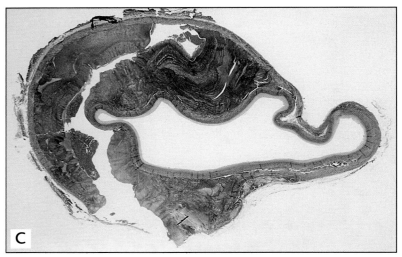

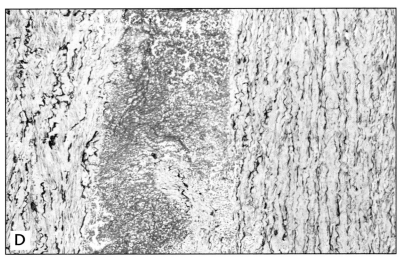

▌Figure 17-21

Aortic dissection. **A,** Ascending aorta and arch opened longitudinally at autopsy of an 85-year-old man with long-standing hypertension who died as a result of aortic dissection. Transverse and longitudinal intimal tear is present along with dissecting hematoma, which ruptured into pericardial sac causing fatal tamponade. Distal to the intimal tear is extensive atherosclerotic plaque. **B,** View from above of aortic root in same patient shown in *panel A* demonstrating extension of the dissection proximally to the level of the aortic valve. **C,** Whole mount of aorta demonstrating aortic dissection with true lumen to the *lower right* and the blood-filled hematoma in the false lumen to the *upper left* (Movat's pentachrome stain). **D,** Histologic section of aorta showing dissection involving the outer media a region of hematoma. Loss of elastin fibers is present in the adjacent medial tissue (Movat's pentachrome stain × 100).

COMPLICATIONS OF AORTIC DISSECTION

Complete rupture of aorta with extravasation of blood into the
 following areas:
 Pericardial sac
 Pleural space
 Mediastinum
 Retroperitoneum
 Wall of pulmonary trunk and/or main right and left pulmonary
  arteries
  Pulmonary artery stenosis
 Atrial and/or ventricular cardiac septum
  Atrioventricular conduction defect
 Lung
 Esophagus
Partial or complete obstruction by medial hematoma of the
 lumen of an artery arising from aorta
 Coronary
  Sudden death
  Acute myocardial infarction
 Innominate and/or common carotid
  Syncope, confusion, stroke
 Innominate and/or subclavian
  Upper limb ischemia, gangrene, paralysis
  Intercostal and/or lumbar
  Spinal cord ischemia-paraplegia
 Celiac
 Renal
  Oliguria
  Infarction/ischemia
 Mesenteric
  Bowel ischemia/infarction
 Common iliac
  Leg ischemia, gangrene, paralysis
 Separation of branch of aorta from aorta
 Aortic regurgitation
 Obstruction of aorta itself (true aortic stenosis)
  By compression of true lumen by medial hematoma
  Intussusception of aorta

Figure 17-22.
Complications of aortic dissection.

REFERENCES

1. Waller BF, Clary JD, Rohr T: Clinical pathologic correlations, nonneo-plastic diseases of aorta and pulmonary trunk: part I. *Clin Cardiol* 1997:20, 730–734.

2. Waller BF, Clary JD, Rohr T: Clinical pathologic correlations, nonneo-plastic diseases of aorta and pulmonary trunk: part II. *Clin Cardiol* 1997:20, 798–804.

3. Waller BF, Clary JD, Rohr T: Clinical pathologic correlations, nonneo-plastic diseases of aorta and pulmonary trunk: part III. *Clin Cardiol* 1997:20, 879–884.

4. Lederle FA, Johnson GR, Wilson SE, *et al.*: Prevalence and associations of abdominal aortic aneurym detected through screeing. *Ann Intern Med* 1997:126:441–449.

5. Ernst CB: Abdominal aortic aneurysm. *N Engl J Med* 1993, 328:1167–1172.

6. Grange JJ, Davis V, Baxter BT: Pathogenesis of abdominal aortic aneurysm: an update and look toward the future. *Cardiovasc Surg* 1997, 5:256–265.

7. Nevitt MP, Ballard DJ, Hallett JW Jr: Prognosis of abdominal aortic aneuryms: a population-based study. *N Engl J Med* 1989, 321:1009–1114.

8. Virmani R, McAllister HA Jr: *Aortitis: Clinical, Pathologic and Radiographic Aspects.* New York: Raven Press; 1986.

9. Schlatmann TJM, Becker AE: Histologic changes in the normal aging aorta. *Am J Cardiol* 1997, 39:13.

INDEX

in myocarditis, 170–172
Bjork-Shiley prosthetic valve, 217, 219, 221
Bone marrow embolism, in pulmonary artery, 130
Bone marrow transplantation, myocarditis after, 178
Bronchial circulation, physiology of, 116
Bronchiole, normal, 117
Bundle branch block, 252
Bundle branch reentry, in cardiomyopathy, 262
Bundle branches, physiology of, 246
Bypass grafting, coronary artery, 76–78
  prosthetics in, 216, 226–227

C

Calcification, prosthetic valve, 222
  pulmonary vascular, 129
Calcium, in pulmonary vascular wall, 129
  in reperfusion after myocardial ischemia, 99
Candidiasis, myocarditis in, 178
Cardiac amyloidosis, 144–145
Cardiac arrhythmias, 245–246, 246–268 See also Arrhythmias
Cardiac chamber abnormalities, in congenital heart disease, 35–38
Cardiac conduction, 246–250
  in transgenic animals, 7–10
Cardiac electrophysiology, 246–250
Cardiac fibroma, 235–236
Cardiac hemangioma, 240, 262
Cardiac hypertrophy, maternal diabetes and, 164
  in transgenic animals, 13–15
Cardiac lipoma, 237
Cardiac lymphoma, 243
Cardiac myxoma, 231–233
Cardiac rhabdomyoma, 234–235
Cardiac sarcoma, 241–242
Cardiac substrate utilization disorders, 162
Cardiac transplantation See Heart transplantation
Cardiac tumors, 230, 231–243 See also Tumors
Cardiac valves See Heart valves; specific valves
Cardiac vessel abnormalities, in congenital heart disease, 35–38
Cardiomegaly, genetic models of, 8
Cardiomyocytes See Myocytes
Cardiomyopathies, 135–136, 137–151
  arrhythmogenic right ventricular, 151
  bundle branch reentry in, 262
  classification of, 135–136
  defined, 135
  dilated, 137–138, 163
  heart transplantation in, 185–186
  histiocytoid, 162
  hypertrophic, 140 See also Hypertrophic cardiomyopathy
  infiltrative, 144–146
  metabolic and hereditary, 138–139, 153–154, 154–167
  mitochondrial, 158–162
  restrictive, 141–143
  toxic and drug-related, 147–151
  tumor-like masses in, 231
Cardiovascular system, genetic models of pathophysiology of, 1–16, 3–16
  tumors of, 230, 231–243 See also Tumors
Carnitine deficiency, 162
Carotid arteries, atherosclerosis in, 65

stenting or, 75
  neovascularization in, 108
Carpentier-Edwards porcine valve, 218
Catecholamine-induced myocarditis, 148
Cerebrovascular accident, prosthetic valves and, 220
Childhood See also Congenital heart disease; Pediatric diseases
  metabolic and hereditary myopathies of, 138–139, 153–154, 154–167
  myocarditis in, 174–176
Chloroquine cardiotoxicity, 146
Cholesterol, in atherosclerosis, 60–61, 61–62
Coarctation of the aorta, 37, 271, 279
  other anomalies and, 32
Cocaine, cardiomyopathy from, 148
Colitis, ischemic, 275–276
Collateral vasculature, in ischemia, 95
  in normal heart, 94
Common atrioventricular canal, 22–23
  complete, 24–25
  incomplete, 24–26
Complete heart block, 251–252
Conal septal hypoplasia ventricular septal defect, 19
Congenital absence, of coronary artery, 58
Congenital heart disease, 18–38 See also Pediatric diseases; specific disorders
  aortic valve, 202–203, 205, 207
  atrial septal defects as, 20–21
  atrioventricular alignments in, 22–29
  chamber, valve, and vessel abnormalities in, 35–38
  conotruncal alignments in, 30–34
  coronary artery anomalies in, 40–58
  defined, 18
  ventricular septal defects as, 19–20
  ventricular tachycardia in, 266
  ventriculoarterial alignments in, 30–34
Connective tissue diseases, heart valve disease in, 212
Conotruncal anomalies, in congenital heart disease, 30–34
Conoventricular/perimembranous ventricular septal defect, 19
Contraction band necrosis, in myocardial ischemia, 86, 91, 100–101
  toxic or drug-related, 148
Conus artery, anomalies of, 42
Cor pulmonale, defined, 122
Cori disease, 156
Coronary angioplasty, percutaneous transluminal, 70–72
Coronary arteries, anomalies of, 39–58, 39–40
  absence as, 58
  aneurysm as, 54–55
  fistula as, 56
  high take-off as, 57
  of origin, 40–53
  tunneled as, 57
  bypass grating of, 76–78
  dilatation of, 54–55
  neovascularization in, 109
  stenting of, in atherosclerosis, 73–75
Coronary atherosclerosis, acute, 67–68
  in heart transplantation, 197–199
  topography of, 79–80, 80–84
Coronary steal phenomenon, anomalies associated with, 41, 56
Coxsackievirus, myocarditis induced by, 168–169, 180–181

Cystic atrioventricular nodal tumor, 239
Cytomegalovirus, after heart transplantation, 194
    myocarditis in, 178

D

Dacron graft, 226
Diabetes, fetal effects of maternal, 164–165
Dilated cardiomyopathy, 137–138
    classification of, 135–136
    heart transplantation in, 186
    pediatric, 163
Dilation lesions, defined, 125
Diphtheria toxin, myocarditis from, 149
Dissection, aortic, 281–283
Dobutamine, toxicity of preparations of, 148
Double-outlet right ventricle, 32–33
Doxorubicin cardiotoxicity, 149–150
Drug abuse, pulmonary talcosis in, 131
Drug-related cardiomyopathy, 147–151
Duchenne muscular dystrophy, cardiomyopathy and, 139
Dysplasia, arrhythmogenic right ventricular, 136, 151, 263
Dystrophin gene, cardiomyopathy and, 139

E

Ebstein's anomaly, pulmonary atresia and, 36
    tricuspid valve disease in, 214
Ectasia, in aortic aneurysm, 274
Embolism, amniotic fluid, 132
    bone marrow, 130
    fat, 131
    pulmonary tumor, 129
Embryonic stem cell technology, in genetic models, 2, 4
Endocardial fibroelastosis, 143
    pediatric, 165–167
Endocarditis, 214–215
    prosthetic valve, 220
Endomyocardial biopsy, in heart transplantation, 187–194
    in myocarditis, 170–172
Endothelial cells, in angiogenesis, 104
Enteroviral myocarditis, 182
Eosinophilia, heart valve disease in, 213
Eosinophilic myocarditis, heart transplantation in, 186
Epstein-Barr virus, in posttransplant lymphoproliferative disorder, 197
ES cells, in genetic models, 2, 4
Extremities, atherosclerosis in, 65

F

Fabry's disease, 145
Fallot, tetralogy of, 30–31
False aneurysm, aortic, 69
Familial hypertrophic cardiomyopathy, genetic models of, 15
Fat embolism, pulmonary, 131
Fatty acid oxidation, in cardiovascular disease, 267–268
Fetal hyperinsulinemia, 164
Fibrillation, atrial, 257
    ventricular, 258, 263
Fibrillin, aortic, 278

Fibrinoid necrosis, in primary pulmonary hypertension, 126
Fibroatheromas, in atherosclerosis, 63
Fibroelastoma, papillary, 238
Fibroelastosis, endocardial, 143
    pediatric, 165–167
Fibroma, 235–236
Fibrosis, in cardiomyopathy, 137, 140–143
    drug-related endocardial, 147
Fibrous caps, in atherosclerosis, 67–68
    pulmonary, 118
Fistula, coronary arterial, 56
Fusiform aneurysm, 273–274

G

Gain-of-function transgenic animals, defined, 1–2
    generation of, 3
    research with, 5–8, 10–11, 13–14
Gangliosidosis, 158
Gangrene, atherosclerosis and, 65
Gene therapy, vascular endothelial growth factor, 111
Genetic diseases See also specific diseases
    aorta in, 278–281
    cardiomyopathy in, 138–139, 153–154, 154–163
    fatty acid oxidation in, 267–268
Genetic models, 1–16
    experiments with, 3–16, 3–16
    principles of, 1–2
Giant cell myocarditis, 179
Glycogen storage diseases, 154–157
Gore-Tex graft, 227
Grafting, coronary artery bypass, in atherosclerosis, 76–78
    prosthetics in, 216, 226–227
Granulomas, sarcoid, 267
Great arteries, transposition of, 30–32
Growth factors, in angiogenesis, 104, 105–108, 111–114

H

Hancock porcine valve, 218
Harken prosthetic valve, 219
Heart, arrhythmias of, 245–246, 246–268 See also Arrhythmias
    disease of See also specific disorders
        congenital See Congenital heart disease
        rheumatic See Rheumatic heart disease
    electrophysiology of, 246–250
    transplantation of See Heart transplantation
    tumors of, 230, 231–243 See also Tumors
    valves of See Heart valves; specific valves
Heart block, complete, 241–252
Heart failure, endomyocardial biopsy in, 172
    heart transplantation in, 184
    myocarditis in, 174–176
Heart rate, resting sinus, 248
Heart transplantation, 184–185, 185–199
    allograft rejection in, 187–192, 195
    autopsy specimens in, 195–199
    disease recurrence in, 186
    donor criteria in, 185
    drug-related myocarditis and, 148
    endomyocardial biopsy in, 172, 187–194

indications for, 184, 185
  myocarditis as, 176
  ventricular fibrillation as, 263
opportunistic infections after, 194, 196
pathology of recipient heart in, 185–186
pediatric, 165
posttransplant lymphoproliferative disorder in, 194, 196–197
Quilty effect in, 193
Heart valves, autograft, 225
  diseases of, 201–202, 202–215
    aortic, 202, 202–207, 212
    congenital, 35-38, 202–203, 207
    endocarditis as, 214–215
    mitral, 208–213, 215
    pulmonary, 213
    tricuspid, 209, 214
  homograft, 224
  prosthetic, 216, 217–225
Heath-Edwards grading system, or secondary pulmonary hypertension, 121
Hemangioma, cardiac, 240, 262
Hemangiomatosis, pulmonary capillary, 127
Hemochromatosis, 145
Hemorrhage, in atherosclerosis, 64
  in reperfusion after myocardial ischemia, 102
Hereditary diseases *See also* specific diseases
  aorta in, 278–281
  myopathies as, 138–139, 153–154, 154–163
High take-off coronary artery, 57
Histiocytoid cardiomyopathy, 162
Homografts, valvular, 224
Hurler syndrome, 157
Hypereosinophilic syndrome, heart valve disease in, 213
Hyperinsulinemia, fetal, 164
Hypersensitivity myocarditis, 148
Hypertension, pulmonary *See* Pulmonary hypertension
Hypertrophic cardiomyopathy, 140
  histologic features of, 264
  maternal diabetes and, 165
  pathophysiology of, 136
Hypoplasia, coronary artery, 58
Hypoplastic left heart syndrome, 37

I

Idiopathic dilated cardiomyopathy, heart transplantation in, 186
Iliac artery, plaque rupture in, 110
Immune compromise, myocarditis in, 178
In situ hybridization, in viral myocarditis, 169, 175, 180–181
Infarction, myocardial *See* Myocardial infarction
  pulmonary, 118
Infections, aortitis as, 277
  endocarditis as, 214–215
  opportunistic, in heart transplantation, 194, 196
    in myocarditis, 178
  viral, cardiac arrest and, 268
    in myocarditis, 168-169, 175, 180–182
Infiltrates, in myocarditis, 173–174
Infiltrative cardiomyopathy, 144–146
Inflammation, in atherosclerosis, 61
Influenza, myocarditis in, 175

Internal mammary artery, in coronary artery bypass grafting, 76–78
International Society for Heart and Lung Transplantation, rejection grading of, 188–190
Interrupted aortic arch, 31
Intima, in aortic aneurysm, 274
  in atherosclerosis, 60–61, 61–64
  in primary pulmonary hypertension, 124
  in pulmonary venous sclerosis, 117
Intravascular lymphomatosis, pulmonary, 130
Intravenous drug abuse, pulmonary talcosis in, 131
Iron encrustation, pulmonary vascular wall, 129
Ischemia, atherosclerosis and, 65
  heart transplantation and, 185, 192
  myocardial *See* Myocardial ischemia
Ischemic colitis, 275–276
Ischemic preconditioning, defined, 86
  experimental, 98

J

Junctional tachycardia, pathophysiology of, 249

K

Kearns-Sayre syndrome, 138

L

Left anterior descending coronary artery, anomalies of, 41–42, 46–53, 58
Left circumflex coronary artery, anomalies of, 41–42, 44, 46–53, 58
Left main coronary artery, anomalies of, 40–53, 58
Left ventricle, aneurysm of, 259
  hypertrophy of, maternal diabetes and, 164
Lipoma, cardiac, 237
Lipomatous atrial septal hypertrophy, 236–237
Löler's disease, 143
Long QT syndrome, 265
Loss-of-function transgenic animals, defined, 1
  generation of, 4
  research with, 6–7, 9–10, 12–13
Lung, circulation in, 115–116
  tissue specimen preparation of, 116
Lymphoma, cardiac, 243
Lymphomatosis, pulmonary intravascular, 130

M

Malalignment ventricular septal defect, 19
Marfan syndrome, 271, 277–278
Medial hypertrophy, in primary pulmonary hypertension, 124
Medtronic FreeStyle prosthetic valve, 225
Medtronic-Hall prosthetic valve, 217
Megakaryocytes, pulmonary, 130
Metabolic myopathies, 153–154, 154–162
Mitochondria, in Kearns-Sayre syndrome, 138
  in mitochondrial cardiomyopathy, 158–162
Mitochondriopathies, pediatric, 158–162
Mitral valve, atresia of, 29